NEW DEVELOPMENTS IN CARDIAC PACING AND ELECTROPHYSIOLOGY

Edited by

I. Eli Ovsyshcher, MD, PhD, FESC, FACC
Professor of Medicine/Cardiology
Soroka University Medical Center &
Faculty of Health Sciences, Ben Gurion University of
the Negev, Beer Sheva, Israel

Published by
Futura Publishing Company, Inc.
135 Bedford Road
Armonk, New York 10504
www.futuraco.com

ISBN #:0-87993-706-8

Foreword

I am pleased to have been asked to write a Foreword for this wonderful book edited by Eli Ovsyshcher. The contents include chapters on basic electrophysiology, atrial fibrillation, the implantable cardioverter-defibrillator, pacing, cardiac resynchronization and new therapeutic approaches. Distinguished experts address each of the specific topics.

This book has appeal to the clinician interested in cardiac arrhythmias since it provides an electrophysiologic foundation for the basis of some arrhythmias, emphasizes atrial fibrillation, the most common sustained cardiac arrhythmia that we treat, and elaborates on the use of the implantable cardioverter-defibrillator, which is becoming a more and more important mainstay in our therapeutic endeavors. The editor does not forget to include the importance of bradyarrhythmias and pacing approaches to terminating tachyarrhythmias. The last two sections deal with new concepts in electrophysiology. Cardiac resynchronization therapy for patients with congestive heart failure has become a major area for clinical investigation and therapeutic application. In fact, the benefits achieved by heart failure patients are so striking that they overshadow many of the time honored medical approaches. A review of this area is of major contemporary importance. The last section covers some new therapeutic approaches to patients with cardiac arrhythmia including syncope, postural tachycardia, atrial fibrillation and the use of rate smoothing for ventricular arrhythmias.

I am certain that the clinician will find this book fun to read and an excellent educational resource. *I recommend it.*

DOUGLAS P. ZIPES, MD, FACC
Distinguished Professor of Medicine, Pharmacology, and Toxicology
Director, Krannert Institute of Cardiology and Division of Cardiology
Indiana University School of Medicine, Indianapolis, IN
President, American College of Cardiology

Preface

This is the second volume of manuscripts resulting from the work of the Dead Sea Symposium, held biennially in Israel. Despite this very troubled era in the region, life, art, science and medicine continue to enrich the area and participate in the activities of the greater world. This volume is an example of what can be assembled even during such turmoil and is a credit to contributions from many areas of the world.

Cardiac stimulation and electrophysiology have come a very long way in the past fifty years. Major contributions can be clearly delineated. It had become gradually accepted over the last quarter of the nineteenth century that graphic techniques were informative and therefore valuable in the analysis and such therapy as was possible in cardiac disease. A vast amount of anatomic and electrophysiologic information was gathered which is today the basis of modern cardiologic practice. Contraction of muscle and especially the heart was found to be accompanied by electrical events which could be recorded by rudimentary techniques from the body surface. By 1903 Einthoven had devised the string galvanometer and simultaneously invented electrocardiography, a tool and technique which, arguably, opened the next century of cardiology and cardiac investigation. Early investigation had demonstrated the normal relationship between contraction of atrium and ventricle and the dissociation and ventricular bradycardia associated with syncope and named the Adams-Stokes disease. While AV dissociation had been recognized clinically before the electrocardiogram, the advent of the electrocardiogram truly clarified the situation. The first effective stimulation of the human heart with therapeutic intention occurred in 1952 when Zoll stimulated the heart across the intact chest wall and perhaps more importantly excited the imagination and expectation of profession and the public. This event began the cascade of innovation and investigation which has resulted in the contemporary field of cardiac stimulation and cardiac electrophysiology. This pacemaker, rudimentary as it was, played an important role in the success of the earliest open heart surgical repair of congenital cardiac anomalies, the prompting of direct myocardial stimulation, the design of the battery external pacemaker, endocardial stimulation in 1958 and implantable pacing in 1960. By 1967 the role of cardiac stimulation in the provocation and termination of ventricular arrhythmias had become clear, and led to the intense electrophysiologic investigations which followed. By 1980 the technique of implantation of a cardioverter defibrillator had been accomplished and in 1981 that of ablation of endocardial lesions and pathways. These discoveries and inventions have opened the modern world of electrophysiology being advanced and enlarged today and in this volume.

The fields continue to evolve progressively. Substantial innovation has occurred over the past decade and indications are that this level of innovation in basic contribution and application to patient therapy will continue. Contributing to this level of innovation is the immensely powerful tool of the randomized trial. Many of the more recent significant contributions have resulted from these studies. These very powerful mathematical tools have driven such studies as CAST, MADIT and AVID to demonstrate facts which otherwise would have been difficult or impossible to ascertain. Such studies continue and will demonstrate much more over the near future. Studies now in progress will push our comprehension even further.

The present volume presents material from basic electrophysiology to the many applications presently involved in therapy. Basic studies evaluate cryoablation and radiofrequency ablation for greater applicability and effectiveness. Ablation of foci and pathways once requiring the most delicate of open heart surgery is now readily and routinely accomplished by relatively minimal catheter ablation. Ablation itself has become one of the most important and frequently applied of the modern cardiac therapies. It is becoming increasingly important in the therapy of atrial fibrillation, the arrhythmia which occupies another section and is the most common arrhythmia and cause of hospitalization and disability. Atrial fibrillation is being intensively investigated and while much treatment remains conventional or is limited to AV node ablation and pacemaker implantation, modification and ablation of foci causing atrial fibrillation is becoming progressively more important therapy. Noncontact mapping is also being presented as a guide to arrhythmia ablation. That modality is increasingly important and able to assist in the analysis of arrhythmias and determination of the means of therapy.

In the now more traditional therapies of cardiac pacing and implantable defibrillation, atrial pacing is a technique of progressively greater importance and its efficacy is being reevaluated and enhanced, as is the means of diagnosing supraventricular arrhythmias with an implanted pacemaker. An important section concerns a potentially major new therapy, ventricular resynchronization. Now in its early evolution and evaluation, biventricular pacing to resynchronize the contraction of the two ventricles for management of heart failure may yet become one of the most important of the new approaches to management of a widespread and devastating cardiac disability. If further investigation and continued application bear out its early hope and benefit occurs reliably, this therapy will open a major new area of pacing therapy. Already the combination of a biventricular pacemaker and an ICD is available to manage the two major complications of congestive heart failure, inefficient ventricular contraction resulting in the failure itself and the sudden death which commonly accompanies this condition as the agonal event.

One of the important papers from a practical perspective deals with extraction of pacing and defibrillating leads. The almost explosive growth of device implantation has been accompanied by increasing lead malfunction, especially of endocardial defibrillator leads, and lead infection. Lead extraction is then required and has become a significant effort in those countries with high levels of implantation. As the indications for device implantation become standardized throughout the world, a topic of another paper, the requirement for lead removal is likely also to increase. That paper is of great practical importance. Another deals with the risks and benefits of driving for a patient with syncope. This is indeed an important topic because of the great prevalence of syncope, its sometime obscure etiology and the need, in very many parts of the world, certainly in the United States for people to drive to work and for shopping. This topic is always interesting and important.

Interventional electrophysiology, pacing and implantable defibrillation and associated issues have come a long way in fifty years, have contributed greatly to medicine and public welfare and continue to have much to contribute.

SEYMOUR FURMAN, MD, FACS, FACC
Professor of Surgery
Professor of Medicine
Albert Einstein College of Medicine of Yeshiva University
Bronx, New York

From The Editor

The last decade has been a period of expansive growth for the electrophysiological management of cardiac arrhythmias. Rapid application of technological advances within clinical practice has been the main focus of these extraordinary developments, rendering the communication and exchange of ideas in this field paramount. Therefore, collective volumes are crucial and decisively important in propagating modern knowledge and technology.

The purpose of this book is to provide its' readers with the latest knowledge in cardiac pacing and electrophysiology. *The book covers a wide variety of topics: basic electrophysiology, and the molecular base of arrhythmias; invasive and noninvasive clinical electrophysiology, and most important of all the clinical aspects of cardiac pacing and defibrillation.* It contains an overview of various methods in the treatment of AF, including new approaches to ablation, the role of pacing in prevention of AF and in the treatment of CHF and dilated cardiomyopathy. The results of recent clinical trials in cardiac pacing, including the prevention and treatment of AF, are also presented. Special sections have been dedicated to resinchronization pacing therapy for heart failure.

Most of the chapters of this book emphasize the *clinical aspects* of pacing and electrophysiology, presenting the impressive contributions by experts in the field. The book also provides a current review of a variety of 'hot' topics, with personal experiences and critical evaluations by the authors, taking into perspective modern pacing and electrophysiology.

We hope that this information will be beneficial to clinicians in selecting and providing appropriate treatment for patients with various cardiac arrhythmias.

I wish to express my gratitude to the authors, all being leaders in their fields, for their willingness to contribute to the creation of this volume (despite the tight time schedule) enabling us to achieve our goal - disseminating this knowledge and information to electrophysiologists, pacemaker specialists, bioengineers, technicians and nurses engaged in all aspects of this field.

I hope you all will find this enjoyable, useful and applicable!

Finally, my sincere thanks to those who inspired and encouraged me in this endeavor, and especially to my beloved Lilly, Masha and Raya for their patient, support and love.

I. ELI OVSYSHCHER, MD, PhD, FESC, FACC

Professor of Medicine/Cardiology

CONTRIBUTORS

CHRISTINE ALONSO, MD
Assistant Professor, University of Rennes I, France

CHARLES ANTZELEVITCH, PHD
Executive Director and Director of Research
Masonic Medical Research Laboratory, Utica, NY, USA

DANIELA ASCHIERI, MD
Department of Cardiology, General Hospital, Piacenza, Italy.

BOAZ AVITALL, MD, PHD, FACC
Professor of Medicine, Director of Clinical and Research Cardiac
Electrophysiology, University of Illinois, Chicago, IL, USA

S. SERGE BAROLD, MD, FRACP, FACC, FACP, FESC
Florida Cardiovascular Institute and Tampa General Hospital,
Tampa, FL, USA

SAROJA BHARATI, M. D.
Director Maurice Lev Congenital Heart and Conduction System
Center, The Heart Institute for Children, Hope Children's Hospital
Advocate Christ Medical Center, Oak Lawn, IL
Professor of Pathology Rush Medical College, Rush University
Rush-Presbyterian-St. Luke's Medical Center, Chicago, IL
Clinical Professor of Pathology Finch University of Health
Sciences Chicago Medical School, North Chicago, IL and Visiting
Professor of Pathology University of Illinois at Chicago, USA

MARK L. BLITZER, MD
Cardiac Electrophysiology and Pacer Laboratory, Hospital of Saint
Raphael and Yale University School of Medicine

A. JOHN CAMM, MD
Professor of Clinical Cardiology, Department of Cardiological
Sciences, St George's Hospital Medical School, London, UK

ALESSANDRO CAPUCCI, MD
Department of Cardiology, General Hospital, Piacenza, Italy.

SERGE CAZEAU, MD
InParys, Saint-Cloud - France

CRISTINA CIAPETTI, MD
Insitute of Internal Medicine and Cardiology, University of Florence, Italy

ANDREA COLELLA, MD
Insitute of Internal Medicine and Cardiology, University of Florence, Italy

STUART J. CONNOLLY, MD
Professor of Medicine, Faculty of Health Sciences, McMaster University, Hamilton, ON, Canada

EUGENE CRYSTAL, MD
Department of Medicine, McMaster University, Hamilton, Ontario, Canada; EP Research Laboratory, Cardiology Department, Soroka University Medical Center and Faculty of Health Sciences, Ben Gurion University of the Negev, Beer-Sheva, Israel

DAWOOD DARBAR, MD
Division of Cardiovascular Medicine, Mayo Clinic, Rochester, MN, USA

JEAN-CLAUDE DAUBERT, MD
Professor of Cardiology, University of Rennes I, Chief of the Department of Cardiology and Vascular Diseases, Centre Hospitalier Universitaire, Rennes, France

E. DZIELICKA, MD
1st Department of Cardiology, Silesian School of Medicine, Katowice, Poland

NABIL EL-SHERIF, MD
Professor of Medicine & Physiology & Director, Clinical Cardiac Electrophysiology Program, State University of New York Health Science Center; Director, Cardiology Division, Veterans Affairs Medical Center, Brooklyn, New York, USA

ILYA FLEIDERVISH, MD, PhD
Koret School of Veterinary Medicine, The Hebrew University, Jerusalem, and EP Research Laboratory, Faculty of Health Sciences, Ben Gurion University of the Negev, Beer-Sheva, Israel

PAUL A. FRIEDMAN, MD, FACC
> Assistant Professor of Medicine, Division of Internal Medicine & Cardiovascular Diseases, Mayo Clinic, Rochester, MN, USA

SEYMOUR FURMAN, MD, FACC, FACS
> Professor of Medicine and Surgery, Albert Einstein College of Medicine, Bronx, NY, USA

I. GALLARDO, MD
> Florida Cardiovascular Institute and Tampa General Hospital, Tampa, FL, USA

HAREL GILUTZ, MD
> Director, ICCU, Cardiology Department, Soroka University Medical Center & Faculty of Health Sciences, Ben Gurion University of the Negev, Beer-Sheva, Israel

INNA GITELMAN, PHD
> Department of Molecular Genetics & Development, Faculty of Health Sciences, Ben Gurion University of the Negev, BeerSheva, Israel

MICHAEL GLIKSON, MD, FACC
> Director, Pacemaker Service, Heart Institute, Chaim Sheba Medical Center, Tel Aviv University, Tel Hashomer, Israel

YURI GOLDBERG, MD
> Research EP Laboratory, Cardiology Department, Cardiac Research Center, Soroka University Medical Center & Faculty of Health Sciences, Ben Gurion University of the Negev, Beer-Sheva, Israel

BLAIR P. GRUBB, MD
> Professor of Medicine & Pediatrics, Division of Cardiology, Medical College of Ohio, Toledo, Ohio, USA

AMIR HALKIN, MD
> Cardiology Department, Tel Aviv Souraski Medical Center, Tel Aviv, Israel

DAVID L. HAYES, MD
> Consultant, Division of Cardiovascular Diseases and Internal Medicine, Mayo Clinic, Professor of Medicine, Mayo Medical School; Rochester, Minnesota 55905, USA.

A. HOFFMANN, MD
1st Department of Cardiology, Silesian School of Medicine, Katowice, Poland.

STEFAN H. HOHNLOSER, MD, FACC FESC
Professor of Medicine, Department of Medicine, Division of Cardiology, J. W. Goethe University Hospital, Frankfurt, Germany

REUVEN ILIA, MD
Professor of Medicine/Cardiology, Chief, Cardiology Department, Soroka University Medical Center, Cardiac Research Center & Faculty of Health Sciences, Ben Gurion University of the Negev, Beer-Sheva, Israel

CARSTEN W. ISRAEL, MD
Department of Medicine, Division of Cardiology, J. W. Goethe University Hospital, Frankfurt, Germany

GAËL JAUVERT MD
InParys, Saint-Cloud - France

EMMANUEL M. KANOUPAKIS, MD
Cardiology Department, Heraklion University, Crete, Greece

W ODZIMIERZ KARGUL, MD, PHD
Department of Electrocardiology, Silesian School of Medicine, Katowice, Polandd

E. KONARSKA-KUSZEWSKA, MD
1st Department of Cardiology, Silesian School of Medicine, Katowice, Poland.

J. KRAUZE, MD
1st Department of Cardiology, Silesian School of Medicine, Katowice, Poland.

ANDRZEJ KUTARSKI, MD, PHD
Department of Cardiology, University Medical Academy, Lublin, Poland

CHU-PAK LAU, MD
> Professor of Medicine, Chief, Cardiology Division, University Department of Medicine, Queen Mary Hospital, Pokfulam, Hong Kong, China

ARNAUD LAZARUS, MD
> InParys, Saint-Cloud – France

CHRISTOPHE LECLERCQ, MD, PHD
> Assistant Professor of Cardiology, University of Rennes I, France

PAUL A. LEVINE, MD
> Vice President & Medical Director, St. Jude Medical-Cardiac Rhythm Management Division, Sylmar, CA; Clinical Professor of Medicine, Loma Linda University School of Medicine, Loma Linda, CA, USA

THORSTEN LEWALTER, MD
> Department of Medicine-Cardiology, University of Bonn, Bonn, Germany

CHARLES J. LOVE, MD
> Associate Professor of Clinical Medicine, Director, Arrhythmia Device Services, Director, Cardiology Information Systems, Division of Cardiology, The Ohio State University Heart Center, Columbus, OH, USA

BERNDT LÜDERITZ, MD, FACC, FESC
> Professor of Medicine, Head, Department of Medicine - Cardiology, University of Bonn, Bonn, Germany

DAVID LURIA, MD
> Clinical Electrophysiology, Heart Institute, Chaim Sheba Medical Center, Tel Aviv University, Tel Hashomer, Israel

H. E. MAVRAKIS, MD
> Cardiology Department, University Hospital, Heraklion, Crete, Greece

MARY E. MCGRORY-USSET, MBA
> Medtronic, Inc., Minneapolis, Minnesota, USA

ANTONIO MICHELUCCI, MD
Insitute of Internal Medicine and Cardiology, University of Florence, Italy

NICOLA MUSILLI, MD
Insitute of Internal Medicine and Cardiology, University of Florence, Italy

W. ORSZULAK, MD
1st Department of Cardiology, Silesian School of Medicine, Katowice, Poland.

I. ELI OVSYSHCHER, MD, PHD, FESC, FACC
Professor of Medicine/Cardiology, EP Research Laboratory and Cardiac Research Center, Department of Cardiology, Soroka University Medical Center & Faculty of Health Sciences, Ben Gurion University of the Negev, Beer-Sheva, Israel

LUIGI PADELETTI, MD
Professor of Medicine, Insitute of Internal Medicine and Cardiology, University of Florence, Italy

PAOLO PIERAGNOLI, MD
Insitute of Internal Medicine and Cardiology, University of Florence, Italy

MARIA C. PORCIANI, MD
Insitute of Internal Medicine and Cardiology, University of Florence, Italy

GIUSEPPE RICCIARDI, MD
Insitute of Internal Medicine and Cardiology, University of Florence, Italy

PHILIPPE RITTER, MD
InParys, Saint-Cloud - France

IRINA SAVELIEVA, MD
Department of Cardiological Sciences, St George's Hospital Medical School, London, UK

MARK H. SCHOENFELD, MD
Cardiac Electrophysiology and Pacer Laboratory, Hospital of Saint Raphael and Yale University School of Medicine

B. ŚMIEJA-JAROCZYŃSKA, MD
Department of Cardiology, Silesian School of Medicine, Katowice, Poland.

MARSHALL S. STANTON, MD
Vice President, Medical Affairs, Cardiac Rhythm Management Division, Medtronic, Inc. Minneapolis, MN, USA

ROLAND X. STROOBANDT, MD
A Z Damiaan Hospital, Oostende, Belgium

MARIA TRUSZ-GLUZA, MD
1st Department of Cardiology, Department of Electrocardiology Silesian School of Medicine, Katowice, Poland

ARVYDAS URBONAS, MD
Electrophysiology Research Laboratory, Department of Medicine, Section of Cardiology, University of Illinois at Chicago, Chicago, USA

DALIA URBONIENE MD, PHD
Electrophysiology Research Laboratory, Department of Medicine, Section of Cardiology, University of Illinois at Chicago, Chicago, USA

PANOS E. VARDAS, MD, PhD, FESC, FACC
Professor of Medicine, Head of the Cardiology Department, Heraklion University Hospital, Crete, Greece

SAMI VISKIN, MD
Cardiology Department, Tel Aviv Souraski Medical Center, Tel Aviv, Israel

HENRY CHEUK-MAN YU
Senior Medical Officer, Director Of Non-Invasive Cardiac Services, Honorary Associate Professor, Division Of Cardiology, Department Of Medicine, The University Of Hong Kong, Queen Mary Hospital, Pokfulam, Hong Kong, China

T. ZAJĄC, MD

1st Department of Cardiology, Department of Electrocardiology
Silesian School of Medicine, Katowice, Poland

ELI ZALZSTEIN, MD

Pediatrics Cardiology, Soroka University Medical Center &
Faculty of Health Sciences, Ben Gurion University of the Negev,
Beer-Sheva, Israel

NILI ZUCKER, MD

Pediatrics Cardiology, Soroka University Medical Center &
Faculty of Health Sciences, Ben Gurion University of the Negev,
Beer-Sheva, Israel

CONTENTS

II. ATRIAL FIBRILLATION

III. IMPLANTABLE CARDIOVERTER-DEFIBRILLATOR

IV. PACING THERAPY

V. CARDIAC RESYNCHRONIZATION THERAPY FOR PATIENTS WITH CONGESTIVE HEART FAILURE

VI. NEW THERAPEUTIC APPROACHES TO PATIENTS WITH CARDIAC ARRHYTHMIA

I. ELECTROPHYSIOLOGY

1.

CELLULAR BASIS FOR THE J, T AND U WAVES OF THE ECG

Charles Antzelevitch, Ph.D.

Masonic Medical Research Laboratory, Utica, NY, USA

Introduction

It was near the turn of the last century that Willem Einthoven first recorded the electrocardiogram (ECG), initially using a capillary electrometer and then a string galvanometer.[1,2] Today, nearly 100 years later physicians and scientists are still learning how to extract valuable information from the ECG and still debating the cellular basis for the various waves of the ECG. In this review, our focus will be on the on the cellular basis for the J, T and U waves of the ECG.   These three waves represent repolarization forces within the ventricles of the heart. The J wave and T wave are thought to arise as a consequence of voltage gradients that develop as a result of the electrical heterogeneity that exists within the ventricular myocardium. The basis for the U wave has long been a matter of debate. One theory attributes the U wave to mechano-electrical feedback. A second theory ascribes it to voltage gradients within ventricular myocardium and a third to voltage gradients between the ventricular myocardium and the His-Purkinje system. Thus, an understanding of the ECG, requires that we have an understanding of the electrical heterogeneity that exists within the heart.

Electrical Heterogeneity

It was not long ago that we used to think of the ventricles of the heart as being comprised of two principal cell types: specialized conducting cells forming the His-Purkinje system and ventricular working muscle cells making up the ventricular myocardium. Studies from a number of laboratories have demonstrated that the ventricular myocardium is comprised of at least three electrophysiologically distinct cell types: epicardial, M and endocardial.[3,4] These three ventricular myocardial cell types differ principally with respect to phase 1 and phase 3 repolarization characteristics. Ventricular epicardial and M, but not endocardial, action potentials display a prominent phase 1, due to a prominent 4-aminopyridine (4-AP) sensitive transient outward current (I_{to}), giving rise to a spike and dome or notched configuration.   These regional differences in I_{to}, first suggested on the basis of action potential data[5], have now been demonstrated using whole

From Ovsyshcher IE. *New Developments in Cardiac Pacing and Electrophysiology.* Armonk, NY: Futura Publishing Company, Inc. ©2002.

cell patch clamp techniques in canine, feline, rabbit, rat, and human ventricular myocytes.(see [3]for references) Recent studies have also shown that the I_{to} –mediated action potential notch is much larger in right vs. left ventricular M and epicardial cells.[6; 7]

M cells are distinguished by the ability of their action potential to prolong more than other ventricular myocardial cell types in response to a slowing of rate and/or in response to agents with Class III actions.[8; 9] These features of the M cell are due to the presence of a smaller slowly activating delayed rectifier current (I_{Ks}), a larger late sodium current (late I_{Na}) and a larger electrogenic sodium-calcium exchange current (I_{Na-Ca}). Histologically, M cells are similar to epicardial and endocardial cells, but electrophysiologically and pharmacologically, they appear to be a hybrid between Purkinje and ventricular cells. M cells displaying the longest action potentials are often localized in the deep subendocardium to midmyocardium in the anterior wall, deep subepicardium to midmyocardium in the lateral wall [8] and throughout the wall in the region of the right ventricular (RV) outflow tracts.[4] Unlike Purkinje fibers, they are not found in discrete bundles or islets. Cells with the characteristics of M cells have been described in the canine, guinea pig, rabbit, pig and human ventricles (see [3] for references)

Contribution of Transmural Heterogeneity to the ECG

Transmural distribution of I_{to} as the basis for the J wave: The presence of a prominent action potential notch in epicardium but not endocardium underlies the development of a transmural voltage gradient during ventricular activation that manifests as a late delta wave (a small secondary R wave (R') following the QRS) or what is more commonly referred to as a J wave [10] or Osborn wave. The J wave and elevated J point have been described in the ECG of animals and humans for over forty years,[11] since Osborn's observation in the early 1950s.[12] A distinct J wave is commonly observed in the ECG of some animal species including baboons and dogs, under baseline conditions and is greatly amplified under hypothermic conditions. [13] An elevated J point is commonly encountered in humans and some animal species under normal conditions. In humans, a prominent J wave in the ECG is considered pathognomonic of hypothermia[14] or hypercalcemia. [15] Direct evidence in support of the hypothesis that the J wave is caused by a transmural gradient in the magnitude of the I_{to}-mediated action potential notch derives from experiments conducted in the arterially-perfused right ventricular wedge preparation. [10] One example is illustrated in Figure 1.

Figure 1. *Hypothermia-induced J wave. Each panel shows transmembrane action potentials from the epicardial (Epi) and endocardial (Endo) regions of an arterially perfused canine left ventricular wedge and a transmural ECG simultaneously recorded A: A small but distinct action potential notch in epicardium*

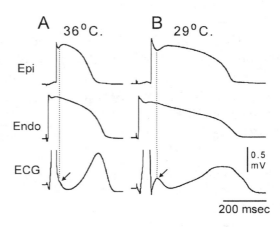

*but not in endocardium is associated with an elevated J-point at the R-ST junction (arrow) at 36°C. **B:** A decrease in the temperature of the perfusate to 29°C results in an increase in the amplitude and width of the action potential notch in epicardium but not in endocardium, leading to a prominent J wave on the ECG (arrow). (Modified from [16], with permission)*

Transmural Dispersion of Repolarization as the Basis for the T wave: Experiments involving the arterially-perfused wedge have also provided new insights into the cellular basis of the T wave suggesting that currents flowing down voltage gradients on either side of the M region are in large part responsible for the T wave (**Figs. 2 and 3**).[17] The interplay between these opposing currents establishes the height and width of the T wave as well as the degree to which either the ascending or descending limb of the T wave is interrupted, leading to a bifurcated or notched appearance. The voltage gradients result from a more positive plateau potentials in the M region than in epicardium or endocardium and from differences in the time-course of phase 3 of the action potential of the three predominant ventricular cell types. Under baseline and long QT conditions, the epicardial response is the earliest to repolarize and the M cell action potential is the last. Full repolarization of the epicardial action potential is coincident with peak of the T wave and repolarization of the M cells coincides with the end of the T wave. The duration of the M cell action potential determines the duration of the QT interval. Under these conditions, the

T_{peak}–T_{end} interval provides an index of transmural dispersion of repolarization, which may prove to be a valuable prognostic tool.[18; 19]

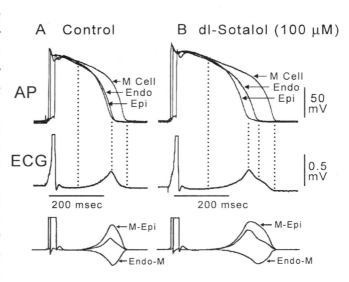

Figure 2. *Voltage gradients on either side of the M region are responsible for inscription of the electrocardiographic T wave.* **Top:** *Action potentials simultaneously recorded from endocardial, epicardial and M region sites of an arterially-perfused canine left ventricular wedge preparation.* **Middle:** *ECG recorded across the wedge.* **Bottom:** *Computed voltage differences between the epicardium and M region action potentials ($\Delta V_{M\text{-}Epi}$) and between the M region and endocardium responses ($\Delta V_{Endo\text{-}M}$). If these traces are representative of the opposing voltage gradients on either side of the M region, responsible for inscription of the T wave, then the weighted sum of the two traces should yield a trace (middle trace in bottom grouping) resembling the ECG, which it does. The voltage gradients are weighted to account for differences in tissue resistivity between M and Epi and Endo and M regions, thus yielding the opposing currents flowing on either side of the M region.* **A:** *Under control conditions the T wave begins when the plateau of epicardial action potential separates from that of the M cell. As epicardium repolarizes, the voltage gradient between epicardium and the M region continues to grow giving rise to the ascending limb of the T wave. The voltage gradient between the M region and epicardium ($\Delta V_{M\text{-}Epi}$) reaches a peak when the epicardium is fully repolarized - this marks the peak of the T wave. On the other end of the ventricular wall, the endocardial plateau deviates from that of the M cell, generating an opposing voltage gradient ($\Delta V_{Endo\text{-}M}$) and corresponding current that limits the amplitude of the T wave and contributes to the initial part of the descending limb of the T wave. The voltage gradient between the endocardium and the M*

region reaches a peak when the endocardium is fully repolarized. The gradient continues to decline as the M cells repolarize. All gradients are extinguished when the longest M cells are fully repolarized. **B:** *D-sotalol (100 uM) prolongs the action potential of the M cell more than those of the epicardial and endocardial cells, thus widening the T wave and prolonging the QT interval. The greater separation of epicardial and endocardial repolarization times also gives rise to a notch in the descending limb of the T wave. Once again, the T wave begins when the plateau of epicardial action potential diverges from that of the M cell. The same relationships as described for panel A are observed during the remainder of the T wave. The d-sotalol-induced increase in dispersion of repolarization across the wall is accompanied by a corresponding increase in the T_{peak}-T_{end} interval in the pseudo-ECG. Modified from* [17] *with permission.*

Figure 3. *Transient shift of voltage gradients on either side of the M region results in T wave bifurcation. The format is the same as in Figure 2. All traces were simultaneously recorded form an arterially perfused left ventricular wedge preparation.* **A:** *Control.* **B:** *In the presence of hypokalemia ($[K^+]_o = 1.5$ mM), the I_{Kr} blocker dl-sotalol (100 uM) prolongs the QT interval and produces a bifurcation of the*

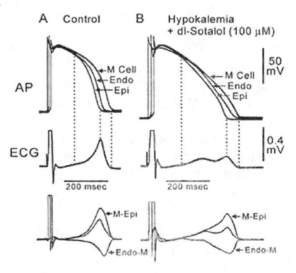

T wave, a morphology some authors refer to as T-U complex. The rate of repolarization of phase 3 of the action potential is slowed giving rise to smaller opposing transmural currents that cross-over producing a low amplitude bifid T wave. Initially the voltage gradient between the epicardium and M regions (M-Epi) is greater than that between endocardium and M region (Endo-M). When endocardium pulls away from the M cell, the opposing gradient (Endo-M) increases, interrupting the ascending limb of the T wave. Predominance of the M-Epi gradient is restored as the epicardial response continues to repolarize and the Epi-M gradients increases, thus resuming the ascending limb of the T wave. Full repolariza-

tion of epicardium marks the peak of the T wave. Repolarization of both endocardium and the M region contribute importantly to the descending limb. BCL = 1000 msec. Modified from [17] with permission.

Role of Electrical Heterogeneity in Inscription of the U wave: A number of theories have been advanced to explain the cellular basis for the U wave. One of these ascribes the U wave to delayed repolarization of the His-Purkinje system.[20] The small mass of the specialized conduction system is difficult to reconcile with the sometimes very large U wave deflections reported in the literature, especially in cases of acquired and congenital long QT syndrome (LQTS). It has previously been suggested that the M cells, more abundant in mass and possessing delayed repolarization characteristics similar to those of Purkinje fibers, may be responsible for the inscription of the "pathophysiologic U wave". [21] More recent findings derived from the wedge clearly indicate that what many clinicians refer to as an accentuated or inverted U wave is not a U wave, but rather a component of the T wave whose descending or ascending limb (especially during hypokalemia) is interrupted (**Figure 3**).[17; 22] A transient reversal in flow of current across the wall due to shifting voltage gradients between epicardium and the M region and endocardium and the M region appear to underlie these phenomena. The data suggest that the "pathophysiologic U wave" that develops under conditions of acquired or congenital LQTS is part of the T wave and that the various hump morphologies represent different levels of interruption of the T wave, arguing for use of the term T2 in place of U to describe these events, as previously suggested by Lehmann et al.[17; 23]

What then is responsible for the normal U wave, the relatively small distinct deflection following the T wave? The repolarization of the His–Purkinje system as previously suggested by Watanabe and co-workers [20] remains a most plausible hypothesis. Repolarization of the Purkinje system is temporally aligned with the expected appearance of the U wave in the perfused wedge preparation.[17] The absence of a U wave in the wedge is likely related to a low density of the Purkinje system in the dog. Unfortunately, direct evidence in support of this hypothesis is lacking, as it is for the other hypotheses concerning the origin of the U wave. Indirect support for the Purkinje hypothesis derives from the recent finding that isoproterenol-induced changes in the repolarization of Purkinje fibers parallel those of the U wave.[24] In healthy humans, isoproterenol abbreviates both QT and

QU intervals, whereas in LQT1 patients (defective I_{Ks}) isoproterenol remarkably prolongs the QT interval but abbreviates the QU interval.[25] Experimental studies involving canine left ventricular M cell preparations and Purkinje fibers demonstrate that isoproterenol abbreviates the action potential of both cell types under normal conditions, but that under conditions mimicking LQT1 (chromanol 293B-induced I_{Ks} block) isoproterenol abbreviates the Purkinje fiber action potential, but markedly prolongs that of the M cell. [24]   The isoproterenol-induced changes in Purkinje action potential duration parallel those of the QU interval, thus providing support for the hypothesis that repolarization of the Purkinje system is responsible for the inscription of the U wave. Evidence in support of a mechano-electrical basis for the U wave also exists, but is likewise indirect.[26]

Acknowledgment

Supported by grants from the National Institutes of Health (HL 47678), the American Heart Association, New York State Affiliate, and the Masons of New York State and Florida.

References

1.   Einthoven W: The galvanometric registration of the human electrocardiogram, likewise a review of the use of the capillary electrometer in physiology. *Pflugers Arch.* 1903;99:472-480

2.   Einthoven W: Uber die Deutung des Electrokardiogramms. *Pflugers Arch.* 1912;149:65-86

3.   Antzelevitch C, Dumaine R: Electrical heterogeneity in the heart: Physiological, pharmacological and clinical implications., in Page E, Fozzard HA, Solaro RJ (eds): *Handbook of Physiology. The Heart.* New York, Oxford University Press, 2002, pp 654-692

4.   Antzelevitch C, Shimizu W, Yan GX, et al: The M cell. Its contribution to the ECG and to normal and abnormal electrical function of the heart. *J.Cardiovasc.Electrophysiol.* 1999;10:1124-1152

5.   Litovsky SH, Antzelevitch C: Transient outward current prominent in canine ventricular epicardium but not endocardium. *Circ.Res.* 1988;62:116-126

6.   Di Diego JM, Sun ZQ, Antzelevitch C: I_{to} and action potential notch are smaller in left vs. right canine ventricular epicardium. *Am.J.Physiol.* 1996;271:H548-H561

7.   Volders PG, Sipido KR, Carmeliet E, et al: Repolarizing K+ currents ITO1 and IKs are larger in right than left canine ventricular midmyocardium. *Circulation* 1999; 99:206-2108.   Sicouri S, Antzelevitch C: A subpopulation of cells with unique electrophysiological properties in the deep subepicardium of the canine ventricle: The M cell. *Circ.Res.* 1991;68:1729-1741

9.   Anyukhovsky EP, Sosunov EA, Rosen MR: Regional differences in electrophysiologic properties of epicardium, midmyocardium and endocardium: *In vitro* and *in vivo* correlations. *Circulation* 1996; 94:1981-1988

10. Yan GX, Antzelevitch C: Cellular basis for the electrocardiographic J wave. *Circulation* 1996;93:372-379

11. Gussak I, Bjerregaard P, Egan TM, et al: ECG phenomenon called the J wave. History, pathophysiology, and clinical significance. *J.Electrocardiol.* 1995;28:49-58

12. Osborn JJ: Experimental hypothermia: respiratory and blood pH changes in relation to cardiac function. *Am.J.Physiol.* 1953;175:389-398

13. West TC, Frederickson EL, Amory DW: Single fiber recording of the ventricular response to induced hypothermia in the anesthetized dog. Correlation with multicellular parameters. *Circ.Res.* 1959;7:880-888

14. Dillon SM, Allessie MA, Ursell PC, et al: Influences of anisotropic tissue structure on reentrant circuits in the epicardial border zone of subacute canine infarcts. *Circ.Res.* 1988;63:182-206

15. Sridharan MR, Horan LG: Electrocardiographic J wave of hypercalcemia. *Am.J.Cardiol.* 1984;54:672-673

16. Yan GX, Antzelevitch C: Cellular basis for the electrocardiographic J wave. *Circulation* 1995;92:1-71(Abstract)

17. Yan GX, Antzelevitch C: Cellular basis for the normal T wave and the electrocardiographic manifestations of the long QT syndrome. *Circulation* 1998;98:1928-1936

18. Antzelevitch C: T peak-Tend interval as an index of transmural dispersion of repolarization. *Eur.J.Clin.Invest* 2001;31:555-557

19. Lubinski A, Lewicka-Nowak E, Kempa M, et al: New insight into repolarization abnormalities in patients with congenital long QT syndrome: the increased transmural dispersion of repolarization. *PACE* 1998;21:172-175

20. Watanabe Y: Purkinje repolarization as a possible cause of the U wave in the electrocardiogram. *Circulation* 1975;51 :1030-1037

21. Antzelevitch C, Nesterenko VV, Yan GX: The role of M cells in acquired long QT syndrome, U waves and torsade de pointes. *J.Electrocardiol.* 1996;28(suppl.):131-138

22. Shimizu W, Antzelevitch C: Sodium channel block with mexiletine is effective in reducing dispersion of repolarization and preventing Torsade de Pointes in LQT2 and LQT3 models of the long-QT syndrome. *Circulation* 1997;96:2038-2047

23. Lehmann MH, Suzuki F, Fromm BS, et al: T-wave "humps" as a potential electrocardiographic marker of the long QT syndrome . *J.Am.Coll.Cardiol.* 1994;24:746-754

24. Burashnikov A, Antzelevitch C: Is the Purkinje system the source of the electrocardiographic U wave? *Circulation* 1999;100:II-386(Abstract)

25. Zhang L, Compton SJ, Antzelevitch C, Timothy KW, Vincent GM, Mason JW: Differential response of QT and QU intervals to adrenergic stimulation in long QT patients with IKs defects. *J.Am.Coll.Cardiol.* 1999;33:138A (Abstract)

26. Surawicz B: U wave: facts, hypotheses, misconceptions, and misnomers. *J.Cardiovasc Electrophysiol.* 1998;9:1117-1128

2

CRYO VERSUS RADIOFREQUENCY ATRIAL TISSUE ABLATION: PATHOLOGY, HISTOLOGY, ATRIAL MECHANICS, AND LONG TERM ELECTROPHYSIOLOGICAL OUTCOMES

Boaz Avitall, MD, PhD, Arvydas Urbonas, MD, Dalia Urboniene MD, PhD

Electrophysiology Research Laboratory, Department of Medicine, Section of Cardiology, University of Illinois at Chicago, Chicago, USA

Introduction

Presently, most of the ablation of atrial fibrillation (AF) in humans is directed at the focal triggers in the pulmonary veins (PVs) using standard 4 mm ablation catheters[1]. However, this is time consuming and laborious procedure. . Although isolating the PVs may cure paroxysmal AF, the cure of persistent and chronic AF will require the application of linear lesions. Recent presentations at ACC 2001 and NASPE 2001 by multiple investigators support the notion that the cure of AF using catheter technology should include the placement of linear lesions, and isolation of the PVs from the left atrium[2,3]. Several investigators have presented additional data further supporting the need to place linear lesions in addition to isolating the PVs during cardiac surgery[4,5]. Radiofrequency (RF) loop catheter, designed for the ablation of AF by creating linear lesions (LL) has been shown to be safe and effective to ablate chronic AF in animal model[6]. However, preliminary results in humans with paroxysmal AF have shown that creation of LL with the RF loop catheter design is associated with low cure rate. Additionally, RF or any other source of tissue heating results in extensive tissue destruction, intense inflammatory response, and the risk of thrombus formation requiring anticoagulation during and following the procedure to prevent stroke[7]. RF ablation also leads to the development of extensive fibrous tissues that impair atrial function[8,9]. To date, only limited attempts were made to evaluate cryoablation of AF in experimental models and humans[10]. In our preliminary studies cryo lesions were discrete with preserved endocardial contours and tissue architecture. These features of cryogenic lesions make cryoablation ideally suited for catheter based MAZE procedures[11,12]. Since RF technology for the ablation of AF has formidable safety and efficacy issues (contact- dependent, thrombogenic, noncontiguous arrhytmogenic lesions, marked fibrous tissue formation), cryoablation may be a promising alternative. We investigated the new Cryo LL technology vs.

From Ovsyshcher IE. *New Developments in Cardiac Pacing and Electrophysiology.* Armonk, NY: Futura Publishing Company, Inc. ©2002.

RF LL and the impact of these technologies on lesion histology, electrophysiological outcome, and atrial mechanical function.

Cryo ablation-mechanism of injury and lesion formation. The destructive effects of freezing tissue are due to a number of factors, which can be grouped into two categories: immediate effects and delayed effects. The immediate cause of injury is the deleterious effect of freezing and re-warming cycles on the cells. The delayed causes in the progressive failure of the microcirculation and ultimate vascular stasis. Intracellular ice disrupts organelles and cell membranes and cell death is unavoidable.

One week after thawing, the periphery of the lesions is sharply demarcated by inflammatory infiltrate, fibrin and collagen stranding, and capillary growth[13]. The final phase in the evolution of a stable cryo lesion is seen by 2-4 weeks. At that time cryo lesion consists mainly of dense fibrous and fat infiltration. The older the lesion, more fibrotic changes are observed. By 12 weeks lesions are completely fibrotic with a normal distribution of blood vessels[14]. The cryo lesion is characterized by sharply circumscribed necrosis, which corresponds to the volume of tissue previously frozen. Recent studies imply that cryosurgery triggers gene regulated cell death-apoptosis. Factors stimulating apoptosis include DNA fragmentation, cytokine release, ischemia, inflammation, elevated calcium level, and macrophage recruitment. Many of aforementioned factors are associated with freezing[15,16,17]. Cryo–lesions show low arrhytmogenic potential as shown in canine model[18,19].

RF ablation-mechanism of injury and lesion formation. RF ablation is currently treatment of choice for many symptomatic cardiac arrhythmias. it is presumed that the primary cause of injury is thermally mediated, resulting in lesion/scar formation. The standard RF technique utilizes sine wave current at frequencies 500 to 1000 kHz. Deeper tissue heating occurs as consequence of heat conduction. In vivo studies demonstrated that lesion size is proportional to RF power delivery because it means higher current density and higher temperature[20].

Cellular effects. Heat induces rise in cytosolic calcium concentration secondary to increase in calcium permeability of the plasma membrane when temperature rises above 45 °C. In addition the activity of sarcoplasmic reticulum ATPase is inhibited at temperatures above 50 °C[21]. RF ablation has also direct effect on microcirculation-causes marked reduction in microvascular perfusion within acute lesion extending up to 6 mm beyond the acute margin and characterized by endothelial injury[22]. It appears to be thermally mediated and most probably occurs at temperatures above 45 °C. Clinical observation suggest direct electrical effect of RF field by inducing poration of cells, increase in membrane permeability, cellular depolarization, and conduction block[23].

RF Lesion.   Macroscopically, within the first few hours after RF application the endocardium appears pale and at times hemorrhagic, especially the surrounded tissue[24]. Underlying tissue is shrunk at the point of electrode contact. There is fibrinous material adherent to the lesion and frequently thrombi are noted.   The endocardial surface frequently is charred, and disrupted. Five days after ablation well-circumscribed areas of coagulation necrosis surrounded by peripheral zone of hemorrhage and inflammation are visible under the microscope[25].   Chronic RF lesions 2 months after ablation are significantly contracted.   Microscopically, the lesions are composed of fibrous scar, granulation tissue, fat cells, cartilage and chronic inflammatory cells[26].

Arrhythmogenicity of atrial radiofrequency (RF) ablation lesions seems to be low.   Analyzing short-term proarrhytmic potential of RF lesions, there was no increase in ambient supraventricular ectopy or ventricular ectopy observed either immediately after or 4 to 9 weeks after RF ablation compared with the baseline Holter recordings[27].   The exceptions are linear lesions created to terminate atrial fibrillation. The so-called skip lesions (isolated areas of nontransmural damage in a region in which an attempt was made to create a line of transmural block) may, in fact, be proarrhythmic, rendering the patient more susceptible to atrial arrhythmias than before ablation[28].

Comparison of clinical applicability of two different modalities: RF ablation vs. Cryo ablation for the ablation of AF.

Radiofrequency. Haines and Mcrury[29] were using sequential right atrial and then left atrial attempts at creating linear RF lesions. They found that AF could not be terminated by a mean of 33 right atrial lesions in any cases but did terminate during left atrial lesions in four of seven dogs. Swartz et al.[30] began performing extensive atrial ablations in patients with AF, aiming to mimic the maze incisions with linear RF applications. They reported that sinus rhythm was restored in 28 of 30 patients with left atrial ablation. The atrial rhythm became progressively more organized as ablation continued but did not revert to sinus until the last lesion had been completed. There is significant risk of thromboembolic events reported ranging from 0.7 to 7%[31]. Several authors have observed the occurrence of atrial flutter (often for the first time) following ablation for or termination of the lesion in a conductive tissues allowing reentry activity around the lesion similar to post surgical scars tachycardia.

Cryo ablation.   To date no cryoablation of Afib by placing LL has been attempted in humans. Animal studies data are also limited. Thibault et al. created lines of conduction block[33] in canine atrial myocardium using 5 cm tip cryocatheter. The cryolesions were discrete, showed preservation of endocardial contours and were covered only by thin layer of thrombus. These results were confirmed by Keane et al.[34] in experiments on goat atrial myocardium. Rodriguez et al compared cryoablation to RF ablation to treat cardiac arrhythmias in dogs and showed that histologically cryo lesions were homogeneous, discrete, preserving endocardial contours and tissue architecture, with minimal cartilage tissue formation and without signs of chronic inflammation, and without evidence of viable myocytes within the lesions. On the other hand, lesions created with RF were less homogenous and still contained cartilage formation, and viable myocytes within the lesions[35]. Cryothermal tissue injury is distinguished from hyperthermic injury by the preservation of basic underlying tissue architecture and minimal thrombus formation[9].

Linear Lesions with the Loop Catheter Design. Our previous studies of RF LL ablation have shown that multielectrode loop catheter technology is capable of creating long (12-19 cm) linear lesions. Recovery of LA mechanical activity was completed within 3 months after ablation, reaching 74% of the pre-ablation LA mechanical function. These results were noted despite the lesion endocardial surface area of 12-15 cm^2.

On palpation, these lesions are very hard and stiff. Trichrome and H&E stained histologic sections of these tissues revealed fibrosis, extensive formation of cartilage in 50% of the lesion depth, and proliferation of connective tissue resulting in the formation of rigid transmural structures within the atria.

RF linear lesions technology: The loop catheter employs fourteen 12-mm long coil electrodes (shown bellow, panel A and B). The electrodes

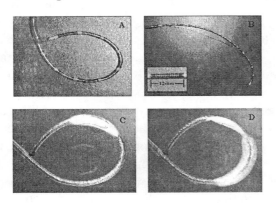

are spaced 2 mm apart such that the ablating section measures 21 cm. When applying RF power through the ablation electrodes the current density is highest at the proximal and distal edges[36]. Therefore, in this catheter thermistors are placed at the edges of each coil electrode so that automatic temperature-controlled RF power delivery could be used. The cryo loop catheter is 9F, 24 cm long stainless steel reinforced flexible tubing that can withstand 200 atmosphere of pressure. The cryo loop catheter uses the same functional principal as the RF loop catheter; it forms an expandable loop by pushing more of the catheter shaft into the sheath (shown above, panels C and D). The cryo section slides within reinforced tubing thus allowing segmental cryo ablation. The application of the cryogen results temperature of –60 to –70 degrees C and the formation of a 4 cm long iced section. By moving the cryogen delivery tubing inside the catheter the iced section moves to create a linear lesion. The resultant gas is vented out of the catheter and properly disposed. This unique catheter design allows for both localized lesion as well as the creation of long linear lesions similar to those formed by the RF loop catheter design. Both cryo and the RF loops have the same stiffness and handling characteristics. The RF LL catheter system with fourteen 12-mm long coil electrodes and Cryo loop catheter the distal tip of the catheter can be retracted to deflect the catheter into loops of various sizes by extending the catheter shaft in or out of the sheath. The stiffness of the loop forces the atrial tissues to conform around the ablation electrodes creating firm electrode-tissue contact.

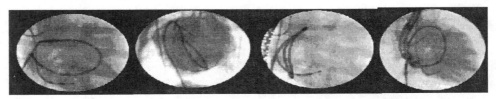

Lesion Locations. Both technologies were placed in the same anatomical positions as shown in the fluoroscopic figure above. The lesions were created at –60° to –70° C applied for 3 minutes and the dogs were allowed to recover for at least 2-month post ablation.

Five anatomical targets in both atria were selected for linear lesion placement. These sites were chosen based upon the maze procedure, and the mechanical characteristics of the loop catheter that adapt to the circumference within a globular chamber:

LAH: A circular horizontal lesion placed under the PV's in the mid LA (panel A above, the fluoroscopic image is in the PA position), above the mitral valve (MV), as indicated by a coronary sinus catheter, the atrial and ventricular electrograms recorded from each of the 14 electrodes on the catheter (this lesion does not isolate the PVs from the LA).

LAV1: LA encircling lesion connecting the medial MV and the intra atrial septum (panel B).

LAV2: LA encircling lesion connecting the lateral MV to the to the superior portion of the intra atrial septum (panel C).

RA Loop: As shown in panel D (LAO image), a circular lesion from the anterior septal tricuspid valve (TV) to the right atrial appendage (RAA) to the superior vena cava (SVC) and back to the inferior vena cava (IVC). An important factor in catheter positioning is the ability to reproduce placement in specific anatomical locations in different hearts. When deflected, the catheter tends to settle in the position with the largest circumference. However, by positioning the sheath at different levels, a variety of different positions can be achieved.

Cryo Linear lesion generation. In previous studies we have shown that LL with RF cause atrial mechanical dysfunction and reduction in atrial size attributed to marked atrial fibrosis and collagen formation.

Ablation with LL using Cryo technology may be potentially safer, create less damage to atrial tissue and preserve the atrial mechanical function after ablation.

We have evaluated the differences between the LL generated with RF and Cryo catheters. The lesion gross appearance, histology and atrial mechanical function of LA after ablation were evaluated in four RF ablated dogs and four cryo ablated dogs. The weight of RF ablated dogs was 31±1.4 kg and for cryo dogs was 33±1.6 kg (p=NS).

In RF dogs LL were created in LA by using RF multi-electrode ablation catheter capable of creating an expanding loops in both atria. Radiofrequency energy was delivered through each electrode. Power was titrated with automatic temperature control to attain an average target temperature of 70°C for 60 seconds. In RF LL group dogs a total 4.3 ± 3.8 lesions were created in the left atrium.

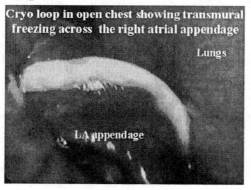

Cryo loop in open chest showing transmural freezing across the right atrial appendage

Lungs

LA appendage

In Cryo LL group a 24 cm long 9F hardened flexible cryo catheter was used with intra chamber pressure of <1 atmosphere. Total of 4.3 ± 2.9 LL were placed in the LA. Temperature was titrated to at least -50°C for 3 minutes (as shown in the panel to the left, a continuous line of ice has formed over the epicardium of the LA appendage at cryo catheter temperature of –60°C). After LL creation, in all the dogs, rhythm status was monitored weekly via surface ECG and telemetry from the intracardiac pacing leads and pacemaker.

Atrial mechanical function and PV Doppler flow patterns was evaluated using transthoracic and transesophageal echocardiography. Transthoracic echocardiography evaluation was preformed weekly to define the time course of mechanical recovery after atrial lesions in all the dogs in NSR. LA and RA mechanical function were evaluated using the same technique as Kou-Gi Shyu et al.[37]. The following were measured: LA systolic and diastolic area; LA area change; left ventricular function (assessed by calculating systolic and diastolic volumes from the two- and four-chamber apical views by single plane ellipse method, and ejection fraction); mitral inflow Doppler parameters (E wave, A wave, A wave time velocity integral, Atrial A wave TVI % to total mitral inflow TVI, and mitral regurgitation grade), and Doppler flow across the LA appendage and PVs. After ablation transthoracic echocardiography data have been collected immediately after ablation, 2 days and weekly thereafter for the 2 months of recovery.

RF vs. Cryo LL Outcomes. The dogs were ablated in NSR, no acute or chronic arrhythmia was recorded, and all the dogs maintained NSR throughout the study period.

Mitral flow characteristics post ablation: Maximal velocity of transmitral flow during LA contraction in RF group dogs decreased at 1 week and stayed stable until 2 mo post ablation (pre ablation transmitral maximal flow was 82 ± 18 cm/s, at 2 months post ablation was 65 ± 18 cm/sec; $p<0.05$) and did not change in cryo dogs (pre 72cm $\pm$ 16 cm/sec, 2 months post 71 ± 12 cm/sec). This is 38% reduction of MV "A" maximal velocity in RF group at 1 week, and 27% reduction at 2months, whereas in Cryo group the reduction noticed after ablation was 1% at 1 week and 2% at 2months.

Left atrial systolic area: Significant reduction of left atrial systolic area was noticed in RF group after ablation. Preablation LA systolic area was 10.2 ± 0.5 cm^2 in Cryo group, and 10.1 ± 1.1 cm^2 in RF group ($p=NS$). At 1 week after ablation, the LA systolic area in cryo dogs decreased to 9.6 ± 1.5 cm^2 , and 9.0 ± 0.5 cm^2 in RF group. A greater decrease of LA systolic area was observed in RF group at 2 months after ablation. The systolic area difference between the two groups at 2 months was 10.1 ± 0.9 cm^2 in Cryo group and 7.9 ± 1.1 cm^2 in RF group ($p<0.02$). Two months after ablation maximal velocity of PV diastolic flow has significantly increased in RF group versus Cryo, indicating impaired LA compliance in the RF dogs. Deceleration time of PV diastolic wave and the ratio of diastolic to systolic waves followed the same pattern[12].

Gross and histopathologic evaluation. Detailed pathologic and histologic evaluation was performed on the RF and Cryo lesions using Hematoxilin, Eosin and trichrome staining. Acutely, unlike the RF lesion the Cryo lesions create intramyocardial hemorrhage with no tissue discoloration, which are seen post RF lesions. Tetrazolium staining provides similar demarcation of the lesions post RF and cryo. More importantly, cryo lesion leaves no clot or char attached to the endocardial surfaces thus reducing the risk of stroke.

At 2 month or more of healing the RF lesions generated at 70°C result in rough surface and marked dense collagen formation on the epicardium as well as transmurally (as shown on the panels A and B bellow). Furthermore, in some of the RF lesions intramyocardial calcium were noted. Tissue contracture is evident, which is likely the cause of the LA size reduction post recovery. In contrast healed Cryo LL lesions generated with single frizzing at -60°C leaves smooth surface fibrous tissue with minimal superficial collagen (Panel B, bellow). Although repeated applications of Cryo over the same tissues does lead to the formation of dense collagen single application at -60°C does not, and at no time we documented intramyocardial calcium.

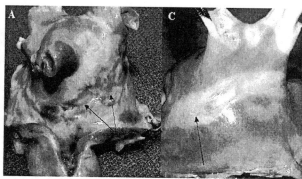

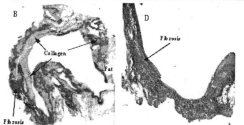

Gross pathology of RF and Cryo Linear Lesions.

Panel A. Healed RF LLs, the ablated tissues are bumpy vs. the remaining atrial tissues. Palpation of this lesion it is very hard and stiff. The rough surface of the LA is in response to 70° C RF heating. The trichrome stained histologic section **(Panel B)** shows transmural contiguous lesion and 50% of the lesion de pth consists of collagen. **Panels C.** Three months after Cryo LL showing smooth soft surface tissues of the LA in response to -60° C. The histologic section consist of transmural contiguous fibrous tissues **(Panel D)**.

Based on the above observations we can conclude that:

1. Cryo linear lesions have minimal effect on left atrial mechanical function. Left atrial size and function are reduced in radiofrequency linear lesions dogs at 2 months of follow-up.
2. Linear lesions both with cryo and radiofrequency impair left atrial compliance with quicker recovery in Cryo group as recorded by thoracic echo.
3. Radiofrequency results in extensive collagen formation, whereas minimal collagen is noted after cryo ablation.
4. Left atrial does not shrink after Cryo ablation.

REFERENCES

1. Haissaguerre M, Jais P, Shah DC, et al. Spontaneous initiation of atrial fibrillation by ectopic beats originating in the pulmonary veins. N Engl J Med 1998; 339(10):659-66.
2. Pappone P, Rosanio S, Tocchi M, et al. Circumferential radiofrequency ablation of pulmonary vein ostia for curing atrial fibrillation: long-term results from a large, single center experience (abstr). J Am Coll Cardiol 2001;37(N.2, suppl.A):A802-5.
3. Melo J, Santiago T, Neves J, et al. Is it worth treating atrial fibrillation during mitral valve reoperations? (abstr). PACE 2001;24(N.1, pII):555, A67.
4. Melo J, Santiago T, Adragão P, Neves J, Abecasis M, Ferreira MM. Surgery for atrial fibrillation using epicardial radiofrequency catheter ablation with and without cardiopulmonary bypass. Results at one year (abstr). J Am Coll Cardiol 2001;37(N.2, suppl A):A124.
5. Sueda T, Imai K, Ishii O, et al. Efficacy of pulmonary vein isolation for the elimination of chronic atrial fibrillation in cardiac valvular surgery. Ann Thorac Surg 2001;71:1189-1193.
6. Avitall B, Helms R, Koblish J, et al. The creation of linear contiguous lesions in the atria with an expandable loop catheter. J Am Coll Cardiol 1999; 33(4):972-84.
7. Epstein MR, Knapp LD, Martidill M. Embolic complications associated with radiofrequency catheter ablation. Am J Cardiol 1996; 77:655-58.
8. Avitall B, Urbonas A, Urboniene D, et al. Time course of left atrial mechanical recovery after linear lesions: normal sinus rhythm versus a chronic atrial fibrillation dog model. J Cardiovasc Electropysiol 2000; 11:1397-1406.
9. Lustgarten DL, Keane D, Ruskin J. Cryothermal ablation: mechanism of tissue injury and current experience in the treatment of tachyarrhythmias. Prog Cardiovasc Dis 1999; 41(6):481-98.
10. Gaita F, Gallotti R, Calo L, et al. Limited posterior left atrial cryoablation in patients with chronic atrial fibrillation undergoing valvular heart sugery. J Am Coll Cardiol 2000; 36(1):159-66.
11. Avitall B, Urboniene D, Urbonas A, Rozmus GP, Lafontaine D, Wales L. New cryo balloon technology for the electrical isolation of the pulmonary veins. PACE 2001; 24(4 pt 2): 542, 15A.
12. Avitall B, Urboniene D, Urbonas A, Rozmus GP. New cryo technology for creation of long contiguous linear lesions: comparison with radiofrequency ablation on left atrial mechanics and lesion morphology. PACE 2001; 24(4 pt 2): 610, 286A.
13. Mikat EM, Hackel DB, Harrison L, et al. Reaction of the myocardium and coronary arteries to cryosurgery. Lab Invest 1977; 37:632-641.
14. Harrison L, Gallagher JJ, Kasell J, et al. Cryosurgical ablation of the AV node-His bundle: A new method for producing AV block. Circulation 1977; 55:463-470.
15. Nagle WA, Bernard L, Soloff A, et al.. Cultured Chinese hamster cells undergo apoptosis after exposure to cold but nonfreezing temperatures. Cryobiology 1990; 27, 439–451.
16. Baust JG, Hollister W, Mathews A, and Van Buskirk R. Gene-regulated cell death follows cryo-surgery [abstract]. Cryobiology 1997; 35, 322.
17. Hollister WR, Mathew AJ, Baust JG, et al. The effects of freezing on cell viability and mechanisms of cell death in an in vitro human prostate cancer cell line. Mol. Urol. 1998; 2, 13–18.
18. Holman WL, Ikeshita M, Douglas JM, et al. Ventricular cryosurgery: Short term effects on intramural electrophysiology. Ann Thorac Surg 1983; 35:386-393.

19.Klein GJ, Harrison L, Ideker RF, et al. Reaction of myocardium to cryosurgery: Electrophysiology and arrhytmogenic potential. Circulation 1979; 59:364-372.

20. Wittkampf FH, Hauer RN, Robles de Medina EO. Control of radiofrequency lesion size by power regulation. Circulation 1989; 80:962-68.

21. Inesi G,Millman M, Eletr S. Temperatue-induced transitions of function and structure in sarcoplasmic reticulum membranes. J Mol 1973; 81:483-504.

22. Nath S, Whayne JG, Kaul S, et al. Effeects of radiofrequency catheter ablation on regional blood flow: Possible mechanism for late electrophysiological outcome. Circulation 1994; 89:2667-2672.

23. Chang DC, Reese TS. Changes in membrane structure induced by electroporation as reviled by rapid-freezing electron microscopy. Biophys J 1990; 58:1-12.

24. Nath S, Haines DE. Biophysics and pathology of catheter energy delivery systems. Prog Cardiovasc Dis 1995; 4:185-204.

25. Huang SK, Bharati S, Graham AR, et al. Closed chest catheter desiccation of AV junction using radiofrequency energy - A new method of catheter ablation. JACC 1987; 9:349-358.

26. Huang SK, Bharati S, Lev M, et al. Electrophysiological and histological observations of chronic AV block induced by close chest catheter desiccation with RF energy. PACE 1987;10:805-16.

27. Johnson TB. Lack of proarrhythmia as assessed by Holter monitor after atrial radiofrequency ablation of supraventricular tachycardia in children. Am Heart J 1996; 132(1 Pt 1): 120-4.

28. Avitall B, Helms RW, Chiang W, et al. Nonlinear atrial radiofrequency lesions are arrhythmogenic: A study of skipped lesions in the normal atria. Circulation 1995;92:I-265A.

29. Mitchell MA, McRury ID, Haines DE. Linear atrial ablations in a canine model of chronic atrial fibrillation: morphological and electrophysiological observations. Circulation 1998, 97:1176-85.

30. Swartz JF, Pellersels G, Silvers J, et al. A catheter-based curative approach to atrial fibrillation in humans [abstr]. Circulation1994; 90:I-335.

31. Epstein MR, Knapp LD, Martidill M. Embolic complications associated with radiofrequency catheter ablation. Atakr Investigation Group. Am J Cardiol 1996;77:655.

32. Jais P, Haissaguerre M, Gencel L, et al. Incidence of common atrial flutter following catheter ablation of atrial fibrillation in the right atrium. Circulation1995; 92:I-266A.

33. Thibault B, Villemaire C, Talajic M, et al. Catheter cryoablation is more effective and potentially safer method too create atrial conduction block: Comparison with radiofrequency ablation. Semin Intervent Cardiol 1997; 2:251-265.

34. Keane D, Zhou L, Ruskin J. Percutaneous cryothermal catheter ablation for the creation of linear atrial lesions. J Med Sci 1998.

35.Rodriguez LM, Leunissen J, Hoekstra A, et al. Transvenous cold mapping and cryoablation of the AV node in dogs: observations of chronic lesions and comparison to those obtained using radiofrequency ablation. J Cardiovasc Electrophysiol 1998; 9(10):1055-61.

36. McRury ID, Panescu D, Mitchell M, et al. Nonuniform heating during radiofrequency catheter ablation with long electrodes: monitoring the edge effect. Circulation 1997; 96(11):4057-4064.

37. Shyu KG, Cheng JJ, Chen JJ, et al. Recovery of atrial function after atrial compartment operation for chronic atrial fibrillation in mitral valve disease. J Am Coll Cardiol 1994; 24:392-8.

3

POST-MI SIGNALING PATHWAYS AS TARGETS FOR NOVEL THERAPEUTIC INTERVENTIONS

Nabil El-Sherif, MD

Cardiology Division, Department of Medicine, State University of New York, Downstate Medical Center and Veterans Affairs Medical Center, Brooklyn, NY, USA

Supported in part by VA MERIT and REAP grants

Introduction

Ventricular remodeling is the process by which ventricular size, shape and function are regulated by mechanical, neurohormonal, and genetic factors.[1,2] Remodeling may be physiological and adaptive during normal growth or pathological due to myocardial infarction, cardiomyopathy, hypertension, or valvular heart disease. Following myocardial infarction (MI), the heart undergoes a complex time-dependent remodeling process that involves structural, biochemical, neurohormonal, and electrophysiologic alterations.[1-3] The acute loss of myocardium results in an abrupt increase in loading conditions that induces a unique pattern of remodeling involving the infarcted border zone and remote noninfarcted myocardium.[4] Post-MI remodeling is associated with time-dependent dilation, distortion of ventricular shape, and hypertrophy of the noninfarcted myocardium. Following a variable period of compensatory hypertrophy deterioration of contractile function may develop resulting in congestive heart failure. The molecular, morphologic, and functional alterations underlying post-MI remodeling bear resemblance to those described in other models of hypertrophy.[3] Those changes have been investigated in detail in our laboratory.[5-14] However, other studies from our laboratory have also emphasized differences in cardiac gene expression in the post-MI heart compared to other overload hypertrophy models. This may suggest stimuli-specific recruitment of distinct signal transduction pathways. Understanding the signal transduction pathways for cardiac remodeling in pressure /volume overload or post-MI experimental models is a key for the design of appropriate therapeutic interventions.

Post-MI Signaling Pathways

Figure 1 illustrates a proposed scheme for post-MI signaling pathways. Many of these pathways were shown to be activated either in response to ischemia/reperfusion stimuli or to a stretch stimulus using different experimental models and sometimes non-cardiac cell systems. However, cell membrane receptors and intracellular signaling proteins are highly conserved between mammalian species and the triggering events for cellular hypertrophy in humans are likely to resemble closely those in the various animal models used. The diagram shows that a cascade of successive transduction steps allows signal

From Ovsyshcher IE. *New Developments in Cardiac Pacing and Electrophysiology.* Armonk, NY: Futura Publishing Company, Inc. ©2002.

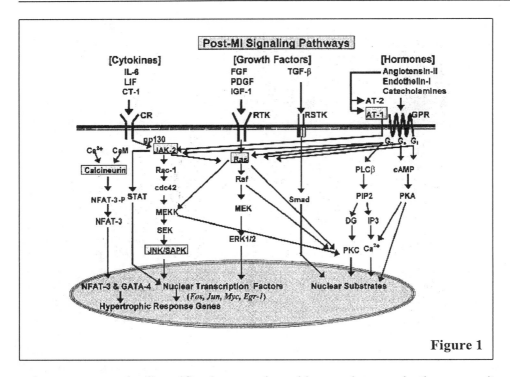

Figure 1

enhancement and diversification at branching points and thus permits combinatorial interactions between multiple pathways. Although, multiple signaling pathways may act in synergistic, antagonistic, or permissive way some key pathways may play a dominant role. There is a plethora of experimental and clinical data that show that the renin-angiotensin system (RAS) plays a major role in post-MI remodeling. More recently the Janus kinase/signal transducer and activator of transcription (JAK/STAT) signaling pathway was found to be prominently associated with activation of the autocrine loop of the heart tissue-localized RAS.[15] The JAK/STAT pathway, originally identified as a major signal transduction pathway of the cytokine superfamily through the gp130 is known also to be activated by several G protein-dependent receptors.[16] The contribution of the 21 kDa guanine nucleotide-binding protein Ras, the mitogen-activated protein kinases (MAPK), and the calcineurin-dependent pathway to postMI remodeling remains largely unexplored even though all of these pathways have been shown to induce hypertrophic signals.

Why reverse/modify remodeling? The diastolic/systolic dysfunction and the negative electrophysiologic alterations of post-MI remodeling have provided the impetus for the various therapeutic strategies that attempt to reverse/modify the remodeling process. Pharmacologic agents that target specific pathophysiologic processes are one major approach. However, the introduction of novel therapeutic modalities entails better understanding of the molecular and functional consequences of post-MI remodeling. The recent success of some non-pharmacologic therapeutic measures, for example, the left ventricle assist device (AVAD) have shown that even in an advanced stage of heart failure, the remodeling process could be reversed with significant improvement of ventricular function.[17]

Electrophysiologic alterations in post-MI remodeled heart

Three weeks post-MI in the rat, remodeled hypertrophy of the noninfarcted myocardium is at its maximum and the heart is usually in a compensated stage. At this stage, we have shown that prolongation of action potential duration (APD) of remodeled myocardium is primarily due to decreased density of both I_{to-f} and I_{to-s}[6] while both the density and kinetics of I_{Ca-L} were not significantly different from control[5] The changes in I_{to-f} and I_{to-s} were explained by decreased expression of mRNAs and proteins of Kv4.2/4.3 and Kv2.1, respectively.[7] We have shown a high incidence of inducible ventricular tachyarrhythmias (VT) in the three-week-old post-MI rat heart, which could be partly explained by inhomogeneity of APD prolongation across the left ventricular wall, favoring circus movement reentry. Further, post-MI remodeled myocytes were shown to generate both early afterdepolarization- (EAD) and delayed afterdepolarization (DAD)-induced triggered activity.[6] In a recent study we showed that regional variations in Kv channel genes expression and K^+ currents are significant determinants of increased electrophysiologic heterogeneity of the post-MI heart.[13] In another study we demonstrated regional alterations in connexin 43 expression which can affect the passive electrical properties of remodeled myocardium.[18]

For many years the observation was made that cardiac hypertrophy from whatever cause is consistently associated with down regulation of K^+ channel genes and K^+ currents. We have recently provided evidence to support the hypothesis that this down regulation in the post-MI heart occurs early and may be dissociated from the slower time course of post-MI remodeled hypertrophy.[11]

Post-MI diastolic and systolic dysfunction

A variable period of compensatory hypertrophy is eventually followed by decompensation and heart failure. The structural, neurohormonal, ionic, and molecular changes associated with the transition from compensated cardiac hypertrophy to decompensated heart failure are currently the subject of extensive investigation. Defects in the regulation and signaling pathways of β-adrenergic receptors, and alterations in calcium handling of the myopathic cardiac muscle have been described. Of the multiple factors involved in diastolic/systolic dysfunction of hypertrophied heart, including the post-MI remodeled heart, the β-adrenergic pathway and the sarcoplasmic reticulum (SR) play major roles. Heart failure is accompanied by an increased adrenergic drive and hence increased plasma catecholamine levels. The elevated circulating catecholamine level downregulates β-adrenergic receptor density and is responsible for the transcriptionally regulated elevation of $G_{\alpha i2}$[19] The diminished positive inotropic effect of β-adrenergic agonists in end-stage human heart failure could be explained only in part by a decreased density of β-adrenoreceptors. Some data lead to the hypothesis of a defect in the signaling pathway beyond the β-adrenoreceptors. This hypothesis is supported by the clinical finding that some alterations can be reversed in patients with end-stage heart failure after long-term therapy with β-blockers.[20]

We have recently shown that three weeks post-MI in the rat, there was evidence of diastolic dysfunction, which was explained by reduced SERCA2 activity.[9] The reduction in SERCA2 activity at this stage was not due to decreased basal levels of both p16-PLB and p17-PLB. The reduced p-PLBs were mainly due to enhanced activity of type 1 phosphatase which dephosphorylates p16-PLB and p17-PLB.

Some investigators strongly believe that the interaction of two ongoing processes in the remote myocardium, i.e. remodeled hypertrophy that develops gradually and peaks before the hypertrophic process is exhausted and the smoldering ongoing apoptosis may underlie the transition to heart failure and marked ventricular dilatation.[21] Other investigators argued that remodeling of interstitial matrix with increased collagen deposition and matrix metalloproteinase activity is a significant factor in diastolic dysfunction and the transition to heart failure.[22]

Therapeutic interventions

The effects of therapies designed to prevent or attenuate post-MI left ventricular remodeling are best considered with reference to the pathophysiological mechanisms involved. Infarct size is a major determinant of ventricular remodeling and both early and late cardiac mortality. Benefit from early myocardial reperfusion has been demonstrated to reduce infarct size and associated improvement in both regional and global ventricular function. This subject is beyond the scope of this review.

Angiotensin converting enzyme (ACE) inhibition – The efficacy of ACE-inhibitors in attenuating left ventricular dilatation after MI was first demonstrated in the rat, and this effect on remodeling was associated with improved survival. A large number of studies have demonstrated a survival benefit when ACE inhibitors have been used in patients with MI and selectively in patients with left ventricular dysfunction or heart failure.[23] The mechanism of improvement with ACE inhibition is related in part to peripheral vasodilatation, ventricular unloading, and the attenuation of ventricular dilatation. There may be additional beneficial effects on the coronary circulation and intrinsic plasminogen-activating system. Importantly, ACE inhibition may have a direct effect on myocardial tissue, preventing the inappropriate hypertrophy stimulated by AngII and other growth factors.

Beta-blockade – The effects of beta-blockade on post-MI left ventricular remodeling have been little studied. Preliminary data suggest that carvedilol may attenuate remodeling, an effect associated with a significant reduction in subsequent adverse events.[24] The effects of ACE inhibition and beta-blockade seem complementary. After MI and in chronic heart failure, ACE inhibition improves remodeling and primarily reduces deaths from progressive heart failure. In chronic heart failure caused by ischemia, beta-blockade with carvedilol can reverse remodeling, which may progress despite standard treatment, including

ACE inhibition. The mortality benefit from beta-blockade in chronic heart failure, which is now clearly established, is due to a reduction in both progressive heart failure and sudden cardiac death.

Endothelin antagonists – ET-1 is the most potent endogenous vasoconstrictor known; in addition, it acts as a potent growth factor and (co)mitogen. There is substantial experimental evidence that ET-1 may contribute not only to sustained vasoconstriction, but also to remodeling within the cardiovascular system . Both myocardial and plasma ET-1 are elevated in heart failure. However, the role played by endogenous ET-1 in the progression of heart failure remains unknown. In an experimental post-MI rat model, bosentin, an ET-1 receptor antagonist, was shown to modestly reduce preload and afterload, resulting in substantially attenuated left ventricular dilatation and causing improved pressure-volume relationships. However, the compensatory hypertrophic response was not altered by ET-receptor antagonism. The Authors concluded that ET-1 does not appear to play a crucial role in the mechanisms of myocardial hypertrophy during the early phase of post-MI failure.[25]

Pharmacologic agents that may impact on the electrophysiologic alterations associated with post-MI remodeling – A key electrophysiologic alteration in post-MI remodeled heart is down regulation of K^+ gene expression and K^+ currents resulting in spatially heterogenous prolongation of APD and increased dispersion of refractoriness. It is therefore not surprising that the post-MI heart is more sensitive to hypokalemia and to the proarrhythmic effects of drugs that depress K^+ currents, especially I_{kr} blockers. On the other hand, some pharmacological interventions have been shown to reduce the incidence of sudden death in post-MI patients, like magnesium and spironolactone, or to reverse the down regulation of I_{to} in experimental post-MI models, like the thyroid hormone analog DITPA.

Magnesium in acute MI – Potassium depletion is known to increase the incidence of arrhythmias, particularly ventricular arrhythmias, in patients with MI. The well-established link between magnesium and potassium leads one to expect that a correlation exists between magnesium deficiency and arrhythmias in infarcted patients. Magnesium is also a cofactor for sodium-potassium adenosine triphosphatase and calcium adenosine triphosphatase, which are important in maintaining membrane stability. The last decade has seen approximately eight large randomized trials of magnesium therapy in acute MI.[26] However, the patient selection criteria in these studies, and the study protocols varied significantly. The beneficial effects of magnesium received a temporary setback by the ISIS-4 study in which no mortality benefit was obtained from the administration of magnesium . The lack of therapeutic effect of magnesium in the ISIS-4 trial can be explained by the late enrollment of patients and the fact that magnesium infusions were delayed 1 or 2 hours after thrombolytic therapy. In a recent study, intravenous magnesium administered to patients in the immediate post-MI period decreased significantly the incidence of arrhythmias, myocardial dysfunction, and death.[26] The mechanisms of the cardioprotective effects of magnesium remain, however, unclear. Various studies have shown that magnesium can decrease the size of myocardial infarction, decrease platelet aggregation, decrease basal tension of the arterioles, decrease peripheral vascular resistance, and increase coronary vasodilatation.[27] It remains unclear whether the cardioprotective effect of magnesium supplementation in patients with acute MI is due to a correction of a hypomagnesemic state or to the increase of magnesium to above normal levels.

Spironolactone – Aldosterone has an important role in the pathophysiology of heart failure.[28] Aldosterone promotes the retention of sodium, the loss of magnesium and potassium, sympathetic activation, parasympathetic inhibition, myocardial and vascular fibrosis, baroreceptor dysfunction, and vascular damage and impairs arterial compliance. Many physicians have assumed that inhibition of the rennin-angiotensin-aldosterone system by ACE inhibitors will suppress the formation of aldosterone. There is increasing evidence to suggest, however, that ACE inhibitors only transiently suppress the production of aldosterone. A recent multicenter study has shown that spironolactone, an aldosterone-receptor antagonist, when used in conjunction with an ACE inhibitor in patients with severe congestive heart failure and low left ventricular ejection fraction, reduces the risk of both death from progressive failure and sudden death.[29] Although the exact cause of the reduction in the risk of death remains speculative, it is suggested that an aldosterone-receptor blocker can prevent progressive heart failure by averting sodium retention and myocardial fibrosis and prevent sudden death from cardiac causes by averting potassium loss and by increasing the myocardial uptake of norepinephrine.[29] Spironolactone may prevent myocardial fibrosis by blocking the effects of aldosterone on the formation of collagen, which in turn could play a part in reducing the risk of sudden death from cardiac causes, since myocardial fibrosis could predispose patients to variations in ventricular conduction times and, hence, to reentrant ventricular arrhythmias.[29]

Thyroid hormone analogs – Downregulation of I_{to} is a key electrophysiologic alteration of post-MI remodeled myocardium. The thyroid hormone has been shown to increase the expression of genes encoding for I_{to}[30] alter the biophysical properties of I_{to} and, hence, abbreviate APD. The effects of thyroid hormone, however, are complicated by a plethora of noncardiac effects that may limit the beneficial effect of this agent. In a recent study in the experimental post-MI rat model, chronic administration of the thyroid hormone analog 3,5-diiodothyropropionic acid (DITPA) has been shown to restore I_{to} expression, and improve the repolarization abnormalities associated with the post-MI heart, with only minor effects on heart rate and metabolism, compared with thyroid hormone.[31] The clinical validity of this therapeutic measure has not been tested.

Calcium antagonists – The role of antagonists of the L-type Ca^{++} channel in the post-MI heart is limited. On the other hand, the role of antagonists of the T-type Ca^{++} channel remains unexplored. Data on the benefit of I_{Ca-T} antagonist in experimental models are sparse. The selective I_{Ca-T} antagonist, mibefradil, was shown to improve survival in a rat model of chronic heart failure, compared to the I_{Ca-L} antagonist amlodipine.[32] Mibefradil has been introduced in clinical trials for the treatment of hypertension and angina pectoris[33] even though it was recently withdrawn from clinical application. The beneficial effects were attributed to a potent coronary and peripheral vasodilatation. T-type Ca^{++} currents are present in neonatal rat myocytes but are not detected in adult rat myocytes. We have recently shown that T-type Ca^{++} channel genes and current are reexpressed in rat post-MI remodeled left ventricular myocytes.[10] Post-MI remodeled myocytes were shown to generate both EADs and DADs.[6] Although the I_{Ca-T} density is smaller compared to that of I_{Ca-L}, it is possible that slight augmentation of intracellular Ca^{++} at certain phases of action potential can predispose to abnormal afterdepolarizations. However, an arrhythmogenic potential of reexpressed T-type Ca^{++} channel gene and current in the post-MI remodeled rat heart and possible antiarrhythmic effects of I_{Ca-T} antagonists remain to be demonstrated.

Novel therapeutic interventions

Drugs that can modulate post-MI remodeling like the calcineurin blocker, cyclosporine; antiapoptotic agents like caspase inhibitors, and pharmacologic blockers of TGF-β1 , the latter plays a critical role in the development of fibrosis are promising targets for future developments.

Cyclosporine – Calcineurin participates in hypertrophic signal transduction in models of cardiac hypertrophy[34] Cyclosporine, a specific inhibitor of calcineurin, has recently been shown to ameliorate the hypertrophic process in a number of animal models [34,35] In a recent study, cyclosporine was shown to prevent pressure-overload hypertrophy in the mice with maintenance of normal left ventricular size and systolic function.[35] The abolition of the hypertrophic response to systolic pressure overload does not seem to result in left ventricular decompensation. In a recent study we investigated the effects of calcineurin inhibition by cyclosporin on key structural, hemodynamic, and electrophysiologic alterations of post-MI remodeling.[14] Hypertrophy and cardiac dimensions were evaluated by echocardiography. Changes in diastolic function were correlated with changes in protein phosphatase 1 activity and the level of p16-phospholamban. The effects on Kv 4.2/4.3 genes expression and transient outward current density were also evaluated. The study showed that calcineurin inhibition by cyclosporin partially ameliorated post-MI remodeled hypertrophy, diastolic dysfunction, and the down regulation of k^+ genes expression and K^+ current with no adverse effects on systolic function or mortality in the first 3-4 weeks post-MI.[14]

Caspase inhibitors – Apoptosis has been reported to occur in and by conditions characterized by ischemia, like MI and stroke, and may be implicated in the progression of heart failure. Caspase family proteases are recognized as key mediators of apoptosis. The role of caspases in the ischemia-reperfused heart has recently been investigated in the rat model. Myocyte DNA fragmentation and caspase activation were inhibited by caspase inhibitors, However, caspase inhibitors did not significantly change the infarct size.[36]

Epilogue

The future challenge must be the primary prevention of MI in patients at high risk for coronary disease. Meanwhile, new therapeutic strategies should be targeted to limit remodeling by controlled modulation of the molecular and cellular factors involved in tissue repair, including hypertrophy, fibrosis, and the capillary microcirculation. In addition to pharmacologic interventions, gene therapy could play an increasing role. The genetic approach to myocardial angiogenesis promises to exert beneficial effects on the post-MI remodeling process.[37] Last, but not least, genetic engineering may permit phenotypic transformation of embryonic stem cells into cardiomyocytes or facilitate cardiomyocyte regeneration and engraftment in regions of fibrosis and thinning to restore wall thickness and myocardial mass.[38]

References

1. Pfeffer JM, Pfeffer MA, Fletcher PJ, Braunwald E. Progressive ventricular remodeling in rat with myocardial infarction. Am J Physiol. 1991; 260: H1406-H1414.
2. Swynghedauw B. Molecular mechanisms of myocardial remodeling. Physiol reviews. 1999; 79: 215-262.
3. Hefti MA, Harder BA, Eppenberger HM, Schaub MC. Signaling pathways in cardiac myocyte hypertrophy. J Mol Cell Cardiol. 1997; 29: 2873-2892 Sutton MG, St J, Sharpe N. Left ventricular remodeling after myocardial infarction. Pathophysiology and Therapy. Circulation. 2000; 101: 2981-2988.
4. Sutton MG, St J, Sharpe N. Left ventricular remodeling after myocardial infarction. Pathophysiology and Therapy. Circulation. 2000; 101: 2981-2988.
5. Gidh-Jain M, Huang B, Jain P, et al. Reemergence of the fetal pattern of L-type calcium channel gene expression in non-infarcted myocardium during left ventricular remodeling. Biochem Biophys Res Commun. 1995; 216: 892-897.
6. Qin D, Zang Z-H, Caref EB, et al. Cellular and ionic basis of arrhythmias in postinfarction remodeled ventricular myocardium. Circ Res. 1996; 79: 461-473.
7. Gidh-Jain M, Hunag B, Jain P, El-Sherif N. Differential expression of voltage-gated K^+ channel genes in left ventricular remodeled myocardium after experimental myocardial infarction. Circ Res. 1996; 79: 669-675.
8. Gidh-Jain M, Huang B, Jain P, El-Sherif N. Alterations in cardiac gene expression during transition to compensated hypertrophy following myocardial infarction. J Mol Cell Cardiol. 1998; 30: 627-637.
9. Huang B, Wang, S Qin D, et al. Diminished basal phosphorylation level of phospholamban in the post-infarction remodeled rat ventricle. Role of *B-*

adrenergic pathway, G_i protein, phosphodiesterase, and phosphatases. Circ Res. 1999 85: 848-855.

10. Huang B, Qin D, Deng L, et al. Reexpression of T-type Ca^{++} channel gene and current in the post-infarction remodeled rat left ventricle. Cardiovasc. Res. 2000; 46: 442-449.

11. Huang B, Qin D, El-Sherif N. Early down-regulation of K^+ channel genes and currents in the postinfarction heart. J. Cardiovasc. Electrophysiol. 2000 ; 11: 1252-1261.

12. Huang B, El-Sherif T, Gidh-Jain M, et al. Alterations of the sodium channel kinetics and gene expression in the post-infarction remodeled myocardium. J. Cardiovasc. Electrophysiol. 2001.2001; 12:218-225..

13. Huang B, Qin D, El-Sherif N. Spatial alteration of Kv channel expression and K+ currents in post-MI remodeled rat heart. Cardiovasc Res 2001; in press.

14. Deng L, Huang B, Qin D, et al. Calcineurin inhibition ameliorates structural, contractile, and electrophysiological consequences of post-infarction remodeling. J Cardiovasc Electrophysiol 2001; 12:1055-1061..

15. Mascareno E, Dhar EM, Siddiqui, MAQ. Signal transduction and activator of transcription (STAT) protein-dependent activation of ANG promoter: A cellular signal for hypertrophy in cardiac muscle. Proc Natl Acad Sci USA. 1998; 95: 5590-5594

16. Heim HM: The Jak-STAT pathway: Cytokine signaling from the receptor to the nucleus. J Recept signal transduction 1999; 19:75-120

17. Frazier OH, Benedict CR, Radovancevic B, et al. Improved left ventricular function after chronic left ventricular unloading. Ann Thorac Surg 1996;62:675-82.

18. Huang B, Qin D. Gidh-Jain M,. et al. Spatial alterations of Kv channel and connexin 43 expression and K^+ current density of post-infarction remodeled left ventricle. Circulation. 1998, 98 (17): I-697.

19. Swynghedauw B, Chevalier B, Charlemagne D, et al. Cardiac hypertrophy, arrhythmogenicity and the new myocardial phenotype II. The cellular adaptational process. Cardiovasc Res 1997;35:6-12.

20. Jakob H, Sigmund M, Beck F, et al. Reduction of $Gi\alpha$ in myocardial biopsies of patients with heart failure under metoprolol treatment. Circulation 1994;90:I-413.

21. Cheng W, Kajstura J, Nitahara JA, et al. Programmed myocyte cell death affects the viable myocardium after infarction in rats. Exp Cell Res 1996;226:316-327

22. Spinale FG, Coker ML, Thomas CV , et a*l*. Time-dependent changes in matrix metalloproteinase activity and expression during the progression of congestive heart failure-relation to ventricular and myocyte function. Circ Res 82:482-485,1998.

23. Pfeffer MA, Braunwald E, Moye LA, et al, on behalf of the SAVE Investigators. Effect of captopril on mortality and morbidity in patients with

left ventricular dysfunction after myocardial infarction: results of the Survival and Ventricular Enlargement Trial. N Engl J Med 1992;327:669-77.

24. Basu S, Senior R, Raval U, et al. Beneficial effects of intravenous and oral carvedilol treatment in acute myocardial infarction: a placebo-controlled, randomized trial. Circulation 1997;96:183-91.

25. Oie E, Bjonerheim R, Grogaard HK, et al. ET-receptor antagonism, myocardial gene expression, and ventricular remodeling during congestive heart failure in rats. Am J Physiol 1998;275(3Pt2):H868-77.

26. Gyamlani G, Parikh G. Kulkami AG. Benefits of magnesium in acute myocardial infarction: timing is crucial. Am Heart J 2000;139:e2

27. Shechter M, Hod H, Kaplinsky E, Rabinowitz B. The rationale of magnesium as alternative therapy for patients with acute myocardial infarction without thrombolytic therapy. Am Heart J 1996;132:483-6.

28. Barr CS, Lang CC, Hanson J, et al. Effects of adding spironolactone to an angiotensin-converting enzyme inhibitor in chronic congestive heart failure secondary to coronary artery disease. Am J Cardiol 1995;76:1259-65.

29. Pitt B, Zannad F, Remme WJ, et al. The effect of spironolactone on morbidity and mortality in patients with severe heart failure. N Engl J Med 1999;341:709-17.

30. Wickenden AD, Kaprielian R, Parker TG, et al. Effects of development and thyroid hormone on K+ currents and K+ channel gene expression in rat ventricle. J Physiol (Lond) 1997;504:271-86.

31. Wickenden AD, Kaprielian R, You X-M, Backx PH. The thyroid hormone analog DITPA restore Ito in rats after myocardial infarction. Am J Physiol 2000;278:H1105-16.

32. Mulder P, Richard V, Compagnon P, et al. Increased survival after long-term treatment with mibefradil, a selective T-channel calcium antagonist, in heart failure. J Am Coll Cardiol 1997;29:416-21.

33. Kobrin I, Bieska G, Charlon V, et al. Anti-anginal and anti-ischemic effects of mibefradil, a new T-type calcium channel antagonist. Cardiology 1998;89(Suppl 1):23-32.

34. Molkentin JD, Lu J-R, Antos CL, et al. A calcineurin-dependent transcriptional pathway for cardiac hypertrophy. Cell 1998;93:215-28.

35. Hill JA, Karimi M, Kutschke W, et al. Cardiac hypertrophy is not a required compensatory response to short-term pressure overload. Circulation 2000;101:2863-9.

36. Okamura T, Miura T, Takemura G, et al. Effect of caspase inhibitors on myocardial infarct size and myocyte DNA fragmentation in the ischemia-reperfused rat heart. Cardiovasc Res 2000;45:642-50.

37. Li J, Brown LF, Hibberd MG, et al. VEGF, flk-1, and flt-1 expression in a rat myocardial infarction model of angiogenesis. Am J Physiol 1996;270:H1803-11.

38. Li RK, Weisel RD, Mickle DA, et al. Autologous porcine heart cell transplantation improved heart function after a myocardial infarction. J Thorac Cardiovasc Surg 2000;119.

4.

NONCONTACT MAPPING TO GUIDE ABLATION OF ARRHYTHMIAS

Paul A. Friedman, MD, Dawood Darbar, MD, Michael Glikson, MD[*]

Division of Cardiovascular Medicine, Mayo Clinic, Rochester, MN, and [*]Department of Cardiology, Sheba Medical Center, Tel Hashomer, Israel

Introduction: Noncontact mapping is based on the physical principle that if a three dimensional probe is placed within a cardiac chamber and both the probe and endocardial surfaces are defined, measurement of the electrical potential present on the probe's surface permits calculation of the endocardial voltage. This allows reconstruction of electrograms at endocardial sites in the absence of physical electrode contact at those locations (virtual electrograms), permitting recording of cardiac electrical activity from thousands of points simultaneously.

The noncontact mapping system (EnSite 3000; Endocardial Solutions, Inc., St. Paul, MN) consists of catheter-mounted multielectrode array (MEA) which serves as the probe, a custom designed amplifier system, and a computer workstation that is used to display three dimensional maps of cardiac electrical activity. The catheter consists of a 7.5 ml balloon mounted on a 9F catheter around which is woven a braid of 64 insulated 0.003 mm diameter wires. Each wire has a 0.025mm break in insulation that serves as a noncontact unipolar electrode. The raw far-field electrocardiographic data from the MEA are acquired and fed into a multi-channel recorder and amplifier system that also has channels for conventional contact catheters, 12 channels for the surface ECG as well as pressure channels. The unipolar MEA signals are recorded using a ring electrode as a reference, which is located on the shaft of the MEA catheter. An electrically based locator signal is also generated by the system to permit non-fluoroscopic navigation of any standard roving contact catheter used for ablation.

The locator system is able to locate any conventional catheter in space with respect to the MEA by passing a 5.68 kHz, low-current "locator" signal between the contact catheter electrode being located and alternately between ring electrodes proximal and distal to the MEA on the noncontact catheter. This creates a potential gradient across the MEA electrodes used to position the source. This locator signal serves 2 purposes. First, it can be used to construct the 3-D computer model of the endocardium (virtual endocardium) that is required for the reconstruction of endocardial electrograms and isopotential maps (Figure 1).

From Ovsyshcher IE. *New Developments in Cardiac Pacing and Electrophysiology.* Armonk, NY: Futura Publishing Company, Inc. ©2002.

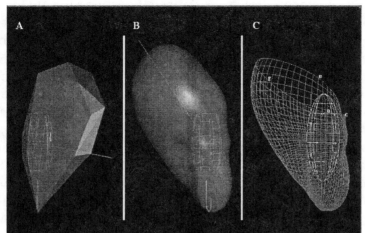

Figure 1. *Creation of the noncontact geometry.   (A)   As a mapping catheter is swept through the chamber to be mapped (left ventricle in this example), each passage of the mapping catheter to a new, more distant location in a given direction from the MEA defines the endocardial boundary.   The green line (locator signal) depicts the position of the mapping catheter relative to the geometry or map. (**B**) Once complete, the geometry is smoothed. (**C**) The geometry of the MEA and chamber (in this case, left ventricle) are defined, so that a map can be generated from a single complex. Further details in text.*

This model is acquired by moving a conventional, contact catheter around the cardiac chamber, building up a series of coordinates for the endocardium, and generating a patient-specific, anatomically contoured model of its geometry.   To accomplish this, the system automatically stores only the most distant points visited by the roving catheter in order to ignore those detected when the catheter is not in contact with the endocardial wall. Geometric points are sampled at the beginning of the study during sinus rhythm, resulting in a contoured, wire-frame model with end–diastolic dimensions (Figure 1). The total time to define the contoured chamber geometry is typically less than 5 minutes.[1] Second, the locator signal can be used to display and log the position of any catheter on the endocardial model. During catheter ablation procedures, the locator system has been used in real-time to navigate the catheter to sites of interest identified from the isopotential color maps, to catalogue the position of RF energy applications on the virtual endocardium, and to facilitate re-visitation of sites of interest by the ablation catheter.

The electrical activity detected by the electrodes on the surface of the MEA is generated by the potential field on the endocardial surface. Once the endocardial geometry has been defined, it is possible to compute endocardial electrograms from the MEA potentials by inverse solution of Laplace's equation, utilizing a boundary element method. [2] The inverse solution considers how a signal detected at a remote point will have appeared at the source, and the boundary element method simplifies application of the inverse solution to resolve a matrix of signals from a source at a known boundary (e.g., the blood-endocardial boundary). The system reconstructs over 3,360 electrograms simultaneously over a computer-generated model of the chamber of interest ("virtual" endocardium). Due to the high density of data, color coded isopotential maps are used to graphically depict regions which are depolarized, and wavefront propagation is displayed as a user controlled three dimensional "movie" (Figure 2). Activation maps can also be created. Additionally, unipolar or bipolar virtual electrograms can be displayed by selection of an area of interest, and displayed as if from point, array, plaque, or circular lasso-type electrodes. The fidelity of virtual electrograms compared to actual contact electrograms has been confirmed in vitro and in vivo, as has the precision of the catheter navigation system.[3,]

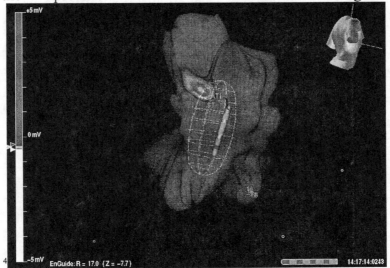

Figure 2: *Single frame from a noncontact "movie" depicting wavefront propagation along the posterior right atrium. Note detailed rendering of complex endocardial cardiac geometry. The position of any mapping catheter can be localized and depicted on the map, as shown above. The colored region on the map indicates depolarized myocardium.*

Clinical Experience

Ectopic Atrial Tachycardia: Noncontact mapping expedites ectopic tachycardia ablation in several ways. Navigation to regions difficult to pinpoint fluoroscopically is facilitated, pertinent structures (such as the His bundle or valve annuli) can be annotated and localized in 3-D space, and the ablation catheter can be accurately and repeatedly re-navigated to predetermined sites in the cardiac chamber. Additionally, the high density parallel data acquisition permits mapping of arrhythmias seen only transiently in the electrophysiology laboratory. Once the geometry is defined, the origin of multiple arrhythmias can be rapidly determined without the need for sequential mapping catheter re-positioning along the endocardium to record new electrogram data. This is particularly useful for patients with atrial tachycardias, as more than one arrhythmia if frequently present. Additionally, catheter contact irritation is avoided during mapping. Due to the intrinsic ability of unipolar electrograms to localize point source arrhythmias, the unipolar-based isopotential maps used in noncontact mapping appear particularly well suited to ectopic tachycardia localization. In a preliminary study in which the noncontact and electroanatomical mapping systems were deployed simultaneously, the site selected using the unipolar noncontact map was more frequently the point of successful ablation than the site selected using the bipolar electroanatomical map.[1]

Atrial flutter: Typical atrial flutter is usually readily-treated utilizing standard ablation techniques. However, noncontact mapping has been used to confirm the anatomic location of the flutter circuit. More importantly, due to its ability to record from multiple sites simultaneously, the technique is uniquely well suited to the identification of gaps in linear lesions, which can be accomplished from a single paced complex without the need to retrace the entire line. Thus, the non-contact mapping system has been used to identify and guide RF ablation to the site of residual conduction following incomplete linear lesion at the isthmus.[5, 6]

The ability of noncontact mapping to verify bi-directional isthmus block during atrial flutter ablation has been confirmed in a study of 12 patients undergoing flutter ablation.[7] In that study, noncontact isopotential maps reliably distinguished conduction delays from complete conduction block, and when a gap in a line of block was present, its location was instantaneously identified. Such a gap could be closed and complete conduction block created by RF application guided by the noncontact system.[5, 7] Moreover, in 33% of patients, localization of a gap using conventional techniques was hampered by the presence of fractionated, low-amplitude signals along the ablation line. Although virtual electrograms were comparable at these sites, the gap was readily by noting the "break out" site of electrical activity across the line on the isopotential map.[7] Additionally, the authors reported that since only a single catheter was needed in the noncontact system, set up time was less than that of placement of the four catheters used for conventional mapping.

Noncontact mapping may be of particular utility in the ablation of atypical (non-sub-Eustachian isthmus-dependent) flutter and post surgical flutter by rapidly defining the circuit. Since atypical flutter may utilize myocardium removed from the usual fluoroscopic landmarks and may include tissues that can be difficult to reach with contact catheters, noncontact mapping has been particularly useful in preliminary reports for the mapping of these arrhythmias.[8] Additionally, since several atypical flutters often coexist in the same patient, the ability to map multiple arrhythmia circuits without the need to recreate a geometry facilitates mapping and expedites ablation. In a study of patients with congenital heart disease and a previous Fontan procedure, noncontact mapping improved recognition of the anatomic and surgical substrate and identified exit sites from zones of slow conduction in all clinical arrhythmias.[9]

Atrial fibrillation: As described above, the two approaches used to treat AF include ablation of focal triggers and creation of linear lesions. Early clinical experience suggests noncontact mapping may play a role in both approaches.

Pulmonary vein foci have been identified as the triggers of paroxysmal and persistent AF.[10] Due to the intermittent and transient nature of pulmonary vein discharges and rapid degeneration to atrial fibrillation, mapping for ablation has been difficult. With its ability to globally map a single complex, noncontact mapping holds unique promise in its ability to identify focal triggers and the bundles of myocardium connecting pulmonary vein to left atrial musculature.[11, 12] We used a dual transseptal puncture technique to place the MEA and a roving catheter in the left atrium in 11 patients with paroxysmal atrial fibrillation (average 2 episodes/week). Acute elimination of culprit pulmonary vein ectopy was achieved in 10 patients. With a median follow up of 10 weeks, arrhythmia recurred in 5 patients. Interestingly, 4 of the 5 patients in whom noncontact mapping was used as a rescue technique after failure of multipolar catheter guided ablation had a recurrence, whereas only one of the 5 patients in whom noncontact mapping was the primary approach experienced recurrent atrial fibrillation (p<0.05).[13] Pulmonary vein "spikes" suggestive of muscle bundles have been described as suitable targets for pulmonary vein ablation.[10] We retrospectively found spikes in the virtual electrograms in 12 of 15 culprit pulmonary veins. Reversal of timing of atrial and pulmonary vein "spike" potentials (premature complexes vs sinus beats) was seen in all 36 episodes of ectopy that initiated atrial fibrillation, and in none of 236 complexes of normal sinus rhythm (p<0.01). However, since the system an endocardial geometry in its calculations, it is likely that only ostial pulmonary vein potentials can be reconstructed.[14]

Noncontact mapping has also been used to guide linear lesion creation for the control of atrial fibrillation. We used noncontact mapping to create right atrial linear lesions in 7 patients with atrial fibrillation.[15] Following initial lesion set creation, 7 conduction gaps were found in 5 of the 7 patients. For four gaps, the noncontact map created while pacing or during sinus rhythm coincided with the predicted gap sites based on review of the three-dimensional catalogue of lesion sites recorded on the virtual endocardium; in the remainder, the noncontact map was superior to the lesion catalogue for localizing the gaps. The ability to assess conduction across the entire length of a long ablation without the need to retrace the line to assess electrograms greatly facilitated lesion assessment. At the end of the procedure, all patients had had complete bi-directional isthmus and intercaval block, demonstrating that this mapping technology can successful guide acute creation of long linear lesions. There were no complications. However, only one patient remained free of AF off of antiarrhythmic drugs, confirming the limited efficacy of linear lesions limited to the right atrium despite acute confirmation of the absence of gaps.

Ventricular tachycardia: The most common cause for clinical ventricular tachycardia is prior myocardial infarction. Catheter ablation of such VTs has been limited by the time required for sequential endocardial activation mapping. The results have been disappointing, with immediate success rates of 71% to 90% but common recurrence.[16]

Successful ablation of VT is critically dependent on locating the diastolic pathway of the reentrant circuit. However, using conventional techniques, as few as 10% of patients may be suitable for catheter mapping and ablation of VT, predominantly because of hemodynamic compromise during VT. Due to its ability to record cardiac activation from a single complex, noncontact mapping can facilitate the mapping of unstable rhythms. Schilling et al. were the first to demonstrate the feasibility of the non-contact catheter for endocardial mapping of human VT.[2] They demonstrated exit sites in 80 (99%) of 81 VTs and VT reentry circuits in 67%. Thirty-eight VTs were ablated with >78% success rate over a follow-up period of 1 year in patients who survived the perioperative period. More recently, Strickberger et al[17] mapped a total of 21 VTs, 12 of which were hemodynamically tolerated and 9 of which were not, using the non-contact mapping system. Isolated diastolic potentials, presytolic areas, zones of slow conduction and exit sites were identified using virtual electrograms and isopotential maps during VT. Among 19 targeted VTs, RF guided by the computerized mapping system and the locator signal was successful in 15.   The ability to rapidly record an unstable VT, then review the map and navigate the catheter to the critical site of the VT circuit during normal rhythm facilitated ablation.

Noncontact mapping has also been used to guide ablation of focal VT in both the right and left ventricles. [18, 19] We successfully ablated right ventricular outflow VT in seven of eight patients, of whom 4 had failed previous ablation and 5 had only transient arrhythmia in the electrophysiology laboratory.   Similar results have been observed in patients with previously failed ablation of idiopathic left ventricular tachycardia.[19]

Conclusions: The non-contact mapping system has several advantages over current mapping techniques. Its high density parallel data acquisition yields high-resolution maps of the entire cardiac chamber from a single beat of tachycardia, enabling registration of transient or hypotensive arrhythmias, and facilitating localization of gaps in long linear lesions. Furthermore, an anatomical representation of the cavity geometry is obtained upon which anatomical structures can be annotated. This three-dimensional virtual chamber can permit radiation-free catheter navigation, facilitate re-visitation of points of interest, and guide linear lesion creation. Additionally, the navigation system can be used with any electrode catheter, permitting operator flexibility in catheter choice. The system has been shown to facilitate ablation of a broad variety of complex ablation procedures including ablation of transient arrhythmias[18] and those resistant to conventional techniques.

REFERENCES

1. Munger TM, Friedman PA, Grice SK, Hammill SC, Packer DL. Feasibility of combined noncontact and electroanatomical mapping for guiding ablation of complex arrhythmias. Journal of the American College of Cardiology 2000; 35:126.
2. Schilling RJ, Peters NS, Davies DW. Feasibility of a noncontact catheter for endocardial mapping of human ventricular tachycardia. Circulation 1999; 99:2543-52.
3. Gornick CC, Adler SW, Pederson B, Hauck J, Budd J, Schweitzer J. Validation of a new noncontact catheter system for electroanatomic mapping of left ventricular endocardium. Circulation 1999; 99:829-35.

4.   Kadish A, Hauck J, Pederson B, Beatty G, Gornick C. Mapping of atrial activation with a noncontact, multielectrode catheter in dogs. Circulation 1999; 99:1906-13.

5.   Friedman PA, Stanton MS. Spot welding the gap in atrial flutter ablation. Circulation (Images in Cardiovascular Medicine) 1999; 99:3206-3208.

6.   Goyal R, Pelosi F, Souza J, et al. Trans-isthmus conduction block in patients with atrial flutter assessed with a non-contact mapping catheter. Circulation 1999:I-282.

7.   Schumacher B, Jung W, Lewalter T, Wolpert C, Luderitz B. Verification of linear lesions using a noncontact multielectrode array catheter versus conventional contact mapping techniques. J Cardiovasc Electrophysiology 2000; 10:791-798.

8.   Paul T, Tebbenjohanns J, Bertram H, Kriebel T, Hausdorf G. Endocardial mapping and radiofrequency catheter ablation of atrial reentrant tachycardia in young patients after surgical correction of congenital heart disease with a novel non-contact mapping system. J Amer Coll Cardiol 2000; 35; Suppl A:516.

9.   Betts T, Roberts P, Allen S, et al. Electrophysiological Mapping and Ablation of Intra-Atrial Reentry Tachycardia After Fontan Surgery With the Use of a Noncontact Mapping System. Circulation 2000; 102:2094-2099.

10.   Haïssaguerre M, Jaïs P, Shah DC, et al. Spontaneous initiation of atrial fibrillation by ectopic beats originating in the pulmonary veins. New England Journal of Medicine 1998; 339:659-66.

11.   Friedman PA, Grice S, Munger TM, Hammill SC, Packer DL. Spot welding the trigger in focal atrial fibrillation ablation. Journal of Cardiovascular Electrophysiology 2000; 11:1061.

12.   Schneider M, Ndrepepa G, Zrenner B, et al. Noncontact mapping-guided catheter ablation of atrial fibrillation associated with left atrial ectopy. Journal of Cardiovascular Electrophysiology 200; 11:475-9.

13.   Friedman PA, Grice SK, Munger TM, et al. Feasibility of ablation of focal atrial fibrillation guided by noncontact left atrial mapping. Journal of the American College of Cardiology 2000; 35:123.

14.   Asirvatham S, Friedman P. Etiology of Electrogram "Spikes" Observed in the Pulmonary Veins. Circulation 2000:--.

15.   Packer D, Asirvatham S, Munger T, et al. Utility of noncontact mapping for identifying gaps in long linear lesions in patients with atrial fibrillation. PACE 2000; 23:673.

16.   Rothman SA, Hsia HH, Cossu SF, Chmielewski IL, Buxton AE, Miller JM. Radiofrequency catheter ablation of postinfarction ventricular tachycardia: long-term success and the significance of inducible nonclinical arrhythmias. Circulation 1997; 96:3499-508.

17.   Strickberger SA, Knight BP, Michaud GF, Pelosi F, Morady F. Mapping and ablation of ventricular tachycardia guided by virtual electrograms using a noncontact computerized mapping system. J Am Coll Cardiol 2000; 35:414-421.

18.   Friedman PA, Grice SK, Munger TM, et al. Utility of noncontact mapping in guiding successful ablation in patients with previously failed ablation procedures. Journal of the American College of Cardiology 2000; 35:126.

19.   Friedman PA, Beinborn DA, Shultz J, Hammill SC. Ablation of noninducible idiopathic left ventricular tachycardia using a non-contact map acquired from a premature complex with tachycardia morphology. PACE 1999.

5.

ENHANCED SUSCEPTIBILITY TO VENTRICULAR ARRHYTHMIAS FOLLOWING MYOCARDIAL INFARCTION: FEASIBILITY OF MURINE MODEL

Yuri Goldberg, MD, *Ilya A. Fleidervish, MD, PhD, Eugene Crystal, MD, Inna Gitelman, PhD, Eli Zalzstein, MD, Nili Zucker, MD, Harel Gilutz, MD, Reuven Ilia, MD, I. Eli Ovsyshcher, MD, PhD

Research Electrophysiology Laboratory and Cardiac Research Center, Cardiology Department, Soroka University Medical Center & Faculty of Health Sciences, Ben Gurion University, Beer-Sheva, Israel; *Koret School of Veterinary Medicine, The Hebrew University of Jerusalem, Rehovot, Israel

Introduction

In the last decade, extensive knowledge of the mouse genome made genetically engineered murine models one of the most promising tools for understanding the mechanisms of heart diseases. They are, however, being relatively rarely used to study the mechanisms of arrhythmias. There are at least two reasons for this. Firstly, implementation of surgical and recording techniques, which are easily applicable in larger species for assessing pathological alterations, is extremely difficult in mice. Secondly, it is not clear whether electrophysiological disturbances in the murine heart are similar to those in larger species, since the electrophysiological characteristics of the normal murine heart are an extreme case amongst mammals. In such, the murine heart has the highest sinus rhythm and shortest action potential duration and ventricular refractoriness[1]. It is not clear whether thin ventricular walls of the murine ventricles possess M-cells[2], which, in larger species, are hypothesized to be the major source of "triggered" arrhythmias. Also, a "critical mass" hypothesis predicts that the murine heart is too small to sustain re-entrant ventricular arrhythmias[3] (but see[4]).

Here, we established and characterized the murine model of post-MI remodeling with the special emphasis on its electrophysiological consequences.

Materials and Methods

Animals. Three month old CD1 mice of either sex, weighing 35–45g each underwent open-chest surgery for ligation of the left coronary artery (14 mice) or sham-operation (16 mice).

From Ovsyshcher IE. *New Developments in Cardiac Pacing and Electrophysiology.* Armonk, NY: Futura Publishing Company, Inc. ©2002.

Preoperative preparation. Mice were anesthetized with a mixture of xylazine and ketamine (5 mg/kg and 100 mg/g, i.p.). A surface 6-lead ECG and echocardiographic imaging (using either M-mode or transesophageal probe) were performed and the mice were allowed to recover. For M-mode echocardiographic study, nine mice were anesthetized as described above, their chests were shaved and they were positioned on the left side. A 12 MHz pediatric transducer with lateral and axial resolution between 0.2 and 0.5 mm was connected to a echocardiographic computer console (Hewlett Packard 5500, Andover, MA). Left ventricular end-systolic and end-diastolic diameters were measured at the level of the papillary muscles. End-diastolic area was defined as the largest LV area and end-systolic as the smallest. In eight animals, transesophageal echocardiography (TEE) has been performed using 30-MHz intravascular ultrasound catheter (Sonicath cv, Mansfield, Boston Scientific Corp, I5007) and standard echocardiographic system (Hewlett Packard Sonos Intravascular). The ultrasound catheter was introduced into the esophagus after the latter was filled with gel. The catheter was carefully advanced until the liver was visualized. Image acquisition was initiated and the catheter manually withdrawn in measured steps of 1 mm with an imaging duration of 5 seconds at each plane. Two to four horizontal planes were obtained. To minimize an error caused by inaccuracy of the measurements and by beat-to-beat variations, for all hearts, between three to six beats were measured using the same transducer position, and the mean values were used for further analysis.

Production of MI. The mice were anesthetized, intubated and ventilated with a tidal volume of 0.2 ml and a respiratory rate of 120 breaths per minute. Adequacy of ventilation was confirmed by blood gases evaluation. Thus, in arterial blood samples taken from the left ventricles of three mice which were held ventilated during a period of fifteen minutes, pO_2 and pCO_2 values were within the normal range (107 ± 20 mmHg and 40 ± 9 mmHg, respectively). After left anterior thoracotomy, left coronary artery was visualized and ligated intramurally ~3 mm from its origin. The ECG was continuously monitored to confirm occlusion (**Figure 1**). Animals were extubated and allowed to recover from the anesthesia. Sham-operated mice underwent identical surgery but did not sustain MI.

Postoperative examination. Sixteen days later, ECG, echocardiography and electrophysiological study (EPS) were performed in both post-MI and sham-operated animals. In EPS, single and double extrastimuli techniques (down to a minimum coupling interval of 30 ms) were used to attempt induction of ventricular arrhythmia. Following echocardiographic and

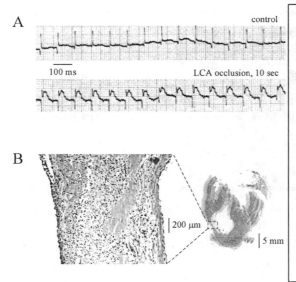

Figure 1. Induction of MI in mice.
A. Lead I of ECG before (top) and 10 sec after (bottom) left coronary artery ligation. Note the significant ST segment elevation that confirmed occlusion of the artery.
B. Morphologic appearance of MI in murine heart, 16 days after left coronary artery ligation. Right, hematoxilin-eosin stained section to show markable thinning of latero-apical free wall of the left ventricle following MI. Left, under higher magnification, the MI area is characterized by intensive replacement of myocardiocytes with inflammatory infiltrates and connective tissue.

electrophysiological recordings, the hearts were removed and rinsed for 1 minute in 0.1 mol/L PBS with 50 mmol/L KCl (pH 7.2) and subsequently fixed overnight at 4°C in 4% paraformaldehyde pre-pared in PBS. Vibratome sections (100 μm) from similar areas of the left ventricles were stained with hematoxiline and eosin. Myocyte widths were measured parallel to the direction of the sarcomeres from unbranched regions of the myocytes near intercalated disks under high magnification.

Statistics. All data are reported as mean ± SE. Comparisons between the groups were made using Student's *t* test.

Results

Left coronary artery ligation was produced in 14 mice. In 9 cases, the MI induction was confirmed histologically. On 16th post-MI day, the infarction area appeared as thinning of the latero-apical free wall of the left ventricle (LV) and it was characterized by intensive replacement of cardiomyocytes with inflammatory infiltrates and connective tissue. As in other species, echocardiographic examination (M-mode in 9 mice and TEE in 4 mice) performed on 16th post-MI day revealed a significant increase in both end-systolic and end-diastolic LV diameters (**Figure 2**; $p < 0.05$; n=9).

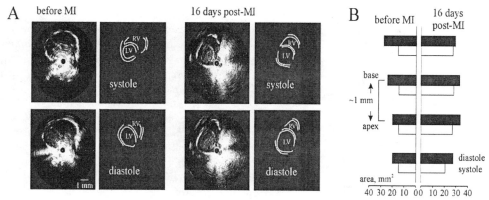

Figure 2. Post-MI dilatation of the LV as revealed by TEE.
A. TEEs from the representative mouse before MI (left) and on 16th day after MI (middle). **B.** *Measurements of diastolic and systolic left ventricular areas in 4 consecutive planes.*

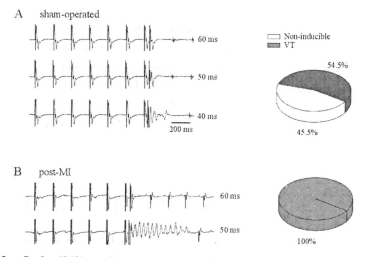

Figure 3. Inducibility of ventricular arrhythmias by programmed epicardial stimulation. **A.** *Left, in a sham-operated mouse, extrastimulus delivered at the edge of refractory period (40 ms) induced a short run of polymorphous VT that stopped spontaneously after 3 beats. Under similar stimulation protocol, brief episodes of VT were induced in 54.5% of sham-operated hearts (right).* **B.** *Left, in a representative post-MI mouse tested using the similar stimulation protocol, single extrastimulus delivered at an interval of 50 ms induced run of VT. The run consisted of 13 beats at cycling of 51±5 ms, and it was 640 msec long. VT was inducible in all post-MI mice (right).*

Macroscopic alterations in geometry of LV chamber, in non-infarcted areas, were accompanied by an increase in myofiber diameter (20.2 ± 5.2 μm vs.15.4 ± 4.0 μm in shams; $p < 0.05$, n = 85 measurements). The QT interval was significantly prolonged in post-MI mice under sinus rhythm (125 ± 19 ms vs. 68 ± 18 ms; $p < 0.05$; n = 6) and under pacing at 300 bpm (106 ± 47 ms vs. 71 ± 40 ms; $p < 0.01$; n = 5). Attempts to induce ventricular arrhythmia by delivering single extrastimulus following the burst of seven stimuli at 5-6 Hz were successful in all post-MI mice, but only in 54.5% of shams **(Figure 3)**. The arrhythmias, a non-sustained VT in inducible cases, consisted of 4-15 beats at cycling of 66 ± 14 ms and lasted for 640 ± 250 ms in post-MI mice.

Discussion

For more than 80 years since Garrey's[3] experiments, there has been a general belief that cardiac tissue smaller than a certain critical mass (originally estimated as 4 cm^2), like murine ventricles, cannot provide an EP substrate for reentry. This concept has been recently revised by Vaidya et al.[4], who using Langendorff-perfused heart preparation demonstrated that the stationary vortex-like reentrant activity is possible in murine ventricles whose surface area is less than 100 mm^2. In the ECG, the activity was manifested as sustained monomorphic tachycardia or polymorphic pattern indistinguishable from ventricular fibrillation[4].

In our hands, burst pacing of sham-operated and post-MI hearts induced only non-sustained polymorphic ventricular activity, lasting no longer than 15 beats. Somewhat longer monomorphic VT (up to 29 s long) has been recently reported in post-MI murine hearts *in vivo*[5]. The differences between our results and data by others[4,5] is unclear. Note, however, that the experiments by Vaidya et al.[4] were done in *in vitro* perfused preparation in presence of electromechanical uncoupler, which might affect the wavelength of potential reentry circuit. Although experimental conditions used by Gehrmann et al.[5] are close to ours, the resulting EP substrate for sustained VT and VF still could be different due to technical differences in MI production.

In the present study, we did not examine the mechanisms of arrhythmias and its substrate. Since both monomorphic and polymorphic VT could be elicited by burst pacing in murine heart (**Figure 3**, refs 4,5), the arrhythmias development, most probably, is dependent on both reentrant and triggered automaticity mechanisms. In a larger species, the latter has been attributed to middle myocardial M-cells[2]. To date, however, there is no evidence on whether M-cells are present in a thin ventricular wall of the murine ventricles. Moreover, it remains unclear whether murine ventricular cardiomyocytes, which posses powerful and unique K^+ channel system, are able to generate early and delayed afterdepolarization the same way as ventricular cells of larger species.

Whatever the mechanisms are of arrhythmias we observed, our data indicate that although the electrophysiological alterations associated with post-MI remodeling in murine heart could facilitate arrhythmogenesis, they differ significantly from those in other species. The results of murine experiments, therefore, should be rather carefully interpreted than directly extrapolated to humans.

References

1.   Berul CI, Aronovitz MJ, Wang PJ, et al. In vivo cardiac electrophysiology studies in the mouse. *Circulation* 1996; 94:2641-8.

2.   Yan GX, Shimizu W, Antzelevitch C. Characteristics and distribution of M cells in arterially perfused canine left ventricular wedge preparations. *Circulation* 1998; 98:1921-7.

3.   Garrey WE. The nature of fibrillary contraction of the heart: its relation to tissue mass and form. *Am J Physiol* 1914; 33: 397-414.

4.   Vaidya D, Morley GE, Samie FH, Jalife J. Reentry and fibrillation in the mouse heart. A challenge to the critical mass hypothesis. *Circ Res* 1999; 85:174-81.

5.   Gehrmann J, Frantz S, Maguire CT, et al., Electrophysiological characterization of murine myocardial ischemia and infarction. *Basic Res Cardiol* 2001; 96:237-50

II.   ATRIAL FIBRILLATION

6.

ANATOMIC BASE FOR ATRIAL FIBRILLATION

Saroja Bharati, M.D.

Maurice Lev Congenital Heart and Conduction System Center, The Heart Institute for Children, Hope Children's Hospital, Advocate Christ Medical Center, Oak Lawn, IL, University of Illinois at Chicago and Rush Medical College, Chicago and Chicago Medical School, Finch University, North Chicago, IL.

Atrial fibrillation is the most common cardiac arrhythmia in the aging population. Pathologically, in chronic atrial fibrillation, the normal architecture of the atria is altered, in practically all hearts examined. These changes, however, are *not specific* for atrial fibrillation, rather, these are relatively non specific changes that may produce other types of atrial arrhythmias as well. There are numerous pathologic findings in the atria including the surrounding conduction system that may alter the normal atrial architecture resulting in atrial fibrillation clinically.[1-12]

At the gross level, the atria are usually hypertrophied and enlarged or aneurysmally dilated with paper thin walls with or without fatty infiltration. Rarely one may find atherosclerotic plaques with or without calcification. At light microscopic level, one may find hypertrophy, atrophy, varying types of degenerative phenomena, such as, focal areas of fibrosis, vacuolar degeneration with practical loss of atrial myocardial cells, and considerable amount of fat. In some, there may be necrosis, acute and/or chronic inflammation, tumor infiltration of the atrial septum. The same findings may be evident in the atrial preferential pathways, approaches to the SA and AV nodes, as well as within the nodes, AV bundle and bundle branches. In still others, there may be narrowing of the SA nodal and AV nodal arteries with or without total occlusion of the large epicardial coronary arteries. It is therefore assumed that the above changes were the anatomic substrate for atrial fibrillation.[1-12] It is also important to note that there may be biochemical, metabolic and physiologic changes that may be associated with the structural changes. Likewise, hormonal imbalances, abnormal neural responses, emotional state, and perhaps other unknown factors that may also induce atrial fibrillation. From our pathological studies, we were able to classify atrial fibrillation in the following manner.[1-12]

From Ovsyshcher IE. *New Developments in Cardiac Pacing and Electrophysiology.* Armonk, NY: Futura Publishing Company, Inc. ©2002.

Classification of Atrial Fibrillation

(I..) Normal aging phenomena as such.

(II.) Acquired heart diseases:

    (a.) Coronary artery disease

    (b.) Hypertensive heart disease

    (c.) Rheumatic heart disease – mitral stenosis

    (d.) Infiltrative diseases of the heart: 1. Fat; 2. Amyloid; 3. Sarcoid.

    (e.) Alcohol

(III.) Atrial Fibrillation Related to Cardiac Surgery

    1. Coronary artery bypass

    2. Atrial septal defect – any type

    3. Mustard or Senning procedure for complete transposition

    4. Atrial septectomy – Blalock Hanlon procedure

    5. Post operative heart disease:

(IV.) Arrhythmias associated with atrial fibrillation

    A. Familial arrhythmias with AV block

    B. Pre-excitation

    C. Congenital AV block in the middle aged

    D. Sick sinus syndrome - tachycardia - bradycardia syndrome

(V.) Congenital:

    (a) Idiopathic dilation of the right atrium

    (b.) Ebstein's anomaly

    (c.) Atrial septal defect – any type of long standing duration

    (d.) Tumors:

        1. Lipoma of the atrial septum

        2. Myxoma

        3. Rhabdomyoma

    (e.) Congenital anomalies of the AV junction — atrio Hisian connection

(VI.) Miscellaneous:

    (a.) Hypothyroidism

    (b.) Hyperthyroism

    (c.) Myotonia dystrophica

    (d.) Kearn-Sayre Syndrome

    (e.) Hypertrophic cardiomyopathy

    (f.) Any disease that affects that the atria from a moderate to considerable extent.

It is emphasized that the above classification is by no means complete, nevertheless, may be found useful clinically.

Normal Aging

The normal aging changes of the atria eventually result in atrophy, hypertrophy, degenerative changes of the myocardial fibers with increase in fat and connective tissue extending near the SA node, AV node and their approaches.[1-12]   It is emphasized that with aging, the left atrium is the first chamber that gets hypertrophied and enlarged thereby making it susceptible for atrial fibrillation. It is to be pointed out that the myocardial fibers of the normal left atrium are arranged in a chaotic fashion and hence normal aging affects the left atrium more than the other chambers of the heart. The loss of myocardial fibers with fibro- fatty degenerative changes in the atria probably alters the transmission of impulses from the SA node to the AV node thereby resulting in atrial fibrillation. The atrial myocardium, in general, show varying stages of degenerative changes accompanied by fat. In addition, at the light microscopic level there are large spaces between the above described pathologic findings in the atria. It is unclear at the moment what occupied the empty spaces. We hypothesize that they may represent the lymphatics or other biochemical phenomena with fluid components.

There is constant increase in connective tissue and fat with aging as such that increases in the elderly gradually. Thus, clinically, with time, there may be intermittent or transient forms of atrial fibrillation to start with that eventually progresses to a permanent form.

Senile Amyloidosis in the Aging Heart

Senile amyloidosis is usually seen in those over the age of eighty. This may be considered a form of primary amyloidosis which is seen with senility and affects the atrial myocardium much more than the ventricular myocardium. Amyloid infiltrates the interstitium and compresses the surrounding myocardial fibers. Amyloid infiltrates the SA node and its approaches, the SA nodal artery, the small blood vessels (arterioles), of the atrium compromising the blood supply to the node and its approaches, the surrounding atrial myocardium, and atrial preferential pathways, thereby resulting in varying types of tachy or bradyarrhythmias.[10,11]

Hypertensive Heart Disease

It is well known that hypertensive heart disease is associated with increase incidence of supra ventricular arrhythmias and atrial fibrillation. Here, the atria are hypertrophied and enlarged associated with moderate to severe coronary artery disease. There is left ventricular hypertrophy as well. Pathologically, there is significant small vessel disease (arteriolosclerosis) in the approaches to the SA node, SA node and the approaches to the AV node. There is also increase in fat and fibroelastosis of the atria and within the AV node to a varying extent. It is also to be noted that the same type of degenerative changes are also present in the distal parts of the conduction system in most cases of hypertensive heart disease associated with chronic atrial fibrillation. In addition, there may be the usual aging changes in the summit of the ventricular septum as well. [2, 5-7]

There is a tendency for atrial fibrillation to occur frequently with hypertensive heart disease and this is accelerated with aging phenomena. Since the peripheral conduction system is equally affected one may also find bundle branch block, especially left bundle branch block, clinically with atrial fibrillation in the elderly.

Coronary Artery Disease
Atrial fibrillation occurs commonly in coronary artery disease which may be seen in the acute or chronic forms of myocardial infarction.[2,5-7,11]

Acute Coronary Insufficiency — Myocardial Infarction
Atrial fibrillation is more commonly seen in acute posteroseptal myocardial infarction than in anteroseptal wall myocardial infarction. The anatomic substrate for atrial fibrillation is usually atrial infarction with or without infarction of the SA node. There may be an associated AV block and infarction of the AV node. The AV nodal artery may be considerably thickened and narrowed.

Chronic Coronary Insufficiency
Atrial fibrillation may be seen with severe coronary artery disease and previous myocardial infarction.

It is again emphasized that in normal aging phenomena (beyond the age of 65 or 70 years) there is a frequent association of hypertensive heart disease, with or without coronary artery disease. In addition, there may be diabetes mellitus. The pathological substrate, however is not distinct for any particular above three entities. [2,5-7,11]

Post-Operative Heart Disease
Atrial fibrillation occurs in various types of post-operative congenital cardiac malformation such as atrial septal defect of a fossa ovalis type, Mustard or Senning procedure for complete transposition and in atrial septectomy

(Blalock-Hanlon procedure). In the Mustard procedure, the entire atrial septum is removed and usually a prosthetic baffle is placed in the atrial septum. In the Senning procedure, several surgical incisions are made in the atrial septum to create flaps for the atrial septal wall. These flaps are then realigned to form the atrial septum. Thus, in both procedures, the atrial septum is considerably altered during surgery.

Pathologically, the atria reveal fibrosis, fat and chronic inflammatory cells. In addition, the SA and AV nodes are isolated from the surrounding atrial myocardium.[6]

Infiltrative Diseases of the Heart
Atrial fibrillation occurs in infiltrative diseases such as amyloidosis and sarcoidosis. Pathologically, there may be infiltration of amyloid in the SA node, atrial septum, atrial preferential pathways, in small vessels (arterioles) with degeneration and atrophy of some of the myocardial cells. This may be accompanied by fat, as well as necrosis of the myocardium. Similar findings may be seen in the AV node and its approaches. [6,9-11]

Atrial Fibrillation Following Coronary Artery By-pass Surgery
Atrial fibrillation occurs quite commonly following coronary artery by-pass surgery, however, an anatomic base to the best of our knowledge has not been delineated. We hypothesize that there may be surgical injury to the SA nodal area, post-operative pericarditis, abrupt beta-blocker withdrawal, or inadequate atrial protection during cardiopulmonary by-pass. It has been documented that older patients were found to be at a greater risk for the development of atrial arrhythmias. [6,7]

Genetic Anomalies of the Atrioventricular Junction

Familial Atrial Arrhythmias with AV Block Associated with Missense Mutation in the Rod Domain of the Lamin A/C Gene
We have studied a family who had adult onset cardiomyopathy with progressive conduction system disease, complete AV block and atrial fibrillation. Several of the family members died suddenly. The atria revealed considerable degenerative changes with tremendous amount of fat and fibrosis. This was associated with similar findings in the SA node and its approaches, AV node and its approaches, AV bundle and the bundle branches. In addition, the ventricular myocardium revealed varying degrees of degenerative changes and fibrosis.[1]

Pre-excitation

It is well known that atrial fibrillation occurs frequently in pre-excitation syndrome. The retrograde conduction through the accessory pathways (Kent bundle) may be responsible for initiation of atrial fibrillation.[2,6]

Congenital AV Block in the Elderly

We have previously demonstrated that atrial fibrillation and/or flutter is associated with congenital AV block of long standing duration. Pathologically, the atria showed considerable fibrosis with fatty infiltration of the bundle and bundle branches. In addition, there was a lack of connection between the atria and the peripheral conduction system. There was extensive fat in the atrial myocardium and absence of AV node. There were varying types of degenerative changes in the atria and the peripheral conduction system. The marked fatty infiltration of the atria probably was responsible for atrial flutter and fibrillation seen clinically. [12]

Tachycardia, Bradycardia Syndrome — Sick Sinus Syndrome

This syndrome is characterized by atrial fibrillation followed by atrial arrest. The anatomic substrate in the elderly with sick sinus syndrome is severe narrowing of the arterioles with acute degeneration and necrosis, fibroelastic proliferation, fat, and focal fibrinoid necrosis. This is associated with fibrosis, elastosis, arteriolosclerosis, chronic pericarditis and degeneration of nerve trunks in the approaches to the SA node. Similar findings were evident in the AV node and its approaches. [6,11]

Congenital Heart Disease

Atrial Septal Defect

Atrial septal defect either of a secundum (fossa ovalis) or ostium primum, or sinus venosus type, may result in atrial fibrillation particularly in later life. In general, the defects are quite large. It is emphasized that in the elderly when there is chronic atrial fibrillation, with atrial septal defect, surgical closure of the defect does not cure the arrhythmias. Indeed, the arrhythmias may get worse and sudden death may occur following closure of the defect. In this disease, there is tremendous enlargement of both the atria. The enlargement of the atria, as such, results in stretching of the myocardial fibers. This is associated with fat and fibrosis thereby forming an anatomic base in atrial fibrillation.[6]

Ebstein's Anomaly
The right atrium is greatly enlarged in most cases of Ebstein malformation of the tricuspid valve. It is not uncommon to find pre-excitation associated with this entity. Here the retrograde conduction through the anomalus bypass pathway may initiate the atrial fibrillation which may accelerate the enlargement of the right atrium.[6]

Tumors of the Heart
Tumor metastasises of primary or secondary nature that infiltrates the atrial septum may cause atrial fibrillation.[2,6]

Atrio-Hisian Connection
The normal right or left atrial myocardium may enter the central fibrous body and join the penetrating part of the AV bundle. The anomalous pathway connection may promote a re-entry phenomenon or retrograde conduction that may initiate atrial fibrillation. This may be accompanied by fat, fibrosis, and total isolation of the AV node from the surrounding atrial myocardium.[6]

Miscellaneous Causes for Atrial Fibrillation
It is well known that atrial fibrillation may occur in neuromuscular disorders, such as, fascio-scapulo- muscular dystrophy, myotonia dystrophica, Kearn-Sayre syndrome and hypertrophic cardiomyopathy. One may find fat with degenerative changes and necrotic changes in and around the SA node, AV node, atrial preferential pathways, AV bundle and bundle branches.[6]

Alcohol
It has been documented that alcohol intake, especially in the elderly triggers the onset of atrial fibrillation. We believe this probably is related to fat and degenerative changes of atrial myocardium extending to the SA node, the AV node and their approaches.[6]

Conclusion

It is to be noted that although one finds varying types of pathologic changes in the atria and the surrounding conduction system, the same type of pathologic findings may also be responsible for other types of atrial arrhythmias such as atrial tachycardia, multi focal atrial tachycardia, paroxysmal supra ventricular tachycardia, and chronic bradycardia–tachycardia syndromes (Sick Sinus Syndrome). Likewise, in chronic atrial fibrillation there is almost always distal conduction system disease.

References

1. Bharati, S, Sasaki, T, Siedman, C, Vidaillet, H: Sudden Death Among Patients with a Hereditary Cardiomyopathy Due to a Missense Mutation in the Rod Domain of the Lamin A/C Gene. (Abstract), J Am Coll Cardiol, 1001; 37:p174A.

2. Bharati S, Bauernfeind R, Josephson M: Intermittent preexcitation and mesothelioma of the atrioventriculr node: a hitherto undescribed entity. J Cardiovasc Electrophysiol, 1995; 6:823-831.

3. Bharati S, Lev M: Pathologic changes of the conduction system with aging. Cardiology in the Elderly, 1994; 2:152-160.

4. Bharati S, Surawicz B, Vidaillet HJ, Jr, Lev M: Familial Congenital Sinus Rhythm Anomalies - Clinical and Pathologic Correlations. PACE, 1992; 15:1720-1729.

5. Bharati S, Lev M: The Pathologic Changes in the Conduction System Beyond the Age of Ninety. Am Heart J, 1992; 124:486-496.

6. Bharati S, Lev M: Histologic Abnormalities in Atrial Fibrillation: Histology of Normal and Diseased Atrium in Atrial Fibrillation. Mechanisms and Management. Edited by Falk RH and Podrid PJ. Published by Raven Press Ltd, 1992; 2:15-39.

7. Lev M, Bharati S: The conduction system in coronary artery disease. In Current Cardiovascular Topics, Ed. by E. Donoso & J. Lipski, Stratton Intercontinental Medical Book Corp., 1978; 1:1-16.

8. Amat-y-Leon F, Racki AJ, Denes P, et al: Familial atrial dysrhythmia with A-V block: intracellular microelectrode, clinical electrophysiologic and morphologic observations. Circulation, 1974; 50:1097-1104.

9. Bharati S, Lev M, Denes P, et al: Infiltrative cardiomyopathy with conduction disease and ventricular dysrhythmia: Electrophysiological and pathological correlations. Am J Cardiol, 1980; 45:163-173.

10. Bharati S, Lev M, Dhingra R, et al: Pathologic correlations in three cases of bilateral bundle branch disease with unusual electrophysiologic manifestations in two cases. Am J Cardiol, 1976; 38:508-518.

11. Kaplan BM, Langendorf R, Lev M, Pick A: Tachycardia-bradycardia syndrome (so-called "sick sinus syndrome"). Pathology, mechanisms and treatment. Am J Cardiol, 1973; 31:497-508.

12. Bharati S, Rosen KM, Strasberg B, et al: Anatomic substrate for congenital atrioventricular block in middle aged adults. PACE, 1982; 5:860-869.

7.

ELECTRICAL REMODELLING IN CHRONIC ATRIAL FIBRILLATION PATIENTS: AN UP-TO-DATE SYNOPSIS

P.E. Vardas, MD, PhD, E.G. Manios, MD, E.M. Kanoupakis, MD, H.E. Mavrakis, MD

Cardiology Department, University Hospital, Heraklion, Crete, Greece

Introduction

A considerable body of experimental and human studies in the past five years have shown shortening of atrial refractoriness and repolarization and abnormal adaptation to rate as well as conduction slowing as a result of rapid atrial rates of certain duration. These changes are referred as atrial electrical remodeling (AER).[1-17]

Short-term rapid atrial rates induce these alterations in atrial electrophysiology via functional changes in ion channels and transporters. However, longer periods of atrial tachycardia result to changes in specific ionic currents density (I_{Ca}, I_{Na}) due to modified expression of the genes that determine the function of the responsible ionic channels.[2, 7-11]

Several studies suggested that AER is involved in the pathogenesis of atrial tachyarrhythmias.[1-4, 7-10] Since it may facilitate initiation, persistence and recurrence of atrial fibrillation (AF), questions regarding the extent and reversibility of AER and finally its prevention in humans, are of special clinical importance.

Acute human studies like that of Daoud et al [4] which showed that several minutes of induced AF shorten atrial effective refractory period (ERP) and that this shortening is reversed within minutes after arrhythmia termination probably, do not reflect the changes in atrial electrical properties after prolonged periods of AF. On the other hand it is difficult to induce and maintain AF in humans for the long time that is required for the development of channel dysfunction and altered gene expression that result in AER. A good way to overcome this handicap is to study patients, which suffer from persistent atrial fibrillation and are subject for electrical conversion to sinus rhythm. Following up these patients and observing the probable changes in their atrial electrical properties in the post cardioversion period should be a sufficient substitute of the lacking direct studies of AER in humans, given that these changes reflect the reversal course from electrical remodeling that was established during AF.

From Ovsyshcher IE. *New Developments in Cardiac Pacing and Electrophysiology.* Armonk, NY: Futura Publishing Company, Inc. ©2002.

What is the recovery course of AER in patients with persistent atrial fibrillation?

A study by Pandozi et al, [12] including chronic AF patients found that atrial ERP was shortened in the immediate post conversion period and was significantly increased one month later in those patients that remained in sinus rhythm. That study was the first that provided evidence about the reversibility of atrial electrical remodeling in humans but it lacked a control group and the interval between ERP evaluations was too long. So the authors could not retrieve detailed information about the recovery process from AER and its full reversibility.

Another study conducted by Franz et al [13] using monophasic action potential recordings (MAP) showed that post conversion patients suffering from persistent atrial fibrillation or flutter had significantly shorter repolarization in comparison with the control group. Also, these authors found that their patients exhibited an abnormal adaptation of repolarization to rate similar to that, which had been observed in the animal studies. These authors did not follow up their patients and thus they couldn't provide evidence about the reversibility of AER. However repolarization shortening remained controversial since, a subsequent study by Kamalvand et al [15] did not confirm shortening of MAP.

Yu et al [16], in a controlled trial that included 19 chronic AF patients converted to sinus rhythm by external defibrillation, studied the recovery course of refractoriness and atrial conduction properties. They found that their patients evaluated 30 min after conversion had atrial ERPs significantly shorter than those of controls. Adaptation of refractoriness to rate was also found abnormal. These authors observed impairment of atrial conduction properties since their patients had longer P wave and right atrial conduction times. The temporal changes of AER in that study were evaluated by repeated electrophysiological studies in four subsequent days. It was found that abnormalities in refractoriness gradually improved and reached a steady state not different from that of the controls in the third day after conversion to sinus rhythm. Conduction abnormalities did not resolve during this interval.

In a recent study [17] that was carried out in our department, 28 drug free, chronic AF patients electrically converted to sinus rhythm were evaluated. Effective refractory period at 500 ms, monophasic action potential at 90% of repolarization (MAPd90) at five cycle lengths (CL, 350,400,450,500,600 ms), and P wave duration were measured three times: within the interval 5-20 min, 24 hours and one month post-conversion. Fifteen subjects with no history of AF and normal atrial structure served as a control group. We observed that ERP increased from

204 ± 20 to 244 ± 31 to 241 ± 24 ms (p<0.001), attaining a level comparable to that of the controls (238 ± 21ms) within 24h. MAPd90 significantly increased (from 175 ± 11 to 190 ± 19 to 191 ± 10 ms at CL 350 ms and 201 ± 21 to 234 ± 20 to 233 ± 23 ms at CL 600ms) also reaching control levels within 24h. MAPd90 exhibited an abnormal adaptation to rate only in the first evaluation. P wave duration was prolonged (137 ± 33 ms) and exhibited a slower course of shortening (130 ± 32 to 123 ± 24 ms, p<0.001), reaching control levels within one month.

In summary data from the above recent studies confirm that AER owing to persistent atrial fibrillation in humans is a reversible feature. They also suggest that refractoriness and repolarization abnormalities resolve rapidly within days after restoration of sinus rhythm while conduction abnormalities exhibit a slower normalization course that is probably completed within a month.

1. Is there a relation of AER with recurrence of AF?

In their classic experimental study Wijffels et al stated, "AF begets AF".[1] Surprisingly, five years later, human studies that directly relate the remodeling process with recurrence of AF are rare.

A small early study by Olsson et al [18] suggested that AF patients in whom postconversion MAPd90 was shorter than 207 ms were likely to relapse, while two recent preliminary reports related fibrillatory cycle length (an indirect indicator of atrial refractoriness) to AF recurrence.[19, 20]

Our findings, in a recent study [17], showed that MAPd90 in the immediate post conversion period contained prognostic information. At short cycle lengths relapsed patients had significantly longer MAPd90 values compared with those who did not relapse. Although this finding looks rather paradoxical it can be explained, at least in part, as a consequence of the inability of chronic AF patients to adapt MAPd90 to rate. The loss of rate adaptation is such that MAPd90 decreases caused by chronic AF are maximal at higher cycle lengths and less at shorter cycle lengths. Probably our relapsed patients exhibited a more abnormal adaptation curve in that they were unable to shorten MAPd90 at short cycle lengths to levels comparable to those of non-relapsed patients.

In our study, we observed most recurrences of AF within the first week post conversion. Taking into account that abnormalities in atrial refractoriness and repolarization in the right atrial appendage were reversed within 24 hours post-conversion our findings suggest that the absolute shortening of refractoriness contributes to the mechanisms, that are responsible for the early recurrence of AF only during the first day after conversion.

More importantly, in our study we found that atrial conduction time is prolonged by chronic AF and exhibits a slower recovery course. We did not find P wave duration to be an independent prognostic factor for recurrence. However, since P wave prolongation coincided with recurrence in most of our patients we believe that our data suggest an important contribution of conduction abnormalities to early recurrences.

It appears evident that factors other than refractoriness shortening should be involved in the remodeling process and that in the genesis of AF the importance of refractoriness shortening alone has been over-estimated. Very recently Garrat et al searched for a "second factor" beyond refractoriness shortening to explain the progressive nature of AF and they did not find paroxysms of AF to have a cumulative effect on inducibility or stability of AF in the goat model.

3. Is sinus node involved in the remodeling process?

Involvement of the sinus node pacemaker in the electrical remodeling process may have important pathophysiological and clinical implications. For example, if sinus dysfunction is a result of atrial electrical remodeling, then it may be a reversible feature and no further treatment for this abnormality would be necessary when it is observed in post-cardioversion AF patients. Furthermore, sinus node function has been implicated in the initiation, perpetuation and recurrence of AF. [21-23]

A reasonable question that arises is whether AF per se can affect the sinus node in the same way as it does the atrial myocardium.

So far, this issue remains largely unresolved since available data are conflicting. n experimental study conducted by Kirchoff and coworkers [24] showed that, although induced non-sustained AF can penetrate the sinus perinodal area and may interact with sinus pacemaker cells, it causes only minor overdrive suppression of automaticity. In contrast, Elvan et al, [5] in a dog study, found that pacing-induced persistent AF induces sinus node dysfunction in parallel with atrial electrical remodeling and that these disorders reverse gradually. Human data are limited, although some studies have shown sinus node dysfunction to follow cardioversion in atrial fibrillation patients. [25,26]

In a study including 12 chronic lone AF patients Kumagai et al [25] assessed the sinus node function on the day after electrical conversion to sinus rhythm. Those authors found that the mean corrected sinus node recovery time (CSNRT) of their patients was significantly longer than that of controls and in nine of them (75%) it was abnormal (>525 ms). Recently Tse et al [26] also studied 11 chronic AF patients ten minutes after electrical conversion to sinus rhythm and found similarly that these patients had significantly longer CSNRT as compared to normal subjects or to patients with paroxysmal AF. In that study abnormal CSNRT was found in 55% of chronic AF patients.

In a recent study that was carried out in our department we investigate the temporal changes in sinus node function in post-cardioversion chronic AF patients and their possible relation with the recurrence rates of AF. [27]

In 37 chronic AF patients internally cardioverted to sinus rhythm, CSNRT was assessed 5-20 min and 24 h after conversion at two pacing cycle lengths (PCL) of 600 ms and 500 ms. Patients were followed up for one month for AF recurrence and Holter recordings were obtained during the first 24h after conversion for assessment of atrial ectopic activity during this interval. Fifteen patients (40.5%) relapsed during follow-up. CSNRT values at PCL 600 ms (371 ± 182 ms) and 500 ms (445 ± 338 ms) were significantly higher than those of control subjects (278 ± 157 ms, p= 0.050, 279 ± 130 ms, p=0.037 respectively). Significant temporal changes in CSNRT were also observed during the first 24 h following conversion (PCL 600 ms: 308 ± 120 ms, p=0.034, PCL 500 ms: 340 ± 208 ms, p=0.017). Similar data were obtained after autonomic blockade. Patients with abnormal CSNRT 5-20 min after cardioversion had higher recurrence rates (50%) as compared to those with normal function (37%), but this difference was not statistically significant.

Patients who relapsed had a significantly (p= 0.001) higher number of atrial ectopic beats per hour (187±132) compared to those that did not (36±39) but there was no significant correlation of this parameter with CSNRT.

Thus our findings do not support a role of sinus node either directly or indirectly in the recurrence of AF. On the other hand, they are compatible with the recently described role of ectopic foci in pulmonary veins and other atrial sites. These focal atrial ectopic beats, which have been convincingly implicated in the initiation, perpetuation and recurrence of AF in humans, are the result of triggered activity rather than abnormal sinus node function. [28-29]

Our data do not prove a significant role of sinus node dysfunction in AF recurrence. Post-cardioversion chronic AF patients exhibit suppressed sinus node function that can be explained as a result of AF induced electrical remodeling, since it resolves with time and is independent of autonomic function.

4. What is the role of calcium blockers and amiodarone in the prevention of remodeling and recurrence of AF?

In the case of chronic AF, the abnormal atrial electrophysiology associated with AER has been attributed to changes in the expression of the genes that determine the function of specific ionic channels especially those of ICa_L.[7,30-32] L-type calcium blockers, such as verapamil or diltiazem, have been proposed as potentially useful drugs for AF patients, since these drugs theoretically could decrease the deleterious calcium cytosolic concentrations that have been implicated as the major contributing factor in the development of AER. [33-35] Although in some studies involving patients with induced short lasting AF verapamil was found to prevent the development of AER, other studies showed that L-type calcium blockers failed to protect patients or experimental animals with long lasting AF from this abnormality. [36,37] Clinical studies that included persistent AF patients who were pretreated with various calcium blockers and subsequently electroverted to sinus rhythm have shown conflicting results,[38-41] since reduction in the recurrence rates was not clearly confirmed. On the other hand, several studies have shown that amiodarone, even under these circumstances,[42-44] is still effective, since a considerable proportion of patients suffering from persistent AF treated with this drug are converted to sinus rhythm and exhibit lower recurrence rates.

Given that the recurrence rate of AF in this subset of patients is > 40% within a month after sinus rhythm restoration, it is of profound importance to know how the various antiarrhythmic drugs can intervene with AER and protect against recurrence of AF. In a prospective trial in our department we studied chronic AF patients randomly assigned to no treatment with antiarrhythmic drug, to treatment with the L-type calcium blocker, diltiazem, or to treatment with amiodarone.[45] Several electrophysiological parameters of the pre- and post-electroversion period were examined, while conversion and recurrence rates (within six weeks after conversion) were measured in order to assess the possible effects of these drugs on AER and whether these actions have any clinical implications.

Compared with controls, amiodarone patients had significantly higher conversion rates (83% vs 100%, p= 0.041) and a higher probability to maintain sinus rhythm after conversion (p=0.037). Patients of amiodarone group had longer fibrillatory cycle length intervals than patients of diltiazem and control groups (180±18 ms vs. 161±17 ms vs. 164±19 ms, p=0.001) and longer effective refractory period (211±22 ms vs. 198±16 ms vs. 194±17 ms, p=0.003) as assessed 5 min after conversion. The recovery course of effective refractory period was similar among groups. Post-conversion density of supraventricular ectopics was significantly lower in amiodarone group patients compared to diltiazem and control groups (25±28 SVC/h vs.110±129 SVC/h vs. 98±95 SVC/h, p=0.001).

The present study does not confirm any significant effect of diltiazem and, in consequence of L-type calcium blockers, on the process of atrial electrical remodeling that is induced by chronic AF. On the other hand oral treatment with amiodarone increases conversion rates and preserves sinus rhythm in chronic AF patients. It exerts these effects by prolonging fibrillatory cycle and atrial effective refractory period and suppressing the ectopics that trigger AF.

Concluding remarks

Recent studies confirm the presence of atrial electrical remodeling in humans, especially in patients, which suffer from prolonged episodes or chronic AF. They elucidate the time course of its reversion and provide evidence about its relation with recurrence in the early post conversion period. Despite this progress however, important questions remain unanswered. So far, research does not adequately support the clinical use of calcium lowering agents, which theoretically may prevent remodeling and subsequently early recurrence of AF.

In humans, worsening of AF with time may not be related only to AF induced refractory period shortening, but it could be related either to electrophysiological remodeling affecting other parameters (conduction velocity, dispersion of refractoriness) or at least for long-term episodes of AF, to structural remodeling (dilation, fibrosis) affecting in turn atrial electrophysiological properties.

References

1. Wijffels MCEF, Kirchoff CJ, Dorland R, Allessie MA. Atrial fibrillation begets atrial fibrillation. A study in awake chronically instrumented goats. Circulation. 1995;92:1954-1968.
2. Morillo C, Klein G, Jones DL, Guiraurdon CM. Chronic rapid atrial pacing: structural, functional, and electrophysiological characteristics of a new model of sustained atrial fibrillation. Circulation.1995;91:1588-95.
3. Goette A, Honeycutt C, Langberg JJ. Electrical remodeling in atrial fibrillation. Time course and mechanisms. Circulation. 1996;94:2968-74.
4. Daoud EG, Bogun F, Goyal R, Harvey M, Man C, Stickberger SA, Morady F. Effect of AF on atrial refractoriness in humans. Circulation. 1996;94:1600-1606.

5. Elvan A, Wylie K, Zipes DP. Pacing-induced chronic atrial fibrillation impairs sinus node function in dogs. Electrophysiological remodeling. Circulation. 1996;94:2953-60.

6. Wijffels MC, Kirchhof CJ, Dorland R, Power J, Allessie MA. Electrical remodeling due to atrial fibrillation in chronically instrumented conscious goats: roles of neurohumoral changes, ischemia, atrial stretch, and high rate of electrical activation. Circulation. 1997;96:3710-20.

7. Gaspo R, Bosch RF, Bou-Abboud E, et al. Tachycardia induced changes in Na+ current in a chronic dog model of atrial fibrillation. Circ Res 1997; 8:1045-1052.

8. Gaspo R, Bosch RF, Talajic M, Nattel S. Functional mechanisms underlying tachycardia-induced sustained atrial fibrillation in a chronic dog model. Circulation. 1997;96:4027-35.

9. Daoud EG, Knight BP, Weiss R, et al. Effect of verapamil and procainamide on atrial fibrillation-induced electrical remodeling in humans. Circulation. 1997;96:1542-50.

10. Tieleman RG, De Langen C, Van Gelder IC et al. Verapamil reduces tachycardia-induced electrical remodeling of the atria. Circulation. 1997;95:1945-53.

11. Fareh S, Villemaire C, Nattel S. Importance of refractoriness heterogeneity in the enhanced vulnerability to atrial fibrillation induction caused by tachycardia- induced atrial electrical remodeling. Circulation. 1998;98:2202-9.

12. Pandozi C, Bianconi L, Villani M, et al Electrophysiological characteristics of the human atria after cardioversion of persistent atrial fibrillation. Circulation. 1998; 98:2860-5.

13. Franz MR, Karasik PL, Li C, Moubarak J, Chavez M. Electrical remodeling of the human atrium: similar effects in patients with chronic atrial fibrillation and atrial flutter. J Am Coll Cardiol. 1997;30:1785-92.

14. Nattel S. Atrial electrophysiological remodeling caused by rapid atrial activation: underlying mechanisms and clinical relevance to atrial fibrillation. Cardiovasc Res. 1999; 42:298-308.

15. Kamalvand K, Tan K, Lloyd G, et al. Alterations in atrial electrophysiology assosiated with chronic atrial fibrillation in man. Eur Heart J. 1999; 20:888-895.

16. Yu W, Lee SH, Tai CT, et al. Reversal of atrial electrical remodeling following cardioversion of long-standing atrial fibrillation in man. Cardiovasc Res. 1999; 42:470-476.

17. Manios E, Kanoupakis E, Chlouverakis G, et al. Changes in atrial electrical properties following cardioversion of chronic atrial fibrillation: relation with recurrence. Cardiovasc Res. 2000; 47:244-253.

18. Olsson SB, Cotoi S, Varnauskas E. Monophasic action potential and sinus rhythm stability after conversion of atrial fibrillation. Acta Med Scand. 1971; 190:381-387.

19. Langberg J, Bollmann A, Pena E, et al. Frequency analysis of the ECG during atrial fibrillation predicts recurrence after internal atrial defibrillation Pacing Clin Electrophysiol 1998; 21 (Abstract)

20. Jung W, Schumacher B, Omran H et al. Predictors of low atrial defibrillation thresholds early and late recurrences of atrial fibrillation after internal atrial defibrillation. J Am Coll Cardiol 1999; 33:142A

21. Page PL. Sinus node during atrial fibrillation. To beat or not to beat. Circulation. 1992; 86:334-336.

22. Nadeu RA, Roberge FA, Billette J. The role of the sinus node in the mechanism of cholinergic atrial fibrillation. Circ Res 1970; 27:129-138.

23. Spach MS, Dolber PC, Heidlage JF. Interaction of inhomogeneities of repolarization with anisotropic propagationin dog atria: a mechanism for both preventing and initiating reentry. Circ Res 1989;65:1612-1631.

24. Kirchoff CJ, Allessie MA. Sinus node automaticity during atrial fibrillation in isolated rabbit hearts. Circulation. 1992; 86:263-271.

25. Kumagai K, Akimitsu S, Kawahira K, Kawanami F, Yamanouchi Y, Hiroki T, Arakawa K. Electrophysiological properties in chronic lone atrial fibrillation. Circulation. 1991; 84:1662-1668.

26. Tse HF, Lau CP, Ayers GM. Heterogeneous changes in electrophysiological properties in the paroxysmal and chronically fibrillating human atrium. J Cardiovasc Electrophysiol. 1999; 10:125-135.

27. Manios E, Kanoupakis E, Mavrakis H, Kallergis E, Dermitzaki D, Vardas P. Sinus pacemaker function after cardioversion of chronic atrial fibrillation: is sinus node remodeling related with recurrence? J Cardiovasc Electrophysiol 2001; 12: 800-6.

28. Haissaguerre M, Jais P, Shah DC et al Spontaneous initiation of atrial fibrillation by ectopic beats originating in the pulmonary veins. N Engl J Med 1998; 339:659-666.

29. Chen S-A, Hsieh M-S, Tai CT et al. Initiation of atrial fibrillation by ectopic beats originating from the pulmonary veins: Electrophysiological characteristics, pharmacological responses and effects of radiofrequency ablation. Circulation. 1999; 100:1879-1886.

30. Yue L, Feng J, Gaspo R, Li GR,Wang Z, Natel S. Ionic remodeling underlying action potential changes in a canine model of atrial fibrillation. Circ Res 1997; 81:512-525.

31. Lai LP, Su MJ, Lin JL, et al. Down regulation of L-type calcium channel and sarcoplasmic reticular Ca2+-ATPase mRNA in human atrial fibrillation without significant change in the m RNA of ryanodine receptor, calsequestrin and phospholamban. J Am Coll Cardiol 1999; 33:1231-7.

32. Bosch R, Zeng X, Grammer J, Popovic K, Mewis C, Kuhlkamp V. Ionic mechanisms of electrical remodeling in human atrial fibrillation. Cardiovasc Res 1999; 44: 121-131.

33. Tieleman RG, De Langen C, Van Gelder IC, et al. Verapamil reduces tachycardia-induced electrical remodeling of the atria. Circulation 1997; 95:1945-1953.

34. Daoud EG, Knight BP, Weiss R, et al. Effect of Verapamil and procainamide on atrial fibrillation-induced electrical remodeling in humans. Circulation 1997;96:1542-1550.

35. Tieleman RG, Van Gelder IC, Crijns HJ, De Kam PJ, Van Den Berg MP, Haaksma J, Van Der Woude HJ, Allessie MA. Early recurrences of atrial fibrillation after electrical cardioversion: a result of fibrillation-induced electrical remodeling of the atria? J Am Coll Cardiol 1998; 31:167-173.

36. Lee SH, Yu WC, Cheng JJ, et al. Effect of Verapamil on long term tachycardia induced atrial electrical remodeling. Circulation 2000; 101:200-6.

37. Benardeau A, Fareh S, Natel S. Effects of Verapamil on atrial fibrillation and its electrophysiological determinants in dog. Cardiovasc Res 2001; 50: 85-96.

38. De Simone A, Stabile G, Vitale DF, et al. Pretreatment with Verapamil in patients with persistent or chronic atrial fibrillation who underwent electrical cardioversion. J Am Coll Cardiol 1999; 34:810-4.

39. Botto GL, Belotti G, Romano M, et al. Verapamil pre-treatment before electrical cardioversion of persistent atrial fibrillation: theVERAF study. Eur Heart J 2001; 22:329 (Abstract).

40. Van Noord T, Van Gelder IC, Tieleman RG, et al. VERDICT: the Verapamil versus Digoxin Cardioversion Trial: A randomized study on the role of calcium lowering for maintenance of sinus rhythm after cardioversion of persistent atrial fibrillation. J Cardiovasc Electrophysiol 2001; 12:766-9.

41. Villani GQ, Piepoli MF, Terracciano C, Capucci A. Effects of Diltiazem pretreatment on direct-current cardioversion in patients with persistent atrial fibrillation: A single-blind, randomized, controlled study. Am Heart J 2000; 140:437-443.

42. Gosselink AT, Crijns HJGM, van Gelder IC et al. Low dose Amiodarone for maintenance of sinus rhythm after conversion of atrial fibrillation or flutter. JAMA 1992; 267: 3289-3293.

43. Capucci A, Villani GQ, Aschieri D, Rosi A, Piepoli MF. Oral Amiodarone increases the efficacy of direct-current cardioversion in restoration of sinus rhythm in patients with chronic atrial fibrillation.Eur Heart J 2000; 21:66-73.

44. Vardas P, Kochiadakis G, Igoumenidis N, Tsatsakis A, Simantirakis E, Chlouverakis G. Amiodarone as a first choice drug for restoring sinus rhythm in patients with atrial fibrillation. Chest 2000; 117: 1538-1545.

45. Manios E,Kanoupakis E,Mavrakis H, Kallergis E, Patrianakos A, Kambouraki D, Dermitzaki D,Vardas P.Effects of Diltiazem and Amiodarone in cardioverted atrial fibrillation patients. Europace 2001;2:B107 (Abstract).

8.

ATRIAL FIBRILLATION AFTER CARDIAC SURGERY: PROPHYLACTIC INTERVENTIONS.

Eugene Crystal, MD, Stuart J. Connolly, MD

Department of Medicine, McMaster University,
Hamilton, Ontario, Canada

Postoperative atrial fibrillation (POAF) is the most common complication of cardiac surgery, occurring in 25 - 40% of patients [1-3]. POAF has also been shown to occur in significant proportion of patients undergoing minimally invasive direct coronary artery bypass surgery (MIDCAB) [4]. Since the development and wide implementation of open-heart surgery, many studies have been done to evaluate etiology of POAF, and possible prophylactic interventions.
This paper summarizes recent developments in understanding of POAF.

Etiology and risk factors

The arrhythmic substrate underlying the development of postoperative AF remains unclear. Electrophysiological testing of right atrial biopsies showed correlation of abnormalities of depolarization, conduction velocities and transmembrane action potentials, with development of POAF [5]. More recent implementation of sophisticated cellular electrophysiology to the evaluation of human atrial tissues collected during cardiac surgery resulted in gradual development of understanding these markers of POAF. One recent study demonstrated that altered expression of connexins, the key component proteins of gap junctions, is a determinant of a predisposition to POAF [6]. In another human study, decreased activity of K currents, regulators of cellular repolarization, indicated significant association with the onset of human POAF [7].
Sympathetic activation in the post-operative period correlates with POAF occurrence, when measured by plasma norepinephrine levels [8]. The efficacy of beta-blockers (BB) also suggest on important role of adrenergic stimultion in the genesis of POAF [9]. However, sympathetic activation is highest during first 24 hours after the surgery, but the typical of onset of POAF is in second and third postoperative day [10]. One study strongly suggested a role of atrial denervation in the development of POAF [11].
Inflammation is other possible trigger. Additional suggestions on the role of inflammatory injury are efficacy of anti-inflammatory drugs in the prevention of POAF [12,13], and correlation with occurrence of pericarditis.

From Ovsyshcher IE. *New Developments in Cardiac Pacing and Electrophysiology.* Armonk, NY: Futura Publishing Company, Inc. ©2002.

Demographic and clinical risk factors for POAF are old age, male sex, prior AF, history of hypertension, decreased left ventricular function, left main disease or multivessel disease, grafting of right coronary artery, left atrial enlargement, valvular disease, obstructive disease in the SA nodal and AV nodal arteries, chronic lung disease, chronic renal failure, pericarditis and other serious postoperative complication [4,14-17]. Intra-operative risk factors associated with development of POAF are prolonged aortic cross-clamp time[17,18], cold blood cardioplegia [19], pulmonary vein venting and bicaval venous cannulation [17].

The many different risk-factors, associated with the development of POAF, suggests multifactorial pathogenesis of this disorder. POAF is probably a result of both substrate (pre-operative heart disease) and trigger (factors associated with operation itself).

Clinical significance

POAF has been repeatedly demonstrated to be a predictor of complicated post-operative course, correlating with an increased incidence of stroke [18,20,21], increased length of hospital stay (LOS) and increased hospital costs [2,17,18,22]. However, episodes of POAF are usually benign. *Is POAF a source, or a sign of associated burden?*

Prevention

Since the association of POAF with poorer outcome has been shown, the issue of prophylaxis becomes important and many studies were published during three last decades. Most studies evaluated interventions by digoxin, verapamil, beta-blockers, sotalol, amiodarone, other pharmacological agents, and, more recently, by pacing.

Two meta-analyses of randomized control trials, published more than a decade ago, demonstrated failure of verapamil and digoxin to reduce occurrence of POAF significantly [9,23], and suggested the efficacy of BB. Many recent trials have evaluated conventional BB, sotalol, and amiodarone.

Beta-blockers

The effectiveness of beta-blockers for the prevention of POAF was proved in multiple controlled trials [24-49]. The attractiveness of beta-blockers is not only efficacy, but also low occurrence of side effects. However, the effect of beta-blockers on total length of stay in controlled randomized trials is unclear. In one recently published study using historical control, the implementation of clinical pathway based on intensive use of beta-blockers, failed to show significant decrease in the occurrence of POAF or in LOS[50].

Beta-blockers are probably the most widely prescribed drugs in patients undergoing CABG because of their anti-anginal properties. In most trials which demonstrated efficacy of beta-blockers in prophylaxis of POAF, the majority of patients were treated with beta-blockers preoperatively. The overall efficacy of against may in part be due to prevention of adverse effects of withdrawal of beta-blockers. In one recent report [51] the positive influence of prophylactic beta-blockers on POAF was confined to the subgroup of patients on beta-blockers preoperatively.

Sotalol

Sotalol, a Class III antiarrhythmic drug with beta-blocker activity, was shown in several randomized controlled trials to be an effective prophylactic agent against POAF [52-58]. In direct comparison against conventional beta-blockers in several trials it had superior efficacy[57,59-61]. However, in addition to usual beta-blocker side effects and contra-indications, sotalol also has proarrhythmic potential, especially in patients prone to ischemia and with decreased left ventricular function. Therefore, the benefit of sotalol as a prophylactic drug over beta-blockers is not clear.

Amiodarone

Amiodarone has also been shown to be an effective prophylactic agent against POAF in several trials [62-70]. In one small report its efficacy was superior to beta-blockers[71]. Despite obvious problems of administration (long oral protocol or complicated intravenous administration), amiodarone is an effective alternative for the patients with contraindications to beta-blockers. Amiodarone also has a excellent safety record in ischemic heart disease patients and those with decreased left ventricular function.

Pacing

Recently atrial pacing has been evaluated for the prevention of POAF [72-82]. Almost all post-cardiac surgery patients have epicardial pacing wires inserted, providing a unique opportunity to test temporary pacing interventions. Study protocols used different locations of pacing electrodes (right atrial, left atrial, bi-atrial pacing). Trials also differed in pacing algorithms; some used simple overdrive at a fixed heart rate, and others used more complex overdrive algorithms. Patients in the control groups usually received atrial demand pacing at rates of 30-45 beats per minute.

Pacing showed a decrease in AF occurrence[83]. No difference was found in a recent meta-analysis of results of different overdriving algorithms. In two recently reported meta-analyses, bi-atrial pacing was statistically significantly more effective[83,84].

Prevention of POAF and LOS.

Only small proportion of trials on prevention of POAF have reported the effect of the treatment on the LOS. In the largest beta-blocker trial [28], despite 20% decrease in POAF, the LOS was not changed significantly. In 5 amiodarone trials[63,64,66,68,85] where the statistics on length of stay were reported, LOS decreased significantly.

The effect of prophylactic therapy against POAF and LOS were subject of two recent reviews [83,86]. Limited to 7 pharmacological trials (amiodarone and sotalol), the first review did not find any significant change in the LOS despite notable changes in occurrence of POAF in treatment groups.

In a more comprehensive meta-analysis including 12 trials [83], the reported decrease in LOS was small (~0.5 day of stay), but significant.

Both studies demonstrated remarkable discrepancy between overall effect on the occurrence of POAF and modest effect on the LOS. One probable explanation is that direct benefit of POAF elimination was counterbalanced by side effects of pharmacological interventions. The other explanation would be that POAF itself does not greatly increase total LOS. Rather it may only be a marker of more complicated disease process.

Conclusion

The evidence that beta-blockers, sotalol and amiodarone all prevent POAF is strong. Despite significant reduction of POAF, the effect of these interventions on LOS is modest. Post-operative pacing is a promising alternative which requires further study.

References

1. Hashimoto K, Ilstrup DM, Schaff HV. Influence of clinical and hemodynamic variables on risk of supraventricular tachycardia after coronary artery bypass. J Thorac Cardiovasc Surg. 1991;101:56-65.
2. Aranki SF, Shaw DP, Adams DH, et al. Predictors of atrial fibrillation after coronary artery surgery. Current trends and impact on hospital resources. Circulation. 1996;94:390-7.
3. Ommen SR, Odell JA, Stanton MS. Atrial arrhythmias after cardiothoracic surgery. N Engl J Med. 1997;336:1429-34.
4. Tamis-Holland JE, Homel P, Durani M, et al. Atrial fibrillation after minimally invasive direct coronary artery bypass surgery. J Am Coll Cardiol. 2000;36:1884-8.

5. Bush HL, Jr., Gelband H, Hoffman BF, et al. Electrophysiological basis for supraventricular arrhythmias: following surgical procedures for aortic stenosis. Arch Surg. 1971;103:620-5.

6. Dupont E, Ko Y, Rothery S, et al. The gap-junctional protein connexin40 is elevated in patients susceptible to postoperative atrial fibrillation. Circulation. 2001;103:842-9.

7. Brandt MC, Priebe L, Bohle T, et al. The ultrarapid and the transient outward K(+) current in human atrial fibrillation. Their possible role in postoperative atrial fibrillation. J Mol Cell Cardiol. 2000;32:1885-96.

8. Kalman JM, Munawar M, Howes LG, et al. Atrial fibrillation after coronary artery bypass grafting is associated with sympathetic activation. Ann Thorac Surg. 1995;60:1709-15.

9. Andrews TC, Reimold SC, Berlin JA, et al. Prevention of supraventricular arrhythmias after coronary artery bypass surgery. A meta-analysis of randomized control trials. Circulation. 1991;84:III236-44.

10. Hogue CW, Jr., Hyder ML. Atrial fibrillation after cardiac operation: risks, mechanisms, and treatment. Ann Thorac Surg. 2000;69:300-6.

11. Davis Z, Jacobs HK, Bonilla J, et al. Retaining the aortic fat pad during cardiac surgery decreases postoperative atrial fibrillation. Heart Surg Forum. 2000;3:108-12.

12. Ghani A, Ahmad F, Zelinger A, et al. Efficacy of Nonsteroidal Anti-Inflammatory Medications for Prevention of Atrial Fibrillation Following Coronary Artery Bypass Graft Surgery. Circulation. 2000;102:II-3873.

13. Yared JP, Starr NJ, Torres FK, et al. Effects of single dose, postinduction dexamethasone on recovery after cardiac surgery. Ann Thorac Surg. 2000;69:1420-4.

14. De Jong MJ, Morton PG. Predictors of atrial dysrhythmias for patients undergoing coronary artery bypass grafting. Am J Crit Care. 2000;9:388-96.

15. Ducceschi V, D'Andrea A, Liccardo B, et al. Perioperative clinical predictors of atrial fibrillation occurrence following coronary artery surgery. Eur J Cardiothorac Surg. 1999;16:435-9.

16. Kolvekar S, D'Souza A, Akhtar P, et al. Role of atrial ischaemia in development of atrial fibrillation following coronary artery bypass surgery. Eur J Cardiothorac Surg. 1997;11:70-5.

17. Mathew JP, Parks R, Savino JS, et al. Atrial fibrillation following coronary artery bypass graft surgery: predictors, outcomes, and resource utilization. MultiCenter Study of Perioperative Ischemia Research Group. Jama. 1996;276:300-6.

18. Creswell LL, Schuessler RB, Rosenbloom M, et al. Hazards of postoperative atrial arrhythmias. Ann Thorac Surg. 1993;56:539-49.

19. Pehkonen EJ, Makynen PJ, Kataja MJ, et al. Atrial fibrillation after blood and crystalloid cardioplegia in CABG patients. Thorac Cardiovasc Surg. 1995;43:200-3.

20. Taylor GJ, Malik SA, Colliver JA, et al. Usefulness of atrial fibrillation as a predictor of stroke after isolated coronary artery bypass grafting. Am J Cardiol. 1987;60:905-7.

21. Almassi GH, Schowalter T, Nicolosi AC, et al. Atrial fibrillation after cardiac surgery: a major morbid event? Ann Surg. 1997;226:501-11; discussion 511-3.

22. Loubani M, Hickey MS, Spyt TJ, et al. Residual atrial fibrillation and clinical consequences following postoperative supraventricular arrhythmias. Int J Cardiol. 2000;74:125-32.

23. Kowey PR, Taylor JE, Rials SJ, et al. Meta-analysis of the effectiveness of prophylactic drug therapy in preventing supraventricular arrhythmia early after coronary artery bypass grafting. Am J Cardiol. 1992;69:963-5.

24. Rubin DA, Nieminski KE, Reed GE, et al. Predictors, prevention, and long-term prognosis of atrial fibrillation after coronary artery bypass graft operations. J Thorac Cardiovasc Surg. 1987;94:331-5.

25. Abel RM, van Gelder HM, Pores IH, et al. Continued propranolol administration following coronary bypass surgery. Antiarrhythmic effects. Arch Surg. 1983;118:727-31.

26. Ali IM, Sanalla AA, Clark V. Beta-blocker effects on postoperative atrial fibrillation. Eur J Cardiothorac Surg. 1997;11:1154-7.

27. Babin-Ebell J, Keith PR, Elert O. Efficacy and safety of low-dose propranolol versus diltiazem in the prophylaxis of supraventricular tachyarrhythmia after coronary artery bypass grafting. Eur J Cardiothorac Surg. 1996;10:412-6.

28. Cybulsky I, Connolly S, Gent M, et al. Beta blocker length of stay study (BLOSS): a randomized trial of metoprolol for reduction of post-operative length of stay. Can J Cardiol. 2000;16:238F.

29. Daudon P, Corcos T, Gandjbakhch I, et al. Prevention of atrial fibrillation or flutter by acebutolol after coronary bypass grafting. Am J Cardiol. 1986;58:933-6.

30. Gun C, Bianco ACM, R.B. F, et al. Beta-blocker effects on postoperative atrial fibrillation after coronary artery by-pass surgery. J Am Coll Card. 1998;CD-ROM of Abstracts from World Cardiology Congress:3801.

31. Ivey MF, Ivey TD, Bailey WW, et al. Influence of propranolol on supraventricular tachycardia early after coronary artery revascularization. A randomized trial. J Thorac Cardiovasc Surg. 1983;85:214-8.

32. Khuri SF, Okike ON, Josa M, et al. Efficacy of nadolol in preventing supraventricular tachycardia after coronary artery bypass grafting. Am J Cardiol. 1987;60:51D-58D.

33. Lamb RK, Prabhakar G, Thorpe JA, et al. The use of atenolol in the prevention of supraventricular arrhythmias following coronary artery surgery. Eur Heart J. 1988;9:32-6.

34. Martinussen HJ, Lolk A, Szczepanski C, et al. Supraventricular tachyarrhythmias after coronary bypass surgery--a double blind randomized trial of prophylactic low dose propranolol. Thorac Cardiovasc Surg. 1988;36:206-7.

35. Matangi MF, Neutze JM, Graham KJ, et al. Arrhythmia prophylaxis after aorta-coronary bypass. The effect of minidose propranolol. J Thorac Cardiovasc Surg. 1985;89:439-43.

36. Matangi MF, Strickland J, Garbe GJ, et al. Atenolol for the prevention of arrhythmias following coronary artery bypass grafting. Can J Cardiol. 1989;5:229-34.

37. Materne P, Larbuisson R, Collignon P, et al. Prevention by acebutolol of rhythm disorders following coronary bypass surgery. Int J Cardiol. 1985;8:275-86.

38. Mohr R, Smolinsky A, Goor DA. Prevention of supraventricular tachyarrhythmia with low-dose propranolol after coronary bypass. J Thorac Cardiovasc Surg. 1981;81:840-5.

39. Myhre ES, Sorlie D, Aarbakke J, et al. Effects of low dose propranolol after coronary bypass surgery. J Cardiovasc Surg (Torino). 1984;25:348-52.

40. Oka Y, Frishman W, Becker RM, et al. Clinical pharmacology of the new beta-adrenergic blocking drugs. Part 10. Beta-adrenoceptor blockade and coronary artery surgery. Am Heart J. 1980;99:255-69.

41. Ormerod OJ, McGregor CG, Stone DL, et al. Arrhythmias after coronary bypass surgery. Br Heart J. 1984;51:618-21.

42. Paull DL, Tidwell SL, Guyton SW, et al. Beta blockade to prevent atrial dysrhythmias following coronary bypass surgery. Am J Surg. 1997;173:419-21.

43. Salazar C, Frishman W, Friedman S, et al. beta-Blockade therapy for supraventricular tachyarrhythmias after coronary surgery: a propranolol withdrawal syndrome? Angiology. 1979;30:816-9.

44. Silverman NA, Wright R, Levitsky S. Efficacy of low-dose propranolol in preventing postoperative supraventricular tachyarrhythmias: a prospective, randomized study. Ann Surg. 1982;196:194-7.

45. Stephenson LW, MacVaugh H, 3rd, Tomasello DN, et al. Propranolol for prevention of postoperative cardiac arrhythmias: a randomized study. Annals of Thoracic Surgery. 1980;29:113-6.

46. Vecht RJ, Nicolaides EP, Ikweuke JK, et al. Incidence and prevention of supraventricular tachyarrhythmias after coronary bypass surgery. Int J Cardiol. 1986;13:125-34.

47. Wenke K, Parsa MH, Imhof M, et al. [Efficacy of metoprolol in prevention of supraventricular arrhythmias after coronary artery bypass grafting]. Z Kardiol. 1999;88:647-52.

48. White HD, Antman EM, Glynn MA, et al. Efficacy and safety of timolol for prevention of supraventricular tachyarrhythmias after coronary artery bypass surgery. Circulation. 1984;70:479-84.

49. Williams JB, Stephensen LW, Holford FD, et al. Arrhythmia prophylaxis using propranolol after coronary artery surgery. Ann Thorac Surg. 1982;34:435-8.

50. Kim MH, Deeb GM, Morady F, et al. Effect of postoperative atrial fibrillation on length of stay after cardiac surgery (the postoperative atrial fibrillation in cardiac surgery study. Am J Cardiol. 2001;87:881-5.

51. Crystal E, Connolly S, Thorpe K, et al. Metoprolol prophylaxis against post-operative atrial fibrillation increases length of hospital stay in patients not on pre-operative beta-blockers: the beta-blocker length of stay (BLOS) trial. Circulation. 2001;104:II-773.

52. Evrard P, Gonzalez M, Jamart J, et al. Prophylaxis of supraventricular and ventricular arrhythmias after coronary artery bypass grafting with low-dose sotalol. Ann Thorac Surg. 2000;70:151-6.

53. Gomes JA, Ip J, Santoni-Rugiu F, et al. Oral d,l sotalol reduces the incidence of postoperative atrial fibrillation in coronary artery bypass surgery patients: a randomized, double-blind, placebo-controlled study. J Am Coll Cardiol. 1999;34:334-9.

54. Jacquet L, Evenepoel M, Marenne F, et al. Hemodynamic effects and safety of sotalol in the prevention of supraventricular arrhythmias after coronary artery bypass surgery. J Cardiothorac Vasc Anesth. 1994;8:431-6.

55. Suttorp MJ, Kingma JH, Tjon Joe Gin RM, et al. Efficacy and safety of low- and high-dose sotalol versus propranolol in the prevention of supraventricular tachyarrhythmias early after coronary artery bypass operations. J Thorac Cardiovasc Surg. 1990;100:921-6.

56. Pfisterer ME, Kloter-Weber UC, Huber M, et al. Prevention of supraventricular tachyarrhythmias after open heart operation by low-dose sotalol: a prospective, double-blind, randomized, placebo-controlled study. Ann Thorac Surg. 1997;64:1113-9.

57. Janssen J, Loomans L, Harink J, et al. Prevention and treatment of supraventricular tachycardia shortly after coronary artery bypass grafting: a randomized open trial. Angiology. 1986;37:601-9.

58. Nystrom U, Edvardsson N, Berggren H, et al. Oral sotalol reduces the incidence of atrial fibrillation after coronary artery bypass surgery. Thorac Cardiovasc Surg. 1993;41:34-7.

59. Abdulrahman O, Dale HT, Levin V, et al. The comparative value of low-dose sotalol vs. metoprolol in the prevention of postoperative supraventricular arrhythmias. Eur Heart J. 1999;20:372.

60. Parikka H, Toivonen L, Heikkila L, et al. Comparison of sotalol and metoprolol in the prevention of atrial fibrillation after coronary artery bypass surgery. J Cardiovasc Pharmacol. 1998;31:67-73.

61. Suttorp MJ, Kingma JH, Peels HO, et al. Effectiveness of sotalol in preventing supraventricular tachyarrhythmias shortly after coronary artery bypass grafting. Am J Cardiol. 1991;68:1163-9.

62. Butler J, Harriss DR, Sinclair M, et al. Amiodarone prophylaxis for tachycardias after coronary artery surgery: a randomised, double blind, placebo controlled trial. Br Heart J. 1993;70:56-60.

63. Daoud EG, Strickberger SA, Man KC, et al. Preoperative amiodarone as prophylaxis against atrial fibrillation after heart surgery. [see comments]. New England Journal of Medicine. 1997;337:1785-91.

64. Dorge H, Schoendube FA, Schoberer M, et al. Intraoperative amiodarone as prophylaxis against atrial fibrillation after coronary operations. Annals of Thoracic Surgery. 2000;69:1358-62.

65. Giri A, White M, Dunn A, et al. Efficacy and safety of ajuvant preoperative oral amiodarone to prevent atrial fibrillation after open heart surgery in elderly patients receiving post-operative beta-blockade. Circulation. 1999;100:2385.

66. Guarnieri T, Nolan S, Gottlieb SO, et al. Intravenous amiodarone for the prevention of atrial fibrillation after open heart surgery: the Amiodarone Reduction in Coronary Heart (ARCH) trial. [see comments]. Journal of the American College of Cardiology. 1999;34:343-7.

67. Hohnloser SH, Meinertz T, Dammbacher T, et al. Electrocardiographic and antiarrhythmic effects of intravenous amiodarone: results of a prospective, placebo-controlled study. Am Heart J. 1991;121:89-95.

68. Lee SH, Chang CM, Lu MJ, et al. Intravenous amiodarone for prevention of atrial fibrillation after coronary artery bypass grafting. Ann Thorac Surg. 2000;70:157-61.

69. Redle JD, Khurana S, Marzan R, et al. Prophylactic oral amiodarone compared with placebo for prevention of atrial fibrillation after coronary artery bypass surgery. Am Heart J. 1999;138:144-50.

70. Treggiari-Venzi MM, Waeber JL, Perneger TV, et al. Intravenous amiodarone or magnesium sulphate is not cost-beneficial prophylaxis for atrial fibrillation after coronary artery bypass surgery. Br J Anaesth. 2000;85:690-5.

71. Solomon AJ, Greenberg MD, Kilborn MJ, et al. Amiodarone versus a beta blocker to prevent atrial fibrillation following cardiovascular surgery. J Am Coll Card. 2001;37:92A.

72. Blommaert D, Gonzalez M, Mucumbitsi J, et al. Effective prevention of atrial fibrillation by continuous atrial overdrive pacing after coronary artery bypass surgery. J Am Coll Cardiol. 2000;35:1411-5.

73. Chung MK, Augostini RS, Asher CR, et al. Ineffectiveness and potential proarrhythmia of atrial pacing for atrial fibrillation prevention after coronary artery bypass grafting. Ann Thorac Surg. 2000;69:1057-63.

74. Daoud EG, Dabir R, Archambeau M, et al. Randomized, double-blind trial of simultaneous right and left atrial epicardial pacing for prevention of post-open heart surgery atrial fibrillation. Circulation. 2000;102:761-5.

75. Fan K, Lee KL, Chiu CS, et al. Effects of biatrial pacing in prevention of postoperative atrial fibrillation after coronary artery bypass surgery. Circulation. 2000;102:755-60.

76. Gerstenfeld EP, Hill MR, French SN, et al. Evaluation of right atrial and biatrial temporary pacing for the prevention of atrial fibrillation after coronary artery bypass surgery. J Am Coll Cardiol. 1999;33:1981-8.

77. Goette A, Mittag J, Friedl A, et al. Effectiveness of atrial pacing in preventing atrial fibrillaion after coronary artery bypass surgery. Pacing Clin Electrophysiol. 1999;23:700.

78. Greenberg MD, Katz NM, Iuliano S, et al. Atrial pacing for the prevention of atrial fibrillation after cardiovascular surgery. J Am Coll Cardiol. 2000;35:1416-22.

79. Kurz DJ, Naegeli B, Kunz M, et al. Epicardial, biatrial synchronous pacing for prevention of atrial fibrillation after cardiac surgery. Pacing Clin Electrophysiol. 1999;22:721-6.

80. Levy T, Fotopoulos G, Walker S, et al. Randomized controlled study investigating the effect of biatrial pacing in prevention of atrial fibrillation after coronary artery bypass grafting. Circulation. 2000;102:1382-7.

81. Orr W, Tsui S, Stafford P, et al. Synchronised Bi-atrial pacing after coronary artery by-pass surgery. Pacing Clin Electrophysiol. 1999;22:755.

82. Schweikert R, Grady T, Gupta N ea. Atrial pacing in the prevention of atrial fibrillation after cardiac surgery: results of the second postoperative pacing study (POPS-2). J Am Coll Card. 1998;31(2):117A.

83. Crystal E, Sleik K, Ginger T, et al. Prevention of atrial fibrillation after cardiac surgery: A meta-analysis. Circulation. 2001;104 (17):II-773.

84. Pinski S, Sgarbossa E. Influence of overdrive atrial pacing on the occurence of atrial fibrillation after cardiac surgery : A meta-analysis. J Am Coll Card. 2001;37:128A.

85. Giri S, White CM, Dunn AB, et al. Oral amiodarone for prevention of atrial fibrillation after open heart surgery, the Atrial Fibrillation Suppression Trial (AFIST): a randomised placebo-controlled trial. Lancet. 2001;357:830-6.

86. Reddy P. Does prophylaxis against atrial fibrillation after cardiac surgery reduce length of stay or hospital costs? Pharmacotherapy. 2001;21:338-44.

9

CIRCUMFERENTIAL PULMONARY VEIN MAPPING AND ABLATION IN FOCAL ATRIAL FIBRILLATION
Breakthrough and Isolation Trial: Mapping and Ablation of Pulmonary Veins (*BITMAP*)-Study

Thorsten Lewalter, MD and Berndt Lüderitz, MD, FESC, FACC

Department of Medicine-Cardiology, University of Bonn, Bonn, Germany

Introduction

As early as 1959 Abildskov and Moe generated in an experimental setting „focal" atrial fibrillation (AF) using Acotinin application to the atrial appendage (1). AF terminated when the site of Acotinine application was isolated from the rest of the atrium myocardium proving the importance of the firing focus for the persistence of this type of AF. Haissaguerre and coworkers were the first who observed ectopic induction of AF in the clinical setting while performing linear lesions in the left atrium ("focally induced atrial fibrillation"). Already in their first observations of this phenomenon they were able to identify the upper pulmonary veins (PV's) as the most frequent location of these arrhythmogenic foci (2). Since then, pulmonary vein (PV) ablation has entered the therapeutic armamentarium as a curative intervention in a subset of patients with focal AF (3,4). Currently various techniques are used to perform such a catheter based trigger elimination. The most widely accepted approach consists of circumferential mapping of the PV ostia with helical shaped mapping catheters and radiofrequency (RF) delivery via a second separate ablation catheter (5,6). Circumferential mapping inside the PV's allows in a subset of veins to localize a circumscript left atrial to PV breakthrough area which offers the chance to limit RF energy delivery to PV segments rather than to perform circumferential ablations (5,6). This "segmental" RF ablation approach may help to reduce the risk of procedural complications like PV stenosis or thrombosis. Various technical and procedural changes and improvements are currently under investigation to enhance the efficacy and overall safety of PV ablation (7).

Breakthrough and Isolation Trial: Mapping and Ablation of Pulmonary Veins (*BITMAP*): Study Design

The BITMAP-Study is a multi-center, non-randomized, single group, treatment-only study to investigate the safety and therapeutic efficacy of a new catheter design (Revelation Helix microcatheter) combining both, circumferential mapping and direct ablation capabilities. The objectives of this study are:

1) To map and ablate the pulmonary vein potentials in the pulmonary veins in patients during the procedure.

2) To demonstrate the safety of RF ablation in the pulmonary veins using the Revelation Helix by measuring the incidence of adverse events reported during the study.

3) To evaluate whether ablated subjects demonstrate a clinically meaningful improvement in functionality as determined at three and six months after treatment by an improved quality of life (Medical Outcomes Trust SF-36 Health Survey).

To evaluate these objectives the following primary outcome measurements are performed during the follow-up period: The time to first reoccurrence of a documented symptomatic AF episode within 6 months after the PV ablation procedure (The documentation of this episode (event recorder/ECG) has to display AF with duration of more than 30 sec). In addition, the incidence of procedural complications related to left atrial RF applications in the pulmonary veins are documented. As secondary outcome measurements the total number of symptomatic AF episodes > 30sec, the time to second reoccurrence of symptomatic AF > 30sec and quality of life assessment using the SF 36 will be explored.

Aside from the absence of a significant structural cardiac disease and relevant left atrial dilatation, the main inclusion criteria are:

1) Patient has documented symptomatic paroxysmal or persistent (no more than 3 months) AF that is refractory to at least one class IC or class III drug. This requires a minimum of 2 ECG documentations of AF.

2) Patient has a history of recurrent AF >2 years.

3) Patient is in normal sinus rhythm at the time of the procedure or can be converted to normal sinus rhythm.

4) Patient has AF originating from the PVs.

The follow-up program includes a patients visit at 1, 3 and 6 months and will be completed at 12 months post-procedure using a telephone call. Aside from resting ECGs, patients are advised to submitt a weekly ECG via telephone or in case of palpitations. To detect changes pulmonary vein anatomy like pulmonary vein stenosis, CT scans are performed at baseline and after 3 months. The complete schedule of follow-up tests is depicted in Table 1.

Table 1: BITMAP-Study: Schedule of follow-up tests

Examination	Baseline	Procedural Measurements	Prior to Hospital Discharge	Month 1	Month 3	Month 6	Month 12
Medical History	X						
Physical Exam	X		X	X	X	X	
Stress Test	X					X	
12 Lead ECG	X		X	X	X	X	
Transesophageal Echocardiogram	X						
Transthoracic Echocardiogram	X		X		X		
PT / PTT / INR	X		X	X	X		
Activated Clotting Time		X					
Quality of Life Questionnaires	X						
Urine or Serum Pregnancy Test (if applicable)	X				X	X	
Cardiac Event Monitor				X	X	X	
Telephone Interview							X
CT scan	CT scan					CT scan	

Case Report: Catheter Ablation in Focal Atrial Fibrillation

As a typical case out of so far 8 patients treated at our center, we report about a 44 years old patient with drug refractory symptomatic paroxysmal AF for several years who was referred to our center for an electrophysiologic study and interventional therapy. Non-invasive and invasive evaluation including left heart catheterisation demonstrated no evidence for structural heart disease. Twenty-four hours Holter-ECG recordings and the pacemaker's detailed onset reports demonstrated frequent premature atrial contractions in part inducing paroxysmal AF as a marker for a focal trigger of this arrhythmia. AV-node ablation as a therapeutic alternative was refused by the patient.

Electrophysiological study and ablation procedure. After the patient's informed consent and approval from the local ethics committee a 4 French fixed-wire catheter with eight 6 mm coiled Platinum electrodes in a looped configuration and an inter-electrode spacing of 2 mm was used for both PV mapping and ablation (Revelation Helix, Cardima, Inc., Fremont, CA, USA; Fig. 1).

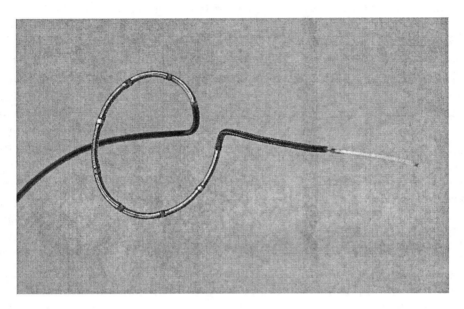

Figure 1: Combined circumferential mapping and ablation catheter (Revelation Helix)
Figure 1 displays the 4 French fixed-wire Revelation Helix microcatheter with eight 6 mm coiled Platinum electrodes in a looped configuration with an inner diameter of 20 mm and an inter-electrode spacing of 2 mm. For distal stabilization, the catheter has a 2 cm long electrically inactive flexible distal tip. The catheter incorporates eight thermocouples for temperature sensing during RF delivery.

One quadripolar 6 French electrode catheter (Bard Angiomed Inc., Tewksbury, MA, USA) was positioned to record the His-bundle signal. An octapolar 6 French catheter, with 2-10-2 mm interelectrode spacing was placed in the coronary sinus (CS) (Bard Inc.). Endocardial bipolar electrograms were recorded with a filter bandwith of 30 to 500 Hz. Electrogram information and a simultaneously registered 12-lead surface electrocardiogram were digitally stored on a Lab computer system (Bard Inc.). Endocardial pacing was performed using a rectangular stimulus of 1-msec duration at twice diastolic pacing threshold amplitude (UHS 20, Biotronik, Lake Oswego, OR, USA). After right atrial mapping and analysing the coronary sinus activation sequence of premature atrial contractions which suggested a left atrial origin, transseptal puncture was performed in standard technique. Venous angiography identified a right upper PV and a common ostium for the left sided PV′s. The right lower PV could not be reached and therefore not mapped or ablated. A Helix Revelation catheter with a 20 mm inner diameter of the distal loop was advanced and positioned inside the right upper PV and the common ostium of the left-sided PV′s.

Short coupled premature atrial contractions originating from both, the left-sided and the right upper PV were notified. During sinus rhythm and fixed rate pacing from the coronary sinus the left atrial to PV breakthrough area was identified in electrode 8, 1, 2, 3 and 4. Unipolar RF application was performed in a temperature-controlled manner using a target temperature of 45-50°C and a maximum power output of 30 watts for 60 seconds (Stockert Inc., Radiofrequency generator). While ablating with electrode 3, after RF energy has sequentially been applied via electrodes 8, 1 and 2, complete PV potential abolition could be documented (Fig. 2). Both left-sided PV′s demonstrated PV potentials which could be successfully abolished by ablating the common PV ostium, however distal PV elimination required three circumferential burns. After PV ablation, a repeated PV angiography did not reveal stenosis or narrowing in any of the ablated veins. The electrophysiological study lasted 6 hours and required a fluoroscopy time of 48 minutes. The procedure was executed without complications.

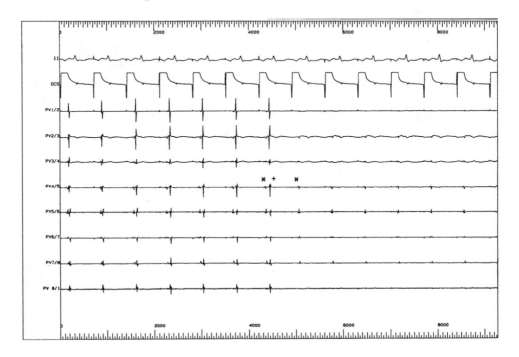

Figure 2: Pulmonary vein potential elimination in the right upper pulmonary vein
Radiofrequency application using a maximum power output of 30 watts at a target temperature of 50°C allowed to persistently abolish the pulmonary vein (PV) potential (+) from the righ upper PV. After PV elimination, the far-field left atrial signal (*) remained detectable inside the PV during coronary sinus pacing.
(Surface ECG lead II, DCS=distal coronary sinus and eight bipolar circumferential recordings from the right upper pulmonary vein: PV 1/2 to 8/1; paper speed: 25 mm/sec).

<u>Summary</u>
Circumferential PV mapping with identification of the left atrial to PV breakthrough area as the target for ostial RF energy delivery represents the most widely accepted ablation technique in the treatment of focal AF. This approach usually requires a minimum of two transseptally advanced catheters, one for circumferential mapping and a separate catheter for ablation.
The *B*reakthrough and *I*solation *T*rial: *M*apping and *A*blation of *P*ulmonary Veins (*BITMAP*) Study investigates the safety and therapeutical efficacy of a new microcatheter design combining both, circumferential mapping and direct ablation capabilities in a single-catheter technique. A follow-up of six months includes transtelephonic ECG monitoring to check for AF recurrencies. A case study illustrates the potential benefits of this approach: Those electrodes picking up early PV potentials during atrial pacing or sinus rhythm can directly be used for radiofrequency delivery necessitating only a single transseptally advanced catheter which may reduce the overall complexity of the procedure. Furthermore, the possibility to limit energy application to those electrodes indicating the left atrial to PV breakthrough avoiding any spatial difference between the mapping and ablation catheter may help to minimize RF applications and potentially reduce the risk of PV stenosis. However, safety and long-term efficacy of this single catheter approach cannot yet definitely be classified and will therefore be evaluated in an ongoing European multicenter study (*BITMAP* study).

References

1. Moe G, Abildskov JA. Atrial fibrillation as a self-sustaining arrhythmia independent of focal discharge. Am Heart J 1959;58:59-70.
2. Haissaguerre M, Jais P, Shah D et al. Right and left atrial radiofrequency catheter therapy of paroxysmal atrial fibrillation. J Cardiovasc Electrophysiol 1996;7:1132-1144.
3. Haissaguerre M, Jais P, Shah D, et al. Spontaneous Initiation of atrial fibrillation by ectopic beats originating in the pulmonary veins. N Engl J Med 1998;339:659-666.
4. Chen SA, Hsieh MH, Tai CT, et al. Initiation of atrial fibrillation by ectopic beats originating from the pulmonary veins. Circulation 1999;100:1879-1886.
5. Haissaguerre M, Shah D, Jais P, et al. Electrophysiological breakthroughs from the left atrium to the pulmonary veins. Circulation 2000;102:2463-2465.
6. Haissaguerre M, Shah D, Jais P, et al. Mapping-guided ablation of pulmonary veins to cure atrial fibrillation. Am J Cardiol 2000;86:9K-19K.
7. Lewalter T, Lüderitz B. Single catheter technique for pulmonary vein mapping and ablation. Cardio News 2001;10:25.

III. IMPLANTABLE CARDIOVERTER-DEFIBRILLATOR

10.

USE OF IMPLANTABLE CARDIOVERTER DEFIBRILLATOR (ICD) THERAPY AND ICD GUIDELINES AROUND THE WORLD

Mary E. McGrory-Usset, MBA, Marshall S. Stanton, M.D.

Medtronic, Inc., Minneapolis, Minnesota, USA

ICD Use Around the World

Implantable cardioverter defibrillators (ICDs) have become an accepted therapy for patients at high risk of ventricular tachyarrhythmias. Worldwide ICD implants have grown significantly in the last five years, with an estimated 33,000 implants in 1996 and 69,000 implants in 2000.[1,2]

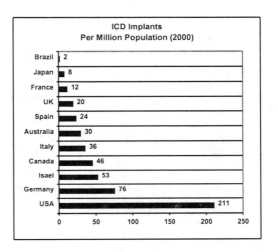

Despite the similarities between many of the ICD published guidelines in various countries, there are significant variations in ICD use around the world, as shown in Figure 1.[1-3] Although the United States has the highest ICD implant per million rate, it is estimated that only one-third of patients who meet the current Class I guidelines have received ICD therapy.[4] If it were assumed that the age distribution and comorbid conditions of the international populations are similar to the United States, the ICD utilization rates in these countries would be significantly lower than the utilization rate in the United States. In addition, these rates of use do not account for potential new patient populations being studied in ongoing clinical trials or who were enrolled in recently completed trials, such as the MADIT II trial.

Published guidelines are an important guide to medical practice, but by themselves do not create behavior change. There are a number of factors that may contribute to low ICD utilization rates and to variations in ICD use by country. Potential factors include: healthcare budgets and policies, the number of available electrophysiologists and implanting centers,

From Ovsyshcher IE. *New Developments in Cardiac Pacing and Electrophysiology.* Armonk, NY: Futura Publishing Company, Inc. ©2002.

physician referral practices, cost-effectiveness of ICD therapy, and acceptance of ICD clinical results.

Current ICD Guidelines

Improved ICD technology, as well as published results of large, prospective, randomized trials, have resulted in many countries developing new ICD guidelines over the last four years. ICDs have been proven to reduce overall mortality between 20 - 31% for secondary prevention patients (AVID, CIDS, CASH trials) and between 30 - 60% for post myocardial infarction (MI) primary prevention patients (MADIT, MUSTT, MADIT II trials) when compared to antiarrhythmic drugs.[5-9] In addition, studies have shown ICDs are up to 99% effective in terminating life-threatening ventricular tachyarrhythmias.[10-12]

Early guidelines supported ICD therapy only for patients who were at the highest risk of sudden cardiac arrest. As ICD technology has improved and evolved in recent years, the risks and costs associated with ICD therapy have been substantially reduced. With newer devices allowing pectoral implants and a concomitant reduction in complications, mortality, and costs, ICD therapy is now considered first-line therapy for patients with life-threatening ventricular tachyarrhythmias.[13-25]

Due to the wealth of clinical data published and major ICD technology advances since 1997, only guidelines published after this date will be reviewed. Guidelines from the following geographic areas and organizations will be described: United States: American College of Cardiology and American Heart Association,[13, 14] Canada: Canadian Cardiovascular Society,[15] and Europe: European Society of Cardiology.[26]

United States Guidelines: American College of Cardiology (ACC) and American Heart Association (AHA)[13]

In 1998, the ACC and AHA published new ICD guidelines using the following classifications:

Class I: Conditions for which there is evidence and/or general agreement that a given procedure is beneficial, useful and effective.

Class II: Conditions for which there is conflicting evidence and/or a divergence of opinion about the usefulness/efficacy of a procedure or treatment.

IIa: Weight of evidence/ opinion is in favor of usefulness/efficacy.

IIb: Usefulness/efficacy is less well established by evidence/opinion.

Class III: Conditions for which there is evidence and/or agreement that a procedure/treatment is not useful/effective and in some cases may be harmful.

The levels of evidence on which each guideline is evaluated on includes:
Level A: Data derived from multiple randomized clinical trials involving a large number of individuals.
Level B: Data derived from one or two randomized studies involving only a small number of patients or from well designed data analysis of nonrandomized studies or observational data registries.
Level C: Consensus opinion of experts is the primary source of condition.

The North American Society of Pacing and Electrophysiology (NASPE) organization endorsed the ACC/AHA ICD guidelines.[27]

The Class I guidelines include:
1. Cardiac arrest due to ventricular fibrillation (VF) or ventricular tachycardia (VT), not due to a transient or reversible cause. (Level A)
2. Spontaneous sustained VT. (Level B)
3. Syncope of undetermined origin with clinically relevant, hemodynamically significant, sustained VT or VF induced at electrophysiological study when drug therapy is ineffective, not tolerated, or not preferred. (Level B)
4. Nonsustained VT with coronary disease, prior myocardial infarction (MI), left ventricular (LV) dysfunction, and inducible VF or sustained VT at electrophysiological study that is not suppressible by a Class I antiarrhythmic drug. (Level B)

The Class IIb guidelines include:
1. Cardiac arrest presumed to be due to VF, when electrophysiological testing is precluded by other medical conditions. (Level C)
2. Severe symptoms attributable to sustained ventricular tachyarrhythmias while awaiting cardiac transplantation. (Level C)
3. Familial or inherited conditions with a high risk for life-threatening ventricular tachyarrhythmias such as long QT syndrome or hypertrophic cardiomyopathy. (Level C)
4. Nonsustained VT with coronary artery disease, prior MI, and LV dysfunction and inducible sustained VT or VF at electrophysiological study. (Level B)

5. Recurrent syncope of undetermined etiology in the presence of ventricular dysfunction and inducible ventricular arrhythmias at electrophysiological study, when other causes of syncope have been excluded. (Level C)

The Class III guidelines include:
1. Syncope of undetermined cause in a patient without inducible ventricular tachyarrhythmias. (Level C)
2. Incessant VT or VF. (Level C)
3. VF or VT resulting from arrhythmias amenable to surgical or catheter ablation; for example, atrial arrhythmias associated with the Wolff-Parkinson-White syndrome, right ventricular outflow tract VT, idiopathic left ventricular tachycardia, or fascicular VT. (Level C)
4. Ventricular tachyarrhythmias due to transient or reversible disorder (e.g., AMI, electrolyte imbalance, drugs, trauma). (Level C)
5. Significant psychiatric illnesses that may be aggravated by device implantation or may preclude systematic follow-up. (Level C)
6. Terminal illnesses with life expectancy $\leq$ 6 months. (Level C).
7. Patients with coronary artery disease with LV dysfunction and prolonged QRS duration in the absence of spontaneous or inducible sustained or nonsustained VT who are undergoing coronary bypass surgery. (Level C)
8. New York Heart Association (NYHA) Class IV drug-refractory congestive heart failure in patients who are not candidates for cardiac transplantation. (Level C)

Canadian Guidelines: Canadian Cardiovascular Society (CCS)[15]

In 1999, the Canadian Cardiovascular Society Consensus Conference on the Prevention of Sudden Death from Ventricular Arrhythmia agreed on the types of patients who would benefit most from ICD therapy. The levels of evidence, guideline grading recommendations and guidelines that were developed are described below:

Level I: Large randomised trials or meta-analysis with clear cut results (and low risk of error). Grade A

Level II: Small randomised trials or meta-analysis with uncertain results. Grade B

Level III: Nonrandomised contemporaneous controls. Grade C

Level IV: Nonrandomised historical controls. Grade C

Level V: No controls, case series. Grade C

Level I – Grade A
1. Patients surviving cardiac arrest or symptomatic sustained VT (not within three days of acute MI and not associated with correctable cause).
   a. Ventricular fibrillation (VF).
   b. Patients with VT causing syncope.
   c. Patients with minimally symptomatic VT with LVEF ≤ 35%.
   d. Patients with minimally symptomatic VT with LVEF > 35% may receive either pharmacological therapy or an ICD.

Level II – Grade B
1. Patients who have had a previous MI with left ventricular dysfunction (LVEF ≤ 35%) and asymptomatic spontaneous nonsustained VT, with sustained VT/VF induced at electrophysiology (EP) study.

Level V – Grade C
1. Patients with long QT syndrome (LQTS) whom have a strong family history of SCD, or LQTS patients without a family history of SCD who have recurrent syncope due to VT despite beta-blocker and pacing therapies.
2. Patients with Brugada syndrome presenting with VT/VF, or a history of syncope and inducible VT at EP study.
3. Patients with arrhythmogenic right ventricular dysplasia (ARVD) and documented sustained VT/VF, or asymptomatic ARVD patients who have a strong family history of SCD.
4. Hypertrophic cardiomyopathy (HCM) patients with sustained VT/VF in the absence of a reversible cause, or asymptomatic HCM patients with a strong family history of SCD.

European Guidelines

The cardiology associations or governments in many European countries developed new ICD guidelines since 1997 or adopted the 1998 ACC/AHA guidelines. These countries include: United Kingdom, Germany, Italy, Spain, Denmark, Austria, and France.[17-23] In addition to individual European countries developing ICD guidelines, the Study Group on Guidelines on ICDs of the Working Group on Arrhythmias and the Working Group on Cardiac Pacing of the European Society of Cardiology (ESC) published ICD guidelines in 2001.[26] The Task Force on Sudden Cardiac Death of the European Society of Cardiology also developed guidelines on sudden cardiac death which include recommendations for the use of ICD therapy.[24] This chapter will highlight the ICD guidelines published by the ESC Study Group. Other European guidelines are similar to these published guidelines.

European Society of Cardiology (ESC) – Study Group on Guidelines on ICDs of the Working Group on Arrhythmias and the Working Group on Cardiac Pacing[26]

The ESC developed ICD guidelines in 2001 and used similar classification definitions and evidence ranking to the ACC/AHA organizations.

Class I guidelines include:

Cardiac arrest:

1. Electrocardiographically documented VT/VF not due to transient or reversible cause. (Level A)

2. VT/VF not electrocardiographically documented, but presumed based on successful external defibrillation and/or inducible VT/VF, and/or other relevant clinical data, and arrhythmia not due to transient, reversible or treatable cause. (Level B)

Electrocardiographically documented ventricular tachycardia without cardiac arrest:

3. Sustained VT with severe haemodynamic compromise (syncope, near-syncope, heart failure, shock or anginal complaints). (Level A)

4. Sustained VT without severe haemodynamic compromise if left ventricular ejection fraction (LVEF) $\leq$ 40%. (Level B)

5. LVEF $\leq$ 40%, 4 days or more after myocardial infarction with inducible VF or sustained VT at electrophysiology study. (Level B)

Syncope without documented ventricular tachyarrhythmia:

6. Inducible VF or VT at electrophysiology study with severe haemodynamic compromise (syncope, near-syncope, congestive heart failure, shock or angina) when drug therapy is ineffective, not tolerated or not preferred, if LVEF $\leq$ 40%. (Level B)

Prophylactic indication:

7. Non-sustained VT 4 days or more after myocardial infarction with a LVEF $\leq$ 40% and inducible VF or sustained VT at electrophysiology study. (Level B)

Class II guidelines include:

Electrocardiographically documented ventricular tachycardia without cardiac arrest:

1. Sustained VT without haemodynamic compromise with LVEF > 40%. (Level C)

2. Patients at high risk for sudden cardiac death awaiting cardiac transplantation and patients with hypertrophic cardiomyopathy with

syncope and/or family history of sudden death at a young age. (Level C)

Syncope without documented ventricular tachyarrhythmia:

3. Inducible VF or VT at electrophysiology study with severe haemodynamic compromise (syncope, near-syncope, congestive heart failure, shock or angina) when drug therapy is ineffective, not tolerated or not preferred, if LVEF > 40%. (Level C)

4. VT/VF non-inducible with cardiac disorder known to be associated with ventricular arrhythmias such as long QT, hypertrophic cardiomyopathy or other diseases when other causes of syncope have been excluded. (Level C)

Prophylactic indication:

5. Familial or inherited conditions such as long QT syndrome, hypertrophic cardiomyopathy, arrhythmogenic right ventricular dysplasia, Brugada syndrome and other apparently genetic disorders, as well as some specific congenital disorders with an approved high risk of sudden cardiac death. (Level C)

Class III guidelines include:

Cardiac arrest:

1. If due to transient, reversible or treatable cause, such as within 48 hours after myocardial infarction, acute ischaemia or Wolff-Parkinson-White syndrome, or monomorphic VT amenable to map-guided surgery or catheter ablation. (Level C)

2. If transient, reversible or treatable cause. (Level C)

Electrocardiographically documented ventricular tachycardia without cardiac arrest:

3. Incessant VT. (Level C)

4. Patients not at high risk, or sustained on non-sustained monomorphic VT amenable to catheter ablation or map-guided surgery. (Level C)

5. Idiopathic monomorphic VT, either sustained or non-sustained. (Level C)

Syncope without documented ventricular tachyarrhythmia:

6. Without cardiac disorder. (Level C)

Prophylactic indication:

7. Coronary artery disease with left ventricular dysfunction and prolonged QRS duration in the absence of spontaneous or inducible sustained or non-sustained VT, who are undergoing coronary bypass surgery. (Level B)

General contraindications:

8. VT/VF associated with terminal illnesses with projected life expectancy $\leq$ 6 months, or significant psychiatric illnesses that may be aggravated by device implantation or may preclude systematic follow-up or NYHA class IV drug-refractory congestive heart failure in patients who are not candidates for cardiac transplantation. (Level C)

9. Patients who have severe neurological sequelae following cardiac arrest. (Level C)

Status of ICD Guidelines in Other Countries

The Brazilian Cardiology Society published ICD guidelines in 2000[25] that are similar to ACC/AHA guidelines. The Japan Circulation Society is in the process of proposing new ICD guidelines, but has not yet finalized their recommendations. The Cardiac Society of Australia and New Zealand's Pacing and EP Working Group are also in the process of developing guidelines. Israel does not have published ICD guidelines at this time.

Summary of ICD Guidelines Around the World

A brief comparison of the guidelines published in the United States Europe, and Canada is shown on Table 1. These published guidelines have many

Table 1. Summary of Class I or II ICD Guidelines for the United States (ACC/AHA), Europe (ESC), and Canada (CCS)

Recommend ICD Therapy for the Following Patients:	ACC/AHA	ESC	CCS
Cardiac arrest due to VT/VF, not due to transient/reversible cause	X	X	X
Cardiac arrest, due to suspected VT, EP testing not possible, or successful defibrillation or inducible VT/VF or other relevant clinical data	X	X	
Spontaneous sustained VT	X	X (w/hemodynamic instability, or LVEF $\leq$ 40% and few symptoms)	X (w/syncope, or if LVEF $\leq$ 35%)
Syncope unknown etiology, hemodynamically significant sustained VT/VF induced at EP study, when drug therapy can not be used	X	X	
Syncope of unknown etiology, with LV dysfunction, and inducible VT/VF at EP study	X		
Symptomatic VT, awaiting cardiac transplant	X	X	

Familial or inherited conditions (LQTS, HCM, Brugada, ARVD) with high risk of life-threatening ventricular tachyarrhythmia	X	X	X
Post-MI, NSVT, LV dysfunction, inducible VT	X	X	X

similarities. Each recommends ICD therapy for patients with documented spontaneous sustained ventricular tachyarrhythmias. In both the European and Canada guidelines, there are additional requirements for patients with spontaneous ventricular tachyarrhythmias to be in a class I or II guideline category. The post-MI patient with non-sustained VT, left ventricular dysfunction, and inducible VT during an EP study is recommended for ICD therapy in the three guidelines. Smaller patient populations with less common forms of heart disease, such as ARVD, HCM, and LQTS are also identified for potential ICD therapy, depending on their level of sudden cardiac arrest risk. Finally, the guidelines for both the United States and Europe have similar contraindication criteria (class III) for ICD therapy.

References

1. Medtronic, Inc. Industry data on file. 2001.
2. Investors Guide to ICDs 2000. Healthcare: Pharmaceuticals, Hospital Supplies & Medical Technology Report, Morgan Stanley Dean Witter; March 2, 2000.
3. U.S. Census Bureau. World Population Profile 2000. www.census.gov; 2001.
4. Ruskin J, Camm A, Zipes D, et al. ICD Utilization based on discharge diagnoses from Medicare and managed care patients. *J Clin Electrophysiology*. 2001;in press.
5. The AVID Investigators. A comparison of antiarrhythmic-drug therapy with implantable defibrillators in patients resuscitated from near-fatal ventricular arrhythmias. *N Engl J Med*. 1997;337:1575-1583.
6. Connolly S, Gent M, Roberts R, et al. for the CIDS Investigators. Canadian Implantable Defibrillator Study (CIDS): a randomised trial of the implantable cardioverter defibrillator against amiodarone. *Circulation*. 2000;101:1297-1302.
7. Moss A, Hall W, Cannom D. Improved survival with an implanted defibrillator in patients with coronary disease at high risk for ventricular arrhythmia. *N Engl J Med*. 1996;335:1933-1940.
8. Buxton A, Lee K, Fisher J, for the Multicenter Unsustained Tachycardia Trial (MUSTT) Investigators. A randomised study of the prevention of sudden death in patients with coronary artery disease. *N Engl J Med*. 1999;341:1882-1890.
9. Guidant Corporation. Press Release: Guidant notified that landmark implantable defibrillator study ends early. November 20, 2001.
10. Saksena S, Investigators for the PCD Investigators. Clinical outcome of patients with malignant ventricular tachyarrhythmia and a multiprogrammable cardioverter-defibrillator implanted with or without thoracotomy: An international multicenter study. *J Am Coll Cardiol*. 1994;23:1521-1530.
11. Zipes D, Roberts D. Results of the international study of the implantable pacemaker cardioverter-defibrillator: A comparison of epicardial and endocardial lead systems. *Circulation*. 1995;92:59-65.

12. Nisam S, Kaye S, Mower M, Hull M. AICD automatic cardioverter defibrillator clinical update: 14 years experience in over 34,000 patients. *PACE* 1995;18:142-147.

13. Gregoratos G, Cheitlin M, Conill A, et al. ACC/AHA guidelines for implantation of cardiac pacemakers and antiarrhythmia devices: A report of the American College of Cardiology/American Heart Association Task Force on Practice Guidelines (Committee on Pacemaker Implantation). *J Am Coll Cardiol.* 1998;31:1175-1209.

14. Gregoratos G, Cheitlin M, Conill A, et al. Executive summary: ACC/AHA Guidelines for implantation of cardiac pacemakers and antiarrhythmia devices. A report of the ACC/AHA Task Force on Practice Guidelines (Committee on Pacemaker Implantation). *Circulation.* 1998;97:1325-1335.

15. Canadian Cardiovascular Society. The Canadian Cardiovascular Society 1999 consensus conference on prevention of sudden death from ventricular arrhythmia. *Can J Cardiol.* 2000;15 (Suppl C).

16. Hauer R, Derksen R, Wever E. Can implantable cardioverter-defibrillator therapy reduce healthcare costs? *Am J Cardiol.* 1996;78(suppl 5A):134-139.

17. National Institute for Clinical Excellence. Guidance on the use of implantable cardioverter defibrillators for arrhythmias. www.nice.org.uk; September 2000.

18. Hohnloser S, Andresen D, Block M, et al. for the Committee of Clinical Cardiology of the German Cardiac Society. *Z Kardiol.* 2000;89:136-143.

19. Italian Societies: ANMCO-SIC-AIAC. Linee guida ANMCO-SIC-AIAC sull'uso appropriato delle metodiche di electtrostimolazione cardiaca definitiva. *Ital Heart J.* 2000;1:551-569.

20. Perez-Villacastin J, Salinas JC, Madrid AH, et al. Guidelines of the Spanish Society of Cardiology. Recommendations for the implantable cardioverter defibrillator. *Rev Esp Cardiol.* 1999;52:1083-1104.

21. Danish Cardiology Society.

22. Austrian Cardiology Society.

23. Society Francaise de Cardiologie. Recommendations de la Societe Francaise de Cardiologie concernant l'electrophysiologie diagnostic et interventionelle, la stimulation cardioque permanente et al defribrillation automatique implantable. *Arch de Maladies du Coeur et des Vaisseaux.* 1999;92.

24. Priori S, Aliot E, Blomstrom-Lundqvist, et al. Task force on sudden cardiac death of the European Society of Cardiology. *Eur Heart J.* 2001;22:1475-1450.

25. Andrade J, Neto A, Braile D, et al. Guidelines for cardioverter defibrillator implantation. *Arz Bras Cardiol.* 2000;74:481-482.

26. Hauer R, Aliot E, Block M, et al. Indications for implantable cardioverter defibrillator (ICD) therapy. *Eur Heart J.* 2001;22:1074-1081.

27. Winters S, Packer D, Marchlinski F, et al. Consensus statement on indications, guidelines for use, and recommendations for follow-up of implantable cardioverter defibrillators. *PACE* 2001: 24:262-269.

11

WELL-TOLERATED SUSTAINED MONOMORPHIC VENTRICULAR TACHYCARDIA AFTER MYOCARDIAL INFARCTION: A BENIGN ARRHYTHMIA OR STILL A CLASS I INDICATION FOR DEFIBRILLATOR IMPLANTATION?

Amir Halkin, MD, *Michael Glikson, MD, **Paul Friedman, MD, and Sami Viskin, MD

Department of Cardiology, Tel Aviv-Sourasky Medical Center, Tel Aviv, *Heart Institute, Sheba Medical Center, Tel Hashomer, Israel, and the **Division of Cardiovascular Medicine, Mayo Clinic, Rochester, MN, USA

Sustained monomorphic ventricular tachycardia (SMVT) that deteriorates to ventricular fibrillation (VF) is the most common mechanism of cardiac arrest in patients with an old myocardial infarction.[1] However, some patients with old myocardial infarction have episodic spontaneous SMVT *without* cardiac arrest or hemodynamic instability. In these patients, SMVT is often a recurrent arrhythmia that is relatively well tolerated.[2] Nonetheless, the risk of ventricular tachycardia (VT) deterioration to VF during any such arrhythmic episode is cause for concern.[3-5] The prevalence of hemodynamically stable SMVT in patients with past myocardial infarction is difficult to estimate because it is dependent on the definition of this arrhythmia as well as on the diagnostic methods used for its detection and the intensity with which they are employed. Nevertheless, this presentation is certainly not uncommon among patients considered for treatment because of ventricular tachyarrhythmias. For example, in the Antiarrhythmics Versus Implantable Defibrillators (AVID) registry (n=4595, 77% with evidence of coronary artery disease), approximately 12% presented with stable sustained VT.[6]

Recent prospective randomized studies have demonstrated that patients with sustained ventricular tachyarrhythmias have higher survival rates if treated with an implantable cardioverter-defibrillator (ICD) instead of – or in addition to – antiarrhythmic drugs.[7-9] However, in these studies patients with SMVT with and without cardiac arrest, as well as patients with VF, were grouped together. Moreover, if the presenting arrhythmia was clinically stable, patients were required to have significant impairment of left ventricular systolic function to qualify for randomization. Finally, the data on long-term survival of patients with well-tolerated VT originates from post-hoc analysis of patient subgroups, and is thus more likely to be biased by confunding factors. Consequently, the advantages of ICD

From Ovsyshcher IE. *New Developments in Cardiac Pacing and Electrophysiology.* Armonk, NY: Futura Publishing Company, Inc. ©2002.

implantation for patients with hemodynamically stable spontaneous SMVT *without* cardiac arrest has not been clearly demonstrated. The 1998 ACC/AHA guidelines on anti-arrhythmic device-therapy regard spontaneous sustained VT, regardless of its etiology or hemodynamic consequences, as a "class I" indication for ICD implantation (i.e., this is a condition for which there was general agreement that the procedure is useful and effective).[10] These guidelines, however, were based on non-randomized studies of a heterogeneous population in which patients with well-tolerated VT represented a relatively small group. No randomized trials of ICD implantation for the primary prevention of sudden death in post-infarct patients who present with stable SMVT have been reported since the 1998 guidelines. Thus, the choice of therapy for such patients must still be based on the assessment of their risk of dying suddenly, relying on data derived from cohort studies and retrospective analyses of randomized trials. Reports of this type have yielded conflicting results concerning the prognosis of patients with stable VT and past myocardial infarction. Some have suggested that the risk of sudden death in this population is low,[2,11] while others have found that the risk approaches,[3,12] or may even exceed,[13] the risk in patients presenting with unstable ventricular tachyarrhythmias.

Brugada et al reported that patients with ventricular tachycardia in the absence of severe heart failure, a history of multiple infarctions or cardiac arrest had a risk of sudden death of only 2.8% at 2 years.[2] Also suggesting a low risk of sudden death, Sarter et al reported a retrospective analysis of outcomes in cohort of 124 patients with coronary heart disease and stable VT.[11] While overall mortality during a period of 3 years (mean) reached 36%, the incidence of sudden death was low (overall annual mortality of about 2.5%). This rate of sudden death reflected the outcome of 78 patients treated with antiarrhythmic drugs. It should be noted however that flaws inherent to the design of this study limit the applicability of its findings. The true cause of death is difficult to determine in retrospective studies. Moreover, more than a third of patients in this study were treated by endocardial resection, with a perioperative mortality exceeding 19%. Thus, in a significant minority of this group the complications of a surgical procedure, now practiced quite rarely, may have artificially reduced the incidence of the primary end-point (sudden death). On the other hand, surgery may have improved the outcome of patients that survived the procedure. In contrast to these studies, other cohort studies and analyses of randomized trials have found that the intermediate-term prognosis of patients with stable VT is poor. In a study by Olson et al, sudden death rates were identical in patients receiving amiodarone for either stable or unstable VT (about 25% during 19 months in both groups).[12] In another study of 50 patients (82% with coronary heart disease) receiving an ICD for stable VT, 22% developed life-threatening ventricular tachycardia necessitating device-therapy during the 17 months following implantation.[3] Data from the randomized, prospective Electrophysiologic Study Versus Electrocardiographic Monitoring (ESVEM) trial[14] suggest that patients with hemodynamically stable SMVT treated with antiarrhythmic drugs have a 4-year incidence of "arrhythmic death" of 31%.[4] The largest report to date on the clinical course of patients with coronary artery disease and stable VT comes from the AVID registry and randomized trial.[13] Raitt et al reported the outcomes of 440 registry patients with stable VT and 1029 patients with unstable VT (of whom 330 were treated in the randomized trial).[13] The prevalence of coronary artery disease and past myocardial infarction were similar in both groups (about 85% and 70%, respectively), but congestive heart failure was more prevalent amongst the patients with unstable VT (45% vs. 34%). Mean left ventricular ejection fraction was slightly lower in the stable VT patients (31% vs. 34%). Patients with unstable VT had an ICD implanted more frequently than the patients with stable VT (49% vs. 32%,). The latter group was more likely to receive antiarrhythmic drugs as single treatment (52% vs. 44%), or to receive no specific treatment at all (16% vs. 7%). After adjusting for baseline clinical variables as well as for ICD implantation, 3-year mortality in the group of patients with stable VT was actually greater than that among patients with unstable VT, although this difference did not attain conventional statistical significance (relative risk 1.25, p=0.06). There is no confirmatory evidence from other trials to suggest that patients with stable SMVT do in fact fare worse than patients with unstable rhythms. However, the results of this study strongly suggest that the absence of symptoms or hemodynamic compromise during SMVT does not signify a stable clinical course in the future. It should be emphasized, however, that the AVID registry provided no data on the mode of death. Since the role of arrhythmic death among patients presenting with well tolerated VT is unknown, one can not assume that their survival would have been drastically improved with ICD implantation.

We therefore recently conducted a study in which we reviewed complete ICD follow up data of 82 pts with ICDs implanted for strictly defined hemodynamically stable VT,   defined on the basis of presenting symptoms, systolic BP> 80, duration > 5 minutes, cycle length>270.

During the follow-up period of 23.6 ± 21.5 months , 15 (18.3%) patients died and 10 (12.2%) developed unstable ventricular arrhythmia. Unstable ventricular arrhythmia was defined as VT/VF with a cycle length (CL) of 100 msec shorter than the clinically stable VT , or 50 msec shorter if the arrhythmia had a cycle length less than 300 msec). Time to unstable arrhythmia was 14.6±14.4 months, and in 8/10 it was the first arrhythmia to occur following ICD imp. Estimated 5 year survival in the whole group was 58%. Estimated 4 year occurrence of any VT and unstable ventricular arrhythmia was 78% (61-88%), and 15% (2-26%), respectively. There were no differences in age, EF, gender, underlying heart disease, cycle length of initial arrhythmia, symptoms or QRS morphology of qualifying VT between patients with and without unstable ventricular arrhythmia. Additionally, baseline electrophysiologic study results could not predict subsequent unstable ventricular arrhythmia.

Therefore, in our study group, patients who presented with hemodynamically stable VT were at risk for subsequent unstable VTs. ICD implantation offered a potential survival benefit in 15% of patients with stable VT who subsequently develop unstable VT/VF over 4 years. No predictors could be found to stratify patients with stable VT into high and low risk groups. One limitation is that we used an ICD-defined endpoint (i.e. treated unstable VTs), which is not identical to arrhythmic death. However, it is not likely that these faster ventricular arrehythmias would be well tolerated in this population with significant structural heart disease.

In summary, due to the lack of efficacy data from randomized trials of specific therapies, controversy still exists regarding the optimal management of patients with old myocardial infarction who have spontaneous hemodynamically sustained monomorphic ventricular tachycardia . However, the available evidence indicates that clinical stability at the time of initial presentation does not predict freedom from faster, likely life-threatening tachyarrhythmias during follow up. Prospective, randomized trials are required to confirm the benefit of ICD implantation over medical or ablative therapy in this population. However, considering the superiority of the defibrillator over medical therapy across a large number of studies of high risk patients (including patient-subsets with coronary artery disease and spontaneous *nonsustained* VT,[15,16]) such a trial may prove difficult to conduct due to physicians' reluctance to subject patients to treatments other than ICD implantation.

References

1. Viskin S, Belhassen B. Noninvasive and invasive strategies for the prevention of sudden death after myocardial infarction. Value, limitations and implications for therapy. Drugs 1992; 44:336-355.

2. Brugada P, Talajic M, Smeets J, Mulleneers R, Wellens HJJ. The value of the clinical history to assess prognosis of patients with ventricular tachycardia or ventricular fibrillation after myocardial infarction. Eur Heart J 1989; 10:747-752.

3. Bocker D, Block M, Isbruch F, et al. Benefits of treatment with implantable cardioverter-defibrillators in patients with stable ventricular tachycardia without cardiac arrest. Br Heart J 1995; 73:158-163.

4. Olshansky B, Hahn EA, Hartz VL, Prater SP, Mason JW. Clinical significance of syncope in the electrophysiologic study versus electrocardiographic monitoring (ESVEM) trial. Am Heart J 1999; 137:878-886.

5. Monahan KM, Hadjis T, Hallet N, Casavant D, Josephson ME. Relation of induced to spontaneous ventricular tachycardia from analysis of stored far-filed implantable defibrillator electrograms. Am J Cardiol 1999; 83:349-353.

6. Anderson JL, Hallstrom AP, Epstein AE, et al. Design and results of the antiarrhythmics vs implantable defibrillators (AVID) registry. The AVID Investigators. Circulation 1999; 99:1692-1699.

7. Conolly SJ, Gent M, Roberts RS, et al. Canadian implantable defibrillator study (CIDS): study design and organization. Am J Cardiol 1993; 72:193F-108F.

8. Cappato R. Secondary prevention of sudden death: the Dutch study, the Antiarrhythmics Versus Implantable Defibrillator trial, the Cardiac Arrest Study Hamburg, and the Canadian Implantable Defibrillator Study. Am J Cardiol 1999; 83:68D-73D.

9. The Antiarrhythmic Versus Implantable Defibrillators (AVID) Investigators. The Antiarrhythmic Versus Implantable Defibrillators (AVID) Investigators. A comparison of antiarrhythmic drug therapy with implantable defibrillators in patients resuscitated from near-fatal ventricular arrhythmias. N Engl J Med 1997; 337:1576-1583.

10. ACC/AHA guidelines for coronary angiography: executive summary and recommendations. A report of the American College of Cardiology/American Heart Association Task Force on Practice Guidelines (Committee of Coronary Angiography). Circulation 1999; 99:2345-2357.

11. Sarter BH, Finkle JK, Gerszten RE, Buxton AE. What is the risk of sudden cardiac death in patients presenting with hemodynamically stable sustained ventricular tachycardia after myocardial infarction? J Am Coll Cardiol 1996; 28:122-129.

12. Olson PJ, Woelfel A, Simpson RJ, Jr., Foster JR. Stratification of sudden death risk in patients receiving long-term amiodarone treatment for sustained ventricular tachycardia or ventricular fibrillation. Am J Cardiol 1993; 71:823-826.

13. Raitt MH, Renfroe EG, Epstein AE, et al. "Stable" Ventricular Tachycardia Is Not a Benign Rhythm : Insights From the Antiarrhythmics Versus Implantable Defibrillators (AVID) Registry. Circulation 2001; 103:244-252.

14. Mason JW. The ESVEM investigators. A comparison of electrophysiologic testing with Holter monitoring to predict arrhythmic drug efficacy for ventricular tachyarrhythmias. N Engl J Med 1993; 329:445-451.

15. Moss AJ, Hall WJ, Cannom DS, et al. for the Multicenter Automatic Defibrillator Implantation Trial Investigators. Improved survival with an implanted defibrillator in patients with coronary disease at high risk for ventricular arrhythmias. N Engl J Med 1996; 335:1933-1940.

16. Buxton AE, Lee KL, Fisher JD, Josephson ME, Prystowsky EN, Hafley G. for the Multicenter Unsustained Tachycardia Trial investigators. A randomized study of the prevention of sudden death in patients with coronary artery disease. N Engl J Med 1999; 341:1882-1890.

12

PREDICTORS OF EFFICIENCY AND SAFETY OF ANTITACHYCARDIA THERAPY IN PATIENTS WITH IMPLANTED CARDIOVERTER-DEFIBRILLATOR

M. Trusz-Gluza, W. Orszulak, Tajac*, E. Konarska-Kuszewska, A. Hoffman, J. Krauze, B. Śmieja-Jaroczyńska, E. Dzielka, W. Kargul*

1st Department of Cardiology, *Department of Electrocardiology
Silesian School of Medicine, Katowice, Poland

Introduction

The implantable cardioverter-defibrillators (ICDs) apart from delivering low and high energy shocks, enable antitachycardia pacing (ATP) in patients with hemodynamically stable ventricular tachycardia (VT). This means of treatment is effective and has advantage of being painless. The use of ATP may reduce the frequency of defibrillation shocks that consequently improve quality of life of the patients and also lengthen battery life. However, antitachycardia pacing cannot terminate the ventricular tachycardia or even lead to acceleration of VT rate. Because of this fact ATP is accompanied by availability of defibrillation [1-4].

The objective of this study was to evaluate the incidence and predictors of ventricular tachycardia termination and acceleration by antitachycardia pacing. The results were assessed during spontaneous episodes of VT.

Methods

Patients. This was a nonradomized retrospective study. The study group consisted of 35 consecutive patients after implantation of ICD device in whom antitachycardia pacing was used during 2 year follow-up. Indications for implantation included sustained ventricular arrhythmias or a history of cardiac arrest due to ventricular fibrillation (VF) unrelated to transient or reversible cause.

Device. All implanted ICDs (Biotronik Phylax 06, XM, AV or MycroPhylax) could perform defibrillation, cardioversion, antitachycardia and antibradycardia pacing and had intracardiac electrograms storage capabilities. Arrhythmia detection was based on heart rate, duration, onset and stability criteria.

Device programming. Antitachycardia pacing was programmed for ventricular tachycardias with rates of 120 to 220 beats per minute. It included three attempts of an autodecrimental RAMP with 5 pulses, 8 ms decrement and the cycle length of 81% of the detected tachycardia. If the

From Ovsyshcher IE. *New Developments in Cardiac Pacing and Electrophysiology*. Armonk, NY: Futura Publishing Company, Inc. ©2002.

ATP was ineffective in VT termination it would be followed by low and high energy cardioversion. For the fast VTs and VF (rate over 220/min) high energy shocks were programmed and confirmed during device implantation. All patients underwent a noninvasive electrophysiological study (EPS) at the predischarge examination (5-7 day after implantation) during which VF was induced (shock on T wave), and terminated. The EPS was also aimed at induction of monomorphic ventricular tachycardia (mVT). If mVT was induced by premature extrastimuli the ATP therapy was delivered. If the therapy was unsuccessful the ATP scheme was modified and the procedure was repeated. In remaining patients ATP was programmed empirically.

Follow-up procedures. Patients after implantation were followed up every 3 months and after every clinical event. Patients were examined and the device was interrogated to determine spontaneous events with RR intervals, stored electrograms and therapy delivered. If ATP scheme was ineffective in spontaneous VT termination it was optimising. The new ATP scheme was based on investigator's experience.

Analysis of tachycardia episodes. The arrhythmias were classified on the basis of the stored in ICD holter memory intracardiac electrocardiograms and RR intervals. VT was diagnosed if it started with sudden change in heart rate interval and RR intervals were regular. Typical clinical symptoms were included in analysis. Sinus tachycardia was stated if the episode occurred during physical exercise without typical symptoms and with slow increase of heart rate. A tachycardia episode was classified as atrial fibrillation (AF) if the RR intervals were irregular (>30ms differences between consecutive beats) and no symptoms of VT were observed. VF or fast VT was diagnosed when recorded RR intervals were shorter than 275ms (220/min).

Pacing success was defined as termination of the mVT upon cessation of the pulse train or spontaneous termination within 5 beats after pacing termination. Acceleration was defined as a decrease in VT cycle length by > 50ms after an ATP attempt. Ineffective antitachycardia pacing was defined as persistence of VT after complete ATP therapy algorithm.

Statistics. Continuous data are presented as mean ± SD. The relationships between clinical variables (presence of coronary heart disease, ejection fraction < 40%), VT cycle length, circadian rhythm of VT, mode of ATP, RR coupling interval and type of antiarrhythmic agent, and successful VT termination and acceleration were tested using a stepwise multivariate logistic regression analysis.

Results

Patients. The study group consisted of 35 patients, 29 men and 6 women with a mean age of 54±12 years (Table 1). The most common underlying disease was coronary heart disease – 71%. Fifteen patients had ejection fraction (EF) below 40% with mean EF 41,5% ranging from 20% to 60%. Monomorphic VT was induced with ATP during predischarge EPS in 22 (63%) patients. In 11 cases the delivered ATP successfully terminated tachyarrhythmias. If ATP was not efficacious a different ATP scheme (more pulses, higher decrement within pulses, shorter cycle length) was

Table 1. Characteristics of study patients and episodes of VT

Patients:	
Age (yrs)	54 ± 12
Sex (M/F)	29/6 (83%/17%)
Heart disease	
- Coronary heart disease	25 (71%)
- Dilated cardiomyopathy	3 (9%)
- RV arrhytmogenic cardiomyopathy	3 (9%)
- Other	4 (11%)
Left ventricular EF < 40%	15 (43%)
Episodes:	
VT cycle length ≥ 340ms	212 (71%)
Onset of tachycardia	
- day	247 (83%)
- night	52 (17%)
Antiarrhythmics	
- sotalol	157 (53%)
- beta-blocker	61 (20%)
- amiodarone	81 (27%)
Antitachycardia pacing	
- ramp	281 (94%)
- burst	18 (6%)
- pacing coupling interval < 80%	26 (9%)
- pacing coupling interval ≥ 80%	273 (91%)

programmed and induction was repeated. In 13 patients mVT was noninducable and ATP was programmed empirically. None of our patients died during the follow-up.

Spontaneous tachyarrhythmia episodes. During follow-up in 35 patients 299 episodes of spontaneous mVT appeared. Characteristics of these episodes are listed in Table 1. The mean number of episodes per patient was 8±10, median 4. Episodes of VF or fast VT treated initially with high energy shock defibrillation (100% were effective) and inappropriate therapy (AF or sinus tachycardia) were excluded from the analysis. ATP was effective in 94.3% of patients (at least once) and in 82% of episodes. Acceleration occurred in 37,1% of patients and in 12,5% of episodes.

Table 2. Predictors of ATP efficacy and safety

TERMINATION	Univariate			Multivariate		
Variable	OR	95%CI	p value	OR	95%CI	p value
Absence of CHD	2,38	1,07- 5,31	0,03	7,69	2,86-20,7	0,001
EF < 40%	2,26	1,28-4,05	0,005	4,70	2,09-10,56	0,002
Antiarrhythmic agent						
- Sotalol	3,24	1,56-6,69	0,01	3,17	1,45-6,95	0,004
VTCL ≥ 340ms	3,67	2,01-6,61	0,0002	2,47	1,25-4,09	0,009

ACCELERATION	Univariate			Multivariate		
Variable	OR	95% CI	p value	OR	95% CI	p value
EF >40%	2,95	1,43-6,09	0,004	2,5	1,16-5,4	0,019
VTCL < 340ms	2,28	0,77-3,61	0,024			

ATP- antitachycardia pacing; CHD - coronary heart disease;
CI - confidence interval; EF - ejection fraction; OR - odds ratio;
VTCL - ventricular tachycardia cycle length.

Predictors of ATP efficacy. Multivariate logistic regression analysis revealed that only lack of coronary heart disease, EF<40%, longer VT cycle length and treatment with sotalol were independent predictors of VT termination (Table 2). Mode of ATP (ramp or burst pacing, pacing coupling interval) and circadian rhythm of spontaneous arrhythmia did not impact the efficacy.

Predictors of ATP safety. Univariate analysis indicated that the risk of VT acceleration by ATP may be higher in faster episodes of arrhythmia and in patients without depressed left ventricular function. However, in the multivariate analysis, only preserved left ventricular ejection fraction predicted the subsequent development of VT acceleration (Table 2).

Discussion

Antitachycardia pacing has many advantages over shock therapy. This therapy is painless and therefore is better tolerated by patients. However, ATP has the potential to accelerate treated VT into unstable arrhythmia, which needs shock for termination. Several studies have assessed the efficacy of ATP [1-6]. Hammill et al. [5] in multicenter study evaluated efficacy of ATP for termination and acceleration of VT in 1240 episodes. This analysis and many others [1,2,5,7] include therapy of VT induced in the electrophysiology laboratory, which may differ from the patient's clinical arrhythmia.

ATP is reported to terminate VT in 60-95% of episodes, with acceleration in 0-26 % of episodes [1-5,8]. The discordance reflects the imperfectly reproducible nature of this phenomenon. Different definitions of acceleration were also used. Our results are similar to those of studies but it should be stressed that an acceleration of VT appeared during follow-up at least once in 37% of patients.

Our analysis showed no difference between efficacy and safety of ramp pacing and burst pacing. Most studies suggest that patient selection rather than pacing method is the most important determinant of ATP success [5,7]. Peinado et al. [6] and Newman et al.[7] found that ATP efficacy was higher and incidence of pacing induced acceleration was lesser in slower monomorphic VT. These results are in agreement with our observation. A higher mVT cycle length was an independent predictor of efficacy in the multivariate model.

The relationship between efficacy and safety of ATP and left ventricular function is controversial. Hammill et al. [5] reported that ATP was more effective in patients with ejection fraction >40%. In our study the opposite relationship was identified. In patients with left ventricular dysfunction VT was more prone to termination and more resistant to acceleration by ATP. Few studies evaluated the impact of antiarrhythmic drug therapy on results of antitachycardia pacing. Hammill et al. [5] did not identify any relationship between antiarrhythmic drug use and the results of VT therapy. In present study, use of sotalol was an independent predictor of successful termination of VT in multivariate analysis. Fries et al. [9] found that ATP was less successful and more proarrhythmic during the morning hours. In our study no circadian variation was observed.

Study limitations. There are several limitations to the present study. It is a retrospective and nonrandomized study and therefore contains all the disadvantages of such a comparative analysis.

Conclusions

In patients with ICD antitachycardia pacing is highly effective, especially in slower episodes of VT, in subjects without coronary heart disease, with lower left ventricular ejection fraction and during treatment with sotalol. Acceleration of VT is not frequent but may occur in about one third of patients. The risk of acceleration appears to be independent of the presence of coronary heart disease, depressed left ventricular function and antiarrhythmic therapy.

References

1. Waldecker B, Brugada P, Zehender M, et al.: Importance of modes of electrical termination of ventricular tachycardia for the selection of implantable tachycardia devices. Am J Cardiol 1986; 57:150-155
2. Brady GH, Troutman C, Poole JE et al.: Clinical experience with a tiered-therapy, multiprogrammable antiarrhythmia device. Circulation 1992; 85:1689-1698
3. Pinski SL, Fahy GJ: The proarrhythmic potential of implantable cardioverter-defibrillators. Circulation 1995; 92:1651-1664
4. Schaumann A, Muehlen F, Herse B et al.: Empirical versus tested antitachycardia pacing in implantable cardioverter-defibrillators. Circulation 1998; 97:66-74
5. Hammill SC, Packer DL, Stanton MS et al.: Termination and acceleration of ventricular tachycardia with autodecremental pacing, burst pacing and cardioversion in patients with an implantable cardioverter-defibrillator. PACE 1995; 18:3-10
6. Peinado R, Almendral J, Rius T et al.: Randomized prospective comparison of four burst pacing algorithms for spontaneous ventricular tachycardia. Am J Cardiol 1988; 82:1422-1425
7. Newman D, Dorian P, Hardy J: Randomized controlled comparison of antitachycardia pacing algorithms for termination of ventricular tachycardia. JACC 1993; 21:1413-1418
8. Leitch JW., Gillis AM, Wyse DG et al.: Reduction in defibrillator shocks with an implantable device combining antitachycardia pacing and shock therapy. JACC 1991; 18:145-151
9. Fries R, Heisel A, Nikoloudakis N et al.: Antitachycardia pacing in patients with implantable cardioverter-defibrillators: Inverse circadian variation of therapy success and acceleration. Am J Cardiol 1991; 80:1487-1489

IV. PACING THERAPY

13

RECHARGEABLE POWER SOURCES IN THE HISTORY OF CARDIAC PACING

Seymour Furman, MD FACS, FACC

Albert Einstein College of Medicine, Bronx, NY 10467

During September 1958 a conference was held at Rockefeller University in New York City under the auspices of Vladimir Zworykin PhD, who had been a major contributor to the invention of television, concerning the then new field of cardiac stimulation which had then been known to have been used clinically only as temporary myocardial stimulation in patients who had acquired complete heart block during open heart surgery for the repair of a congenital cardiac defect. While transvenous pacing had been used twice it was neither represented nor considered at the conference. Indeed, the existence of fixed, acquired heart block requiring long term pacing was hardly known or considered. Pacing was deemed, at that time, to be required briefly, consistent with the operative experience then dominant. Zoll proposed the exclusive use of brief application of external transcutaneous pacing when necessary during an episode of extreme bradycardia or asystole, while several others proposed radio frequency stimulation via the intact skin and still others long term maintenance of wire leads to the myocardium through the otherwise intact skin. Potential implantable devices were conceded to require an energy source adequate to power an electronic circuit and stimulate the heart over the long term. No such energy source was considered then to be in existence.[1]

During the second half of that year two seminal events in the history of cardiac pacing did occur, neither represented nor considered, at the Rockefeller University Conference. The first had been the successful initial use of clinical transvenous pacing on July 16, and another patient on August 8, 1958 (before the conference was held) and the subsequent use of long term transvenous pacing with an external pulse generator.[2] The second was the unsuccessful clinical implantation of a rechargeable bipolar cardiac pacemaker on October 8, 1958 (shortly after the conference)[3]. Both, more than anything discussed at the Conference, were the precursors of the future of cardiac pacing and indeed, implanted cardioversion-defibrillation.

From Ovsyshcher IE. *New Developments in Cardiac Pacing and Electrophysiology.* Armonk, NY: Futura Publishing Company, Inc. ©2002.

While implantation of a pacemaker by thoracotomy was the dominant approach for 5-7 years thereafter, transvenous stimulation, first temporary and thereafter permanent transvenous stimulation has become almost the exclusive route. Rune Elmqvist, the designer of the pacemaker implanted on October 8, 1958 considered the dilemma of the power source and elected the use of a pair of nickel-cadmium cells (in Europe referred to as an accumulator) capable of being repeatedly recharged by radio-frequency transmission of energy through the intact skin. The intention was to use this rechargeable unit for long term pacing as no primary (non-rechargeable) cell suitable for such long term use was considered to be available. Two pulse generators were implanted successively on the same day, October 8, 1958, both soon failed and the patient was left without any pacing, though redesign of the pulse generator, the leads and probable commercialization, continued. Nevertheless, another group had announced that they were proceeding with the manufacture of an implantable pulse generator powered by primary mercuric-zinc-oxide cells, predicted to function for five years and no other rechargeable pulse generator was then designed.

During 1955 a Swedish electrical engineer developed severe myocarditis attributed to eating infected oysters. Intermittent heart block followed, with rates between about 40 and 70/min and with recurrent syncope on a daily basis. Digitalis was administered, which only increased the frequency and severity of the syncope. Work became difficult and then impossible. Diagnosed as AV block with Stokes-Adams episodes, his wife increasingly despaired of his survival. She read in the press of pacing techniques being evaluated and importuned her husband's cardiologist to apply them. Those techniques involved myocardial wires and an external pulse generator. Dr. Ake Senning, the cardiac surgeon at the Karolinska Hospital in Stockholm, was approached but decided that such an approach would be unsatisfactory because of the risk of recurrent infection. He and Rune Elmqvist, himself a physician and engineer who designed medical equipment, had been considering an implantable pulse generator. Urged on by the impetus of Arne Larsson's grave illness and Mrs. Larsson's ceaseless pressure, Elmqvist designed and built two identical models of an implantable rechargeable (nickel cadmium powered) pulse generator. Two stainless steel myocardial sutures were used as the bipolar electrode. During the morning of October 8, 1958 Senning implanted the pacemaker by thoracotomy. It failed after about six hours. The second, identical unit was implanted later the same day and functioned for about eight days, when it too failed.

Larsson, who had by this time stabilized to fixed complete heart block and thereafter had fewer syncopal episodes, was left without a pacemaker until a mercury zinc powered unit was implanted by thoracotomy November 4, 1961. Wife and husband, he with his 28th pacemaker remain alive during December 2001.   Three additional Elmqvist designed rechargeable unipolar units, with a flat disc electrode, were later implanted.   February 3, 1960 in Montevideo, Uruguay Drs. Roberto Rubio and Orestes Fiandra implanted one in a 40 year-old woman, who survived with a functioning device for nine months until she died of sepsis from the original implantation surgery.[4] At least two models were implanted in London, UK, by Harold Siddons, one March 31, 1960 which functioned approximately ten months and a second, the date of which is uncertain, but functioned for only 22 hours.[5]   As the leads and electrodes of the first two and later three implants were different, the early failure of the first two pulse generators may have been lead and not pulse generator related.

On June 6, 1960 the first pacemaker designed with primary (mercuric-oxide zinc) cells, predicted to last five years before requiring replacement was implanted.[6]   On November 7, 1960 and then May 5, 1961 two additional groups implanted their primary cell pacemakers. Had the five year prediction been borne out there might not have been any significant additional research into power sources, especially as the survival of patients with complete heart block was unknown, but believed to be brief.   Within a year two circumstances were clarified, one was that these pulse generators were failing much more quickly than one year (much less five years) and that patients seemed to be stabilized and able to look forward to substantial survival, a condition which has, over the years, been demonstrated to be accurate.

Many other power sources were sought, including biogalvanic electricity, the electricity of glucose oxidation, other primary cells and a reevaluation of rechargeability.   These investigations continued into the 1970s. One clinical model was commercialized until the demonstration of the long term stability and utility of the lithium iodine cell, first clinically implanted in 1972. The following designs were evaluated over the years. Three models were reported in 1965, in two the pulse generators were intended to be attached directly to the heart so that only electrodes would be required, but no lead.

Bonnabeau et al at the University of Minnesota designed an asynchronous (VOO) unit with either one or two commercial nickel cadmium cells each with an output of 1.25 volts and capable of delivering 2.5 mA against a 500 0hm load. Three different varieties of electrodes were used. One type consisted of two rigid pins 5 mm long and 1 mm wide; the second a tapering pin 3 mm long and 2 mm in diameter and a flat oval electrode 10 by 5 mm; the third type was two platinum-iridium coil spring electrodes similar to that previously used in Medtronic epicardial leads. The generator produced 2 ms duration square wave pulses to stimulate the heart at a rate of 70 per minute. The epoxy pulse generator 20x40 by 10 mm thick was covered with silicone rubber and surrounded by a polyester suture skirt 4 mm wide embedded in the silicone rubber, to be sewn to the right ventricular epicardial surface. This device was never used clinically.[7]

Fig. 1. The University of Minnesota pulse generator with two pin electrodes was implanted onto the right ventricular epicardial surface with 5-6 non absorbable sutures through the silicon-polyester suture skirt, with strain relief by Ivalon sponge. The electrodes are introduced with stab wounds into the myocardium.

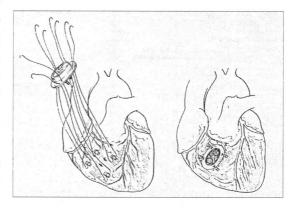

In 1964 a project to develop a rechargeable pacemaker using six commercially available nickel cadmium cells was undertaken by Silver and Byron at the City of Hope Hospital and the Hycon Co. both in Southern California. Recharge was accomplished with a 5 Khertz signal through the intact skin. The impulses were 2 ms in duration. One recharging schedule was ten minutes daily and one hour additionally per month, though others were evaluated. The unit was asynchronous (VOO) in operation. Potted in epoxy it was 7 cm in diameter and 2.2 cm thick. The myocardial electrodes used during 16 pig experiments were of the Chardack variety which fractured frequently. Three months after dog implantation a unit failed because of fluid incursion which caused shorting of the circuit. There is no record of clinical utilization.[8]

Another nickel cadmium rechargeable unit intended for suture to the right ventricular epicardial surface was developed at Montefiore Hospital and Medical Center in the Bronx, NY in cooperation with the Electric Storage Battery Co of Yardley, PA. A single commercial nickel cadmium cell, stimuli were at 70 per minute. Recharge was, by a 500 hertz radio frequency signal through the intact skin. The pulse duration was initially set to be 2 ms, but later reduced to 0.5 ms when experimentation demonstrated the stimulation value of such brief duration pulses. The unit, discoid in shape, potted in epoxy and covered with silicone rubber weighed thirty grams and was attached to the dog right ventricular myocardium with six sutures of Flexon stainless steel suture each of which acted as an electrode. The ground electrode was a platinum disc epicardial electrode 4 mm in diameter. Later designs for transvenous implant were evaluated. No clinical use was done.[9]

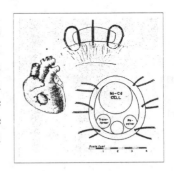

Fig. 2. This 30 gram pulse generator is sutured to the right ventricular epicardial surface with six stainless steel sutures previously loaded into the generator. Each suture acted as a stimulating electrode. The indifferent electrode is a plate on the generator surface held against the epicardial surface.

Two efforts achieved clinical utilization and one commercialization as well. The one which approached but did not achieve commercial distribution was developed at Penn State University by Tyers and Brownlee beginning in 1970 and using a single 1000 mA silver mercury oxide rechargeable cell produced by the T.R. Mallory Co. This cell had sufficient capacity to operate for several years without recharging so that prolonged longevity without frequent recharging was possible. The unit was 7.6 x 3.8 x 1.3 cm in size and implanted experimentally and clinically by thoracotomy and transvenous approaches. Prolonged evaluation and evolution occurred so that both VOO and VVI modes were developed. Recharging was by radio frequency transmission with as little as several minutes per day required for full charge.[10] The unit might have achieved widespread commercial application, but by the time of its full demonstration of functionality the simultaneously introduced lithium iodine cell had revolutionized pacemaker power sources and, remains dominant to this day. The Brownlee-Tyers collaboration was, however, productive and innovative. Recognizing that the failure of most then contemporary pulse generators was caused by fluid incursion, they designed a hermetically sealed device. As the mercury zinc cell emits hydrogen when producing electricity a hydrogen absorbing compound termed a "getter", capable of absorption for 20-40 years was introduced into the casing. The effort introduced other innovations such as telemetry of pacemaker function, including battery charge status, lead impedance and hermeticity status, which have continued in use. Ten of these units were eventually clinically implanted and functioned for four years without failure.[11] With the dominance of the lithium iodine cell in cardiac pacing, the program was ended.

Fig. 3. The Brownlee-Tyers hermetically sealed pulse generator (right) adjacent to a last generation mercury-zinc, non-hermetic, non-programmable unit with a maximum longevity of 30 months (left) and an early hermetically sealed lithium iodine, non-programmable unit with an average longevity of eight years (center). The lithium iodine unit was smaller, simpler to implant, more reliable and required less intervention than either of the other two. The illustration is of the last of the old, an early version of the new and a technically sophisticated effort, superceded by technology.

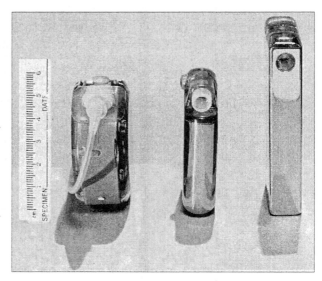

Several other designs were experimentally attempted but without achieving clinical utilization. The last and by far the most successful of the rechargeable pacemakers was that initially developed at the Applied Physics Laboratory at Johns Hopkins University by Fischell who was conversant with the developments in rechargeable cells used in the space program and determined that a nickel cadmium cell could be manufactured with far greater reliability than the mercury oxide cells then in use with an estimated life less than two years, typical of the power sources for implantable pacemakers of 1968. The rechargeable design did not produce hydrogen during electricity production and so could be hermetically sealed in metal avoiding ingress of body fluids and protect against microwave oven radiation, then considered a serious pulse generator threat. The need to charge the implanted unit from outside the body by radio frequency transmission and to avoid overcharging and consequent overheating and burns from within the body (which did actually occur during use from a defect in the system) it was essential that operation of the external recharging module be controlled by the telemetered state of charge of the cell.[12]   A highly durable bipolar endocardial lead was developed with a very reliable Luer-lok type connector requiring a 720 degree twist to connect. The estimated longevity of the unit, which required 90 minutes of recharging once weekly, was twenty years. A corporation was formed to finish development and commercialize. It was initially implanted in a patient on February 10, 1973. Eventually 10,022 pacemakers were implanted, with the last on October 19, 1984. While the other units described (except the silver mercury zinc) had all failed of use because of technical difficulties, this model was technically sophisticated and extremely reliable. It's main difficulty was the need for weekly recharging and many, possibly most, patients with these pacemakers opted for replacement by a lithium unit when lithium had demonstrated durability and reliability, though some of the rechargeable's developers have not accepted this possibility.[13] Indeed, as one of the author's patients with this rechargeable inquired after sitting in the clinic, presumably talking to other patients who still had the mercury units with an eighteen month service life, "Why must I recharge my pacemaker for an hour and a half every week while the others only need an operation, every year and a half?" During fall 1997 approximately 1300 units were still functioning in patients, many then more than 20 years.   In the fall of 2001 the manufacturer reports that requests for repair and replacement of the external recharger module still occur.

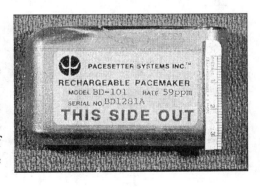

Fig. 4 The only commercialized rechargeable pacemaker. The lead was to be connected by a screw mechanism on the top right of the generator. The unit was non-programmable and required weekly recharging. Longevity was in the overall range or in excess of that achieved by lithium iodine powered generators.

While the very first implantable pulse generator of October 1958 was rechargeable and at least half a dozen later rechargeables were designed and to some extent tested, with one reaching widespread clinical use, in the end these units fell to a superior technology, the lithium iodine cell. The mercury-zinc cell pacemaker standard of a very large pulse generator, electrolyte leakage and body fluid incursion destroying the circuit and two year longevity, would have been displaced by the rechargeable pacemaker. With the hermetically sealed lithium iodine pacemaker in 1972 with relatively trouble free longevity of ten or more years, the best of rechargeability yielded to a superior technology.

References

1. Jeffrey K: Conference on Artificial Pacemakers and Cardiac Prosthesis: Sponsored by The Medical Electronics Center of the Rockefeller Institute, 1958. PACE 1993; 16:1445-1482.
2. Furman S, Schwedel JB: An intracardiac pacemaker for Stokes-Adams seizures. N Eng J Med 1959; 261:943-948.
3. Elmqvist R, Senning A: An implantable Pacemaker for the Heart. In: Smyth CN (ed): Proceedings of the Second International Conference on Medical Electronics, Paris, 24-27 June 1959. London: Iliffe & Sons, 1960, pp. 253- 254..
4. Fiandra O: The first pacemaker implant in America. PACE 1988; 11:1234-1238.
5. Siddons H: Cardiac pacing: Results with three different techniques. Ann Roy Coll Surg Eng 1965; 37:155-159.
6. Chardack WM, Gage AA, Greatbatch W: A transistorized, self-contained implantable pacemaker for the long-term correction of complete heart block.: Surgery 1960; 48:643-654.
7. Bonnabeau RC, Ferlic RM, Lillehei CW: A new rechargeable epicardial cardiac pacemaker. J Thorac Cardiovasc Surg 1965; 50:857-862.
8. Silver AW, Root G, Byron FX, et al.: Externally rechargeable cardiac pacemaker. Ann Thorac Surg 1965; 1:380-388.
9. Furman S, Raddi WJ, Escher DJW, et al.: Rechargeable pacemaker for direct myocardial implantation. Arch Surg 1965; 91:796-800.
10. Tyers GFO, Brownlee RR, Hughes HC, et al.: Development of an optimal rechargeable cardiac pacemaker. J Surg Res 1976; 20:405-411.
11. Tyers GFO, Brownlee RR: Current Status of Pacemaker Power Sources. Ann Thor Surg 1978; 25:571-587.
12. Love JW, Lewis KB, Fischell RE, et al.: Experimental testing of a permanent rechargeable cardiac pacemaker. Ann Thorac Surg 1974; 17:152-156.
13. Stertzer SH, DePasquale NP, Cohn LI, et al.: Evaluation of a Rechargeable Pacemaker System. PACEs 1978; 1:186-188.

14

THE RESULTS OF ATRIAL PACING TRIALS

Irina Savelieva, MD, A. John Camm, MD

Department of Cardiological Sciences, St George's Hospital Medical School, London, United Kingdom

Introduction

The considerable limitations of antiarrhythmic drug therapy, catheter-based techniques, and stand alone atrial defibrillators together with increasing prevalence of atrial fibrillation (AF)[1-4] stimulated a search for alternative non-pharmacologic modes of treatment and encouraged further investigation of mechanisms responsible for initiating and maintaining of the arrhythmia. Rapidly accumulating new experimental and clinical evidence has led to recognition that the development of AF requires both an underlying anatomic and/or electrophysiologic substrate and a trigger to precipitate the onset of the arrhythmia. These findings prompted interest in preventative atrial pacing which may reduce the incidence of AF by either eliminating the triggers and/or by modifying the substrate of the arrhythmia.

Electrophysiologic Background for Pacing in Atrial Fibrillation

I. Inter- and intraatrial conduction delay - a potential for preventative pacing to modify the substrate of the arrhythmia. An important consequence of experimental studies of the electrophysiologic properties of fibrillating atria has been delineation of the role of reentry as a common constituent of the mechanism of the arrhythmia which has recently been summarized in a comprehensive review.[5] Intra-atrial conduction delay, shortening of the atrial effective refractory period, prolonged dispersion of refractoriness and loss or reversal of rate adaptation of the effective refractory periods facilitate the occurrence and perpetuation of reentry. Experimental data substantiate the importance of regional conduction delay for reentrant atrial tachyarrhythmias and AF. Areas with consistently prolonged activation times have been identified in the low right atrium, septum (Bachmann's bundle), and posterior triangle of Koch.[6-8] Critically timed atrial premature complexes (APC) falling into the atrial relative refractory period (when inhomogeneous conduction and increased dispersion of refractoriness are often present) may initiate reentry. Activation times in these regions may be decreased by appropriate pacing

From Ovsyshcher IE. *New Developments in Cardiac Pacing and Electrophysiology.* Armonk, NY: Futura Publishing Company, Inc. ©2002.

from specific, often multiple sites, resulting in a reduction of atrial conduction delay by providing the multidirectional excitation and preventing atrial tachyarrhythmias[8].

II. Data from the implantable devices – a potential for preventative pacing to suppress triggers. A substantial progress in the memory function of implantable pacemakers and ICD has enabled monitoring and accurate detection of the modes of onset of AF. Analysis of the distribution of potential triggers showed that APCs and bradycardia were responsible for triggering 70-84% of AF episodes, and short-long sequence accounted for 20% of onsets of the arrhythmia.[9] In nearly half patients there was a combination of triggers including bradycardia, APCs, and re-initiation.

In a recent Atrial Fibrillation Therapy (AFT) study, of 372 patients with paroxysmal AF, only third of whom met the conventional bradycardia indications for pacemaker implantation, 43% of AF episodes were triggered by APCs, 22% occurred during preceding bradycardia, and 27% were classified as re-initiation of the arrhythmia. The recognition of patterns of ectopic activity and underlying rhythm preceding the onset of AF has encouraged the development of novel atrial pacing algorithms designed to prevent initiation of the arrhythmia on the individual basis, notably, Medtronic Jewel AF, Gem III AT, and AT500 series.

Multisite Atrial Pacing: Modification of the Substrate for AF

I. Acute effects of multisite atrial pacing on inducibility of AF. Experimental and clinical evidence has strongly implicated site dependent non-uniform conduction in the initiation of AF and has suggested that atrial pacing may prevent AF due to improved synchronized depolarization of the atria.[6,7,8] Pacing at Bachmann's bundle, the right posterior interatrial septum, and the distal coronary sinus has also been shown to increase high right atrial (HRA) effective refractoriness and reduce the conduction delay caused by high right atrial extrastimuli.[10] In a series of acute tests, pacing at the os of the coronary sinus, dual-site pacing from both HRA and coronary sinus os, or biatrial pacing (right and left atrium - via distal coronary sinus) prevented the inducibility of AF by an APC from the HRA.[10-13] In these studies, dual-site pacing and biatrial pacing rendered AF non-inducible in 56% to 67% of patients.[10,13] In contrast, HRA pacing resulted in maximal shortening of effective refractory period, prolonged dispersion of refractoriness and increased regional and global conduction delay, and was associated with the highest rate of recurrence of AF, especially in patients with prolonged global atrial activation (P ≥120 ms).[13]

However, single-site atrial pacing from the triangle of Koch abolished recurrences of AF in 30% of patients with refractory arrhythmia as compared with right atrial appendage pacing.[14] Although single-site pacing from the coronary sinus proven to prevent the inducibility of AF in the acute test due to a decrease in dispersion of activation times, there is a pre-excitation of the left atrium with a delay in the right atrium which may attenuate the effect of pacing on suppression of the arrhythmia.

Biatrial pacing has been shown to reduce both the conduction delay and electrogram prolongation at the right posterior septum caused by APCs from the high right atrium.[15] Furthermore, there is experimental evidence for possible benefit of triple-site pacing from two right atrial sites and the left atrium, in terms of decreasing total atrial activation time and enhancing multidirectional excitation.[8]

II. Clinical studies of multisite atrial pacing for prevention of AF.

In their early report, Saksena et al[16] showed that in patients with drug-refractory AF single-site atrial pacing from the HRA or coronary sinus os prevented the recurrence of AF in 62% of patients and increased arrhythmia-free intervals from 9 days at baseline to 143 days after institution of pacing therapy. Dual-site atrial pacing (DAP) resulted in further increases in the proportion of patients without AF (89%) and in prolongation of the mean arrhythmia-free interval. At 1 year, 78% of patients remained in sinus rhythm, and 56% did not have symptomatic recurrences of the arrhythmia after 3 years of follow-up. These effects of atrial pacing translated into a reduction in the need of direct or pharmacologic cardioversion by 33% and a cautious decrease in antithrombotic and antiarrhythmic therapy by 33% and 16%, respectively.

The Dual-Site Atrial Pacing for Prevention of Atrial Fibrillation (DAPPAF) trial prospectively enrolled 120 patients with documented recurrent symptomatic AF and bradycardias requiring cardiac pacing and randomly assigned them to DAP from the right atrium and coronary sinus HRA pacing, and support pacing at 40 bpm for 6-month periods after a 2-week period for optimisation of drug and pacing therapies.[17] After completion of the randomized phase or if symptomatic recurrences of AF or adverse effects occur, patients were crossed over to the other arms. The time to the first symptomatic recurrence of AF and quality of life were the main outcome measures. Although the time to the first recurrent AF episode trended to be longer with DAP compared with support but not HRA pacing modes, in the subgroup analysis of patients with relatively frequent episodes of AF (weekly events to 2 events in 3 months) who received antiarrhythmic drug therapy with class I or III antiarrhythmic agents, DAP was significantly superior compared with HRA and support pacing in prolongation of the time to recurrence of AF (hazard ratios 0.46, $p = 0.004$, and 0.623, $p = 0.006$, respectively), as it was if the time to recurrence the arrhythmia and adherence to pacing mode were combined (hazard ratios 0.687, $p < 0.03$, and 0.582, $p < 0.001$, respectively) with comparable safety. However, the trend to improved quality of life, noted with overdrive pacing modes, was not statistically significant.

DAP has also proven to be effective for preventing AF and was superior to single-site pacing in patients without bradycardia. In the New Indication for Preventive Pacing in Atrial Fibrillation (NIPP-AF) study of 22 patients with ≥2 documented symptomatic AF episodes within 3 months before enrollment and no conventional indications for pacing, all receiving sotalol, dual-site overdrive pacing from the HRA or the right atrial appendage and the coronary sinus os significantly prolonged the time to the first symptomatic recurrence of AF confirmed by an ECG event recorder, with a 3.2-fold relative risk of having an event 'off pacing' and reduced total AF burden from $45 \pm 34\%$ to $22 \pm 29\%$ but provided no effect on quality of life and symptom control.[18] Arrhythmia recurrences were documented by an event recorder, pacemaker datalogs, and 24-hour Holter monitoring. The relative risk of having any AF event was also 1.55-fold greater without pacing. In 19 patients in whom HRA pacing phase was completed, there was no difference in the primary and secondary endpoints compared with 'off pacing' phase. The results of these trials have demonstrated that clinical benefit of atrial pacing may derive from multiple mechanisms, including effects on the substrate, e.g., bradycardia-associated increased dispersion of atrial refractoriness most likely in the DAPPAF patients, and suppression of triggers of the arrhythmia, such as a 33% reduction in atrial premature beats observed in the NIPP-AF patients without bradycardia.

Biatrial pacing may be performed by simultaneously pacing both atria above the intrinsic rate or by sensing one atrium and pacing the other (atrial resynchronization). Daubert et al,[19] using an atrial resynchronization pacing algorithm showed a significant reduction in global atrial activation time and the frequency of AF recurrences. At 9 years, 55 (64%) of 86 patients remained in sinus rhythm, including 28 (33%) patients without documented recurrences.[20] The SYNBIAPACE study (SYNchronous BI-Atrial PAC(E)-ing) demonstrated a trend towards prolongation of the time to first recurrence of AF during biatrial pacing whereas right atrial pacing did not confer any benefit on the arrhythmia-free interval.[21] For technical reasons insufficient number of adequately paced patients were included in this study.

Overdrive and Rate Stabilization Atrial Pacing Algorithms: Suppression of Arrhythmia Triggers

Recognition of bradycardia and short-long sequences as potential triggers for AF have led to early attempts to prevent AF merely by constantly increasing the lower pacing rate. Although this pacing mode has been shown to suppress the recurrence of arrhythmia in 14 (65%) patients and significantly reduced the number of arrhythmia episodes and their total and maximal duration in the remaining patients, it has been associated with poor tolerance.[22] Therefore, specific algorithms have been developed to provide atrial pacing at a rate which is maintained only slightly higher than intrinsic rate.

The Dynamic Atrial Overdrive (DAO) pacing algorithm is based on rate acceleration after a sensed atrial event, overdrive pacing at a plateau level followed by deceleration with rate smoothing until the first sensed atrial event occurs, to ensure that the pacemaker constantly controls the atrial depolarization. Recently completed Atrial Dynamic Overdrive Pacing Trial (ADOPT A) was a randomised crossover trial which enrolled nearly 400 patients with sinus dysfunction and symptomatic paroxysmal or persistent AF with ≥2 episodes within the month prior to DDDR pacemaker implantation (Trilogy DR or Integrity AFx DR, St Jude Medical) with a facility of DAO pacing.[23] About half patients received class III or I antiarrhythmic drugs. With DAO algorithm 'ON', the percentage of atrial pacing was 92.9% compared with 67.9% when DAO was inactive.

During a 6-month follow-up, the combination of DDDR + DAO pacing suppressed symptomatic atrial arrhythmias compared with DDDR pacing alone and was associated a 67% reduction in the burden of organized atrial arrhythmias (atrial tachycardia, atrial flutter), defined as the percentage of days during which these arrhythmias occurred. However, atrial rhythms with organized atrial activity constituted only a small proportion of all symptomatic atrial tachyarrhythmias (9.6%). Although there was a trend towards reduction in AF burden by 25% (from 2.493% to 1.869%), this tendency was lost after 6 months of follow-up.

The AFT trial enrolled 372 patients with paroxysmal AF, only 34% of whom had conventional bradycardia indications for pacing.[24] Class III antiarrhythmic drugs were prescribed in 57% patients, class IA or IC in 23% and 20% patients, respectively. The results of phase 2 of the study in which patients were assigned to one of the three pacing regimes (DDD 40 vs DDD(R) 70 or DDD(R) 85 bpm) showed no difference between the groups. However, during phase 3, the combination of DDD pacing at 70 bpm with preventative pacing algorithms resulted in a significant 30.4% reduction in the primary end-point: the mean AF burden decreased from 3.3 to 2.3 hours/day, with the median AF burden decreased from 0.78 to nearly 0 hours/day. The duration of sinus rhythm increased by 68% (from 828 vs 40 min), and the number of recurrences of AF episodes of more than 7 minute duration decreased from 60% to about 30%, reflecting a 78.1% reduction. The preventative pacing algorithms, aimed to interrupt or to minimize triggers for AF, included pace conditioning based on dynamic overdrive pacing to provide almost constant atrial capture (>95% time in atrial pacing), suppression of APCs and APC-induced pauses, and post-exercise rate response limiting the speed of a post-exercise decrease in heart rate.

The preliminary results of the AF Prevention by OVErdrive (PROVE) study have shown that overdrive pacing combined with an Automatic Rest Rate function (Talent DR 213 pacemaker, Ela Medical) decreased the number of fall-back mode switches by 34%, reduced the overall duration of arrhythmia episodes by 48% and increased the time of atrial pacing to 84%. However, it did not modify the total number of arrhythmia episodes.[25] The Pacing In Prevention of Atrial Fibrillation (PIPAF) trial is an on-going study of the dynamic overdrive pacing algorithm with the time to first recurrence of AF and the reduction in the cumulative arrhythmia duration as end-points.[26]

Conclusions

Multi-factorial aetiology and multiple pathophysiologic mechanisms of AF suggest the need for a multidimensional approach targeting at patients who benefit most from antiarrhythmic drug therapy, ablation techniques, pacing therapies, or combination of these methods known as "hybrid therapy". Atrial pacing studies have shown that patients with advanced inter- and intra-atrial block, and symptomatic, drug-refractory AF may benefit from 'atrial resynchronization' pacing. There may be additional benefits associated with the use of particular sites of pacing and with the use of particular pacing algorithms. Importantly, dual-site atrial pacing appears to have a synergistic relationship with antiarrhythmic class I and III drug therapy, supporting the benefit of a "hybrid" therapy approach.

Novel pacing algorithms for prevention and termination of atrial arrhythmias incorporated in implantable cardioverter-defibrillators and pacemakers are currently under investigation and may offer a valuable alternative to antiarrhythmic drug therapy in patients with severe left ventricular dysfunction at high risk of proarrhythmias or worsening heart failure. An important issue is that the majority of these trials excluded patients with severe organic heart disease, making it unclear whether this vulnerable population benefit from novel non-pharmacologic therapies.

Furthermore, limited selection of appropriate end-points for demonstration of the efficacy and safety of device therapies for prevention and/or termination of atrial arrhythmias may be a cause of divergent results in recently reported studies.[27] Time to the first symptomatic recurrence of AF may not be a reliable measure of the device efficacy as it has recently been shown that the time to the first recurrence of the AF is not associated with the time between recurrences of the arrhythmia.[28] Dual chamber ICD and pacemakers with extended memory and more electrogram storage may allow more precise assessment of burden of the arrhythmia and the efficacy of atrial pacing therapies, therefore, determine a primary end-point which is more reliable than the time to first recurrence of the arrhythmia.

References

1. Lévy S, Breithardt G, Campbell RWF, et al.: Atrial fibrillation: current knowledge and recommendations for management. Working Group Report. Eur Heart J 1998;19:1294-1320.
2. Defaye P, Dournaux F, Mouton E, for the AIDA Multicenter Study Group.: Prevalence of supraventricular arrhythmias from the automated data stored in the DDD pacemakers of 617 patients: the AIDA study. PACE 1998;21:250-255.
3. Best PJ, Hayes DL, Stanton MS.: The potential usage of dual chamber pacing in patients with implantable cardioverter defibrillators. PACE 1999;22:79-85.
4. Santini M, Ricci R.: Atrial fibrillation coexisting with ventricular tachycardia: a challenge for dual chamber defibrillators. Heart 2001;86:253-254.

5. Allessie MA, Boyden PA, Camm AJ, et al.: Pathophysiology and prevention of atrial fibrillation. Circulation 2001;103:769-777.

6. Papageorgiou P, Monahan K, Boyle NG, et al.: Site-dependent intraatrial conduction delay: relationship to initiation of atrial fibrillation. Circulation 1996;94:384-389.

7. Lee SH, Lin FY, Yu WC, et al.: Regional differences in the recovery course of tachycardia-induced changes of atrial electrophysiological properties. Circulation 1999;99:1255-1264.

8. Becker R, Klinkott R, Bauer A, et al.: Multisite pacing for prevention of atrial tachyarrhythmias: potential mechanisms. J Am Coll Cardiol 2000;35:1939-1946.

9. Hoffmann E, Janko S, Hahnewald S, et al.: The atrial fibrillation therapy (AFT) trial: novel information on dominant triggers of paroxysmal atrial fibrillation. Circulation 2000;102:II-481-II-482 (Abstract).

10. Yu WC, Chen SA, Tai CT, et al.: Effects of different atrial pacing modes on atrial electrophysiology: implicating the mechanism of biatrial pacing in prevention of atrial fibrillation. Circulation 1997;96:2992-2996.

11. Papageorgiou P, Anselme F, Kirckhof CJ, et al.: Coronary sinus pacing prevents induction of atrial fibrillation. Circulation 1997;96:1893-1898.

12. Gilligan DM, Fuller IA, Clemo HF, et al.: The acute effects of biatrial pacing on atrial depolarization and repolarization. PACE 2000;23:1113-1120.

13. Prakash A, Saksena S, Hill M, et al.: Acute effects of dual-site right atrial pacing in patients with spontaneous and inducible atrial flutter and fibrillation. J Am Coll Cardiol 1997;29:1007-1014.

14. Padeletti L, Porciani MC, Michelucci A, et al.: Prevention of short term reversible chronic atrial fibrillation by permanent pacing at the triangle of Koch. J Intervent Cardiac Electrophysiol 2000;4:575-583.

15. Delfault P, Saksena S, Prakash A, Krol RB.: Long-term outcome of patients with drug-refractory atrial flutter and fibrillation after single- and dual-site right atrial pacing for arrhythmia prevention. J Am Coll Cardiol 1998;32:1900-1908.

16. Saksena S, Prakash A, Ziegler P, et al, for the DAPPAF Investigators.: The Dual-site Atrial Pacing for Prevention of Atrial Fibrillation (DAPPAF) trial: improved suppression of atrial fibrillation with dual-site atrial pacing and antiarrhythmic drug therapy. J Am Coll Cardiol 2001;38:598-599.

17. Lau CP, Tse HF, Yu CM, et al, for the New Indication for Preventive Pacing in Atrial Fibrillation (NIPP-AF) Investigators.: Dual-site atrial pacing for atrial fibrillation in patients without bradycardia. Am J Cardiol 2001;88:371-375.
18. Daubert C, Mabo PH, Berder V, et al.: Atrial tachyarrhythmia associated with high degree interatrial conduction block: prevention by permanent atrial resynchronization. Eur J Cardiac Pacing Electrophysiol 1994;1:35-44.
19. D'Allonnes GR, Pavin D, Leclercq C, et al.: Long-term effects of biatrial synchronous pacing to prevent drug-refractory atrial tachyarrhythmia: a nine-year experience. J Cardiovasc Electrophysiol 2000;11:1081-1091.
20. Mabo P, Daubert JC, Bouhour, et al.: Biatrial synchronous pacing for atrial arrhythmia prevention: the SYNBIAPACE study. PACE 1999;22:755 (Abstract).
21. Garrigue S, Barold SS, Cazeau S, et al. Prevention of atrial arrhythmias during DDD pacing by atrial overdrive. PACE 1998;21:1751-1759.
22. Carlson MD, Gold MR, Ip J, et al, for the ADOPT Investigators.: Dynamic atrial overdrive pacing decreases symptomatic atrial arrhythmia burden in patients with sinus node dysfunction. Presented at the AHA Sessions, Anaheim, CA, 2001.
23. The Hotline Sessions of the 23rd European Congress of Cardiology. Eur Heart J 2001;22:2033-2037.
24. Funck RC, Adamec R, Lurje L, et al, on behalf of the PROVE Study Group: Atrial overdriving is beneficial in patients with atrial arrhythmias: first results of the PROVE study. PACE 2000;23:1891-1893.
25. Anselme F, Saoudi N, Cribier A.: Pacing in prevention of atrial fibrillation: the PIPAF studies. J Intervent Cardiac Electrophysiol 2000;4:177-184.
26. Camm AJ, Levy S, Saksena S, Wyse DG.: Don't you agree or what part of the problem don't you understand? J Intervent Cardiac Electrophysiol 2000;4:559-660.
27. Kaemmerer WF, Rose S, Mehra R.: Distribution of patients' paroxysmal atrial tachyarrhythmia episodes: implications for detection of treatment efficacy. J Cardiovasc Electrophysiol 2001;12:121-130.

15.

DIAGNOSIS OF SUPRAVENTRICULAR TACHYARRHYTHMIAS BY AUTOMATIC MODE SWITCHING ALGORITHMS OF DUAL CHAMBER PACEMAKERS

S. Serge Barold*, Carsten W. Israel **, Roland X. Stroobandt ***, Chu-Pak Lau ****, I. Gallardo *.

* Florida Cardiovascular Institute and Tampa General Hospital, Tampa, FL, ** JW Goethe University Hospital, Frankfurt, Germany, *** A Z Damiaan Hospital, Oostende, Belgium, **** University of Hong Kong.

Most contemporary dual chamber pacemakers come equipped with automatic mode switching (AMS) algorithms to control the paced ventricular rate if supraventricular tachyarrhythmias (SVT) are detected by the devices.[1-9] Beyond this, AMS episodes may be stored by the device to provide information about the incidence and type of SVT in the individual patient. This chapter will focus on the fundamental principles of SVT detection by dual chamber pacemakers because correct device SVT diagnosis is the key to reliable AMS performance. Optimal SVT detection calls for a high atrial sensitivity and short atrial blanking periods.

Basic Concepts. The atrial channel must be insensitive during certain parts of the pacing cycle to avoid two potential problems.
1. <u>Near-field double sensing of atrial activity</u>. The duration of the atrial blanking period initiated by a paced or sensed atrial event is designed to prevent undesirable near-field atrial sensing or double counting of atrial events. Double atrial counting (double sensing of P waves and possible detection of polarization after atrial pacing) may occur if the atrial blanking period is too short.[10-12] (Fig 1). This problem is especially important with dual-site atrial pacing for the prevention of atrial fibrillation. In this setting, double counting of atrial activity will occur when the atrial blanking period < atrial conduction time between the 2 atrial pacing sites particularly in the presence of severe intra- and interatrial conduction delay or block.
2. <u>Far-field R-wave sensing or VA crosstalk.</u> Far-field R-wave sensing by the atrial channel generally occurs because a high atrial sensitivity is needed to detect atrial fibrillation with a signal amplitude which is substantially smaller than that in normal sinus rhythm.[4, 7, 13, 14] Indeed, for proper AMS function, a device should be programmed at maximal atrial sensitivity or with a sensing safety margin of 300 - 350 % (for a P wave

From Ovsyshcher IE. *New Developments in Cardiac Pacing and Electrophysiology*. Armonk, NY: Futura Publishing Company, Inc. ©2002.

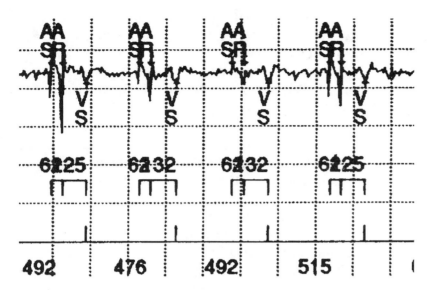

Figure 1. *Double sensing of the P wave (stored atrial electrogram of SVT episode) by Medtronic Kappa 700 pacemaker programmed to nominal settings. AS = Atrial sensed event, AR = atrial sensed event in the atrial refractory period.*

amplitude of 2.0 mV, atrial sensitivity should be programmed to 0.5 mV or higher- i.e. < 0.5 mV) to avoid atrial undersensing during atrial fibrillation.[13] Therefore the elimination of VA crosstalk by reducing atrial sensitivity carries the risk of atrial undersensing during SVT. There are 2 forms of VA or reverse crosstalk according to their timing in the pacemaker cycle: A). *VA crosstalk in the postventricular atrial refractory period (PVARP)*: Atrial sensing of ventricular signals (usually from a paced ventricular beat) occurs in the unblanked portion of the PVARP beyond the initial postventricular atrial blanking period (PVAB).[15-20] Far-field sensing within the PVARP can be corrected by decreasing atrial sensitivity provided the atrial signals during SVT can be sensed at the lower sensitivity or by programming the PVAB to a longer value. A long PVAB predisposes to atrial undersensing especially atrial flutter. B). *VA crosstalk in the AV delay:* the atrial channel may sense the spontaneous QRS complex within the unblanked terminal portion of the AV delay.[2, 3, 20] Partial blanking of the AV delay was designed to enhance sensing of atrial fibrillation. At high atrial sensitivity, the atrial channel can sense the deflection of spontaneous ventricular depolarization registered in the atrial before the ventricular channel (programmed at a lower sensitivity than the atrial channel). This creates an atrial sensed-ventricular sensed AV interval close to zero (fig 2).

If this form of far-field R-wave sensing cannot be eliminated by reprogramming atrial sensitivity, the paced AV delay can be shortened to ensure continual ventricular pacing. Shortening the paced AV delay cannot prevent far-field R-wave sensing from VPCs but counting these signals should not interfere with AMS function unless VPCs develop into ventricular tachycardia. Alternatively ventricular sensitivity can be increased to permit earlier near-field ventricular sensing before far-field R-wave sensing by the atrial channel. In this respect the Frontier (St. Jude) biventricular pacemaker, presently under clinical investigation in the US, is designed with a special timing cycle to prevent VA crosstalk within the AV interval.[5] This interval is called the "preventricular atrial blanking period" though it is a timing cycle and not really a true blanking period. The preventricular atrial blanking is programmable between 0 and 62 ms. The algorithm cancels (for the purpose of AMS) counting of far-field R waves detected by the atrial channel. The preventricular blanking is initiated whenever a P-wave or sensed atrial signal (such as a far-field R

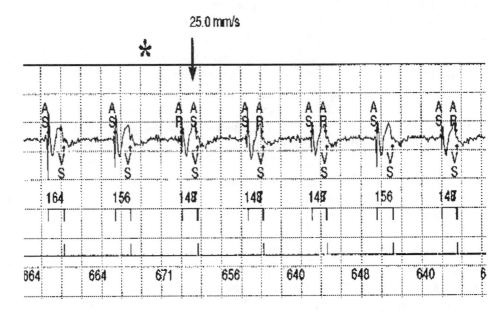

Figure 2. Stored atrial electrogram of SVT by Medtronic Kappa 700 pacemaker. There is far-field R wave oversensing in the terminal part of the AV delay provoked by automatic atrial sensitivity adjustment which was programmed to 0.18 mV. AS and AR abbreviations are the same as in fig 1. VS = ventricular sensed event.

wave) is detected either inside or outside the unblanked refractory period of the atrial channel. If a ventricular depolarization is detected by the ventricular channel within the preventricular atrial blanking period, the P-wave or atrial signal that initiated the preventricular atrial blanking will be invalidated for counting purposes. In other words, it will not trigger an atrial output pulse and it will not be included in the calculation of the atrial rate for the purpose of AMS. Thus the algorithm cancels the preventricular atrial blanking period as soon as the ventricular channel senses the ventricular electrogram as a near field event after a sensed atrial event. Testing for VA crosstalk. The propensity for VA crosstalk during the unblanked PVARP should be tested during ventricular pacing and sensing. For VA crosstalk after ventricular pacing, the sensed AV delay is shortened to permit continual ventricular capture. The pacemaker is then programmed to the highest atrial sensitivity and the largest ventricular output (voltage and pulse duration). These settings should be evaluated at several pacing rates to at least 110-120 ppm because faster ventricular pacing rates impair dissipation of the afterpotential or polarization voltage at the electrode-myocardial interface. Such parameters enhance the afterpotential and therefore generate a voltage superimposed on the tail end of the paced QRS complex. The combined voltage from these two sources may be sensed as a far-field signal by the atrial channel. In devices with a programmable PVAB, the testing procedure if positive for VA crosstalk can be performed at various durations of the PVAB until VA crosstalk is eliminated. VA crosstalk related to the tail-end of the spontaneous QRS complex should be tested in devices where by design the PVAB after sensing is shorter than after ventricular pacing. VA crosstalk within the AV delay is evaluated by programming the highest atrial sensitivity and a slow lower rate with a long AV delay to promote spontaneous sinus rhythm and AV conduction.

Atrial flutter: 2:1 lock-in response and special algorithms. The duration of the atrial blanking periods may prevent detection of atrial flutter. If AV interval + PVAB > atrial cycle length, the pacemaker will exhibit 2:1 atrial sensing if unblanked AV interval < atrial flutter cycle.[2, 3, 5, 21] Sensing of alternate atrial signals is also called the 2:1 lock-in response. For example, if AV interval = 140 ms and PVAB = 120 ms, the pacemaker cannot sense atrial flutter at a rate of 280/min (cycle length = 214 ms) on a 1:1 basis because 140 + 120 or 260 > 214 ms. (concealed or blanked atrial flutter). If PVAB is nonprogrammable, restoration of 1:1 atrial sensing would require programming the AV interval to 90 ms. Now, the sum of the AV interval + PVAB or 90 + 120 or 210 becomes shorter than the atrial flutter cycle length of 214 ms. The pacemaker will now sense atrial flutter on a 1:1 basis and activate AMS. Restoration of AMS function by shortening the AV delay to circumvent a fixed PVAB, produces unfavorable hemodynamics for long-term pacing if the AV interval remains permanently short in the absence of SVT. For this reason, a design that allows substantial shortening of the sensed AV interval only with increasing sensed atrial rates (so-called "rate-adaptive AV delay"), optimizes sensing of atrial flutter, and yet preserves a physiologic AV interval at rest and low levels of exercise.[2] During SVT when sensed AV interval + PVAB = 30 + 120 = 150 ms, this combination allows sensing of atrial flutter with short cycle lengths.

Dedicated algorithms for atrial flutter detection. Supplemental or parallel algorithms for the detection of atrial flutter unrecognized by the primary AMS algorithm have been designed to circumvent the 2:1 lock-in response. No data have yet been published on the sensitivity and specificity of these special atrial flutter detection algorithms. In the Medtronic Kappa 700 and 701 pacemakers, the Blanked Flutter Search™ algorithm is automatically activated whenever the device senses a high atrial rate consistent with atrial flutter and a possible 2:1 lock-in situation, i.e., if 8 consecutive atrial cycles are shorter than twice [AV interval + PVAB] and shorter than twice the tachycardia detection interval.[2, 5, 22] The algorithm "shifts" all atrial blanking times by prolonging one PVARP cycle only (Fig 3). This disrupts synchronization of every second atrial flutter wave with the atrial blanking times. If the Blanked Flutter Search™ algorithm does not disclose atrial flutter, it is automatically deactivated for 90 sec.

The Pulsar max™ system (Guidant Co.) offers an "atrial flutter response". This algorithm starts another atrial refractory period ("AFR window") of 260 ms (equivalent to an atrial rate of 230 bpm) if atrial events are sensed within the PVARP beyond the PVAB.[23] Any atrial signal sensed within the PVARP triggers another 260 ms atrial refractory period (concept of retriggerable atrial refractory periods). As long as the pacemaker senses an atrial rate > 230 bpm , successive AFR windows are continually initiated and ventricular pacing becomes independent of atrial sensing, thereby establishing AMS. The atrial flutter response therefore provides instantaneous AMS. However, if every second atrial flutter potential occurs during the blanked portion of the PVARP, the atrial flutter response cannot detect the SVT and 2:1 tracking will persist.

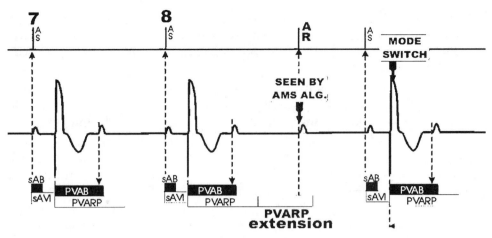

Figure 3. *Medtronic blanked flutter search and automatic mode switching. PVAB = postventricular atrial blanking period. PVARP = postventricular atrial refractory period, sAB = atrial blanking period initiated by atrial sensing, sAVI = AV delay initiated by atrial sensing. The PVARP extension permits the detection of the true atrial interval shown as AR-AS. ALO = algorithm. AR and AS abbreviations are the same as in Fig 1. See text for details.*

Detection of Atrial Tachyarrhythmias. SVT detection should be highly sensitive to prevent rapid tracking of SVT and highly specific to prevent loss of AV synchronous pacing from inappropriate AMS during sinus rhythm. Manufacturers have designed a variety of AMS algorithms based on the following concepts.

1. Calculation of a matching or mean atrial rate. The "running average" of the atrial rate or mean atrial rate (MAR) was developed to provide AMS with high specificity and to prevent frequent mode oscillations back and forth in the presence of intermittent atrial undersensing.[2, 4-7] The device continuously calculates the MAR interval and compares it with the actual sensed atrial interval. If the MAR interval exceeds the sensed atrial interval, it shortens by a fixed value (e. g. 39 ms). If the MAR interval is shorter than the sensed atrial cycle, it lengthens by either the same (unbiased MAR calculation) or a different value (biased MAR calculation). Thus the MAR represents an artificial atrial rate and a moving value that bears a constantly changing relationship to the true or sensed atrial rate. AMS will occur when the MAR reaches the programmed tachycardia detection interval (TDR). This algorithm is used in the Medtronic Thera DR and Kappa 400 pacemakers and the St. Jude Trilogy DR+/Affinity family.[2, 3, 5, 7, 24] In the biased concept used

clinically, undersensing of occasional atrial signals related to blanking periods or intermittent signal drop-out does not prevent or significantly delay SVT detection. Such algorithms are resistant to sudden changes in atrial rate making them effective against intermittent atrial undersensing. Several detected long As-As intervals secondary to undersensing can be compensated with just one short As-As interval enabling SVT detection even if as much as 50 % of atrial signals are unsensed. MAR calculating algorithms are highly specific for SVT. They do not trigger inappropriate AMS in response to occasional far-field R wave oversensing, short runs of SVTs or atrial premature beats. Because the process is gradual, the rapidity of AMS will depend on the preexisting sinus rate, the SVT rate itself, and the programmed TDR . It is easier for the MAR to reach the TDR when SVT occurs in the setting of a higher resting sinus rate than from a sinus bradycardia. This is because the MAR interval starts from a shorter baseline duration on its gradual way to reach the TDR interval. MAR algorithms achieve AMS slowly so that patients may become symptomatic during the delay phase from SVT onset to AMS. Depending on the sinus rate before SVT, there is a minimum delay between SVT onset and AMS of 2.5 to 10 sec when the SVT is tracked at the upper rate limit. Intermittent atrial undersensing may further delay AMS.

Long-short cycles. If alternating sensed atrial cycle lengths are shorter and longer than the TDR interval (e.g.farfield R wave oversensing, supraventricular bigeminy), inappropriate SVT detection may result in biased MAR calculating systems.[2] The algorithm of the Medtronic Thera and Kappa 400 devices substract 24 ms from the MAR interval with shorter atrial cycles and adds only 8 ms to the MAR interval with longer atrial cycles. This process eventually allows the MAR interval to reach the TDR interval and AMS becomes established. Thus, although this algorithm is helpful in detecting an irregular tachycardia with detection gaps (atrial beats undetected in the blanking period or one associated with intermittent undersensing), it may also induce AMS in circumstances without SVT.

2. Number of beats above a tachycardia detection rate ("rate and count"). The pacemaker detects SVT by counting sensed atrial signals occurring at a rate above the programmed TDR.[5] Every short atrial cycle increases the counter by one until the required number of short cycles triggers AMS. Rate and count algorithms designed to count only consecutive short cycles, reset the counter to zero if an atrial cycle lengthens beyond the TDR interval before the number of short cycles required for SVT detection is reached. In rate and count algorithms that utilize non-consecutive short atrial cycles for SVT detection , an atrial cycle > TDR

interval only decreases the counter by one without resetting it to baseline or zero. AMS performance in "rate and count" algorithms is highly dependent on atrial sensing and device programming. Every short atrial cycle increases the counter by one until the required number of short cycles is reached triggering AMS. The sensitivity and specificity of rate and count algorithms for SVT detection depend primarily on the inclusion or exclusion of non-consecutive short atrial cycles into the algorithm. Algorithms using only consecutive sensed atrial cycles < TDR interval are highly immune to VA crosstalk because the alternation of short and normal atrial cycles prevents inappropriate SVT detection. Intermittent atrial undersensing may severely delay or prevent AMS by continually resetting the counter to 0. In contrast, rate and count algorithms using non-consecutive atrial intervals are better suited in an environment of intermittent atrial undersensing but intermittent oversensing may more easily cause inappropriate AMS. AMS may be rapid if the required number of short cycles <TDR interval is low (e. g. 5 beats), but delayed if the programmed number of short cycles is high. However, inappropriate AMS is frequent with sensitive rate and count criteria, and mode oscillations secondary to intermittent atrial undersensing (with marked variation of the ventricular cycles) are more frequent than with other SVT detection algorithms.

3. "x out of y" concept. The "x out of y" concept was introduced to reduce the consequences of intermittent atrial undersensing on the delay to achieve AMS.[22, 25, 26] The algorithm resembles some rate and count algorithms that depend on sensing non-consecutive short cycles for AMS activation. Consecutive and non-consecutive "run and count" algorithms as well as "x out of y " algorithms basically use a number of beats above a certain rate for activation. However, a "rate and run" algorithm using non-consecutive short cycles cannot go below a ratio of 0.5, i. e. a minimum of > 50% of atrial cycles must be short. If every second atrial cycle is short, there will be no SVT detection (counter always +1 and then -1). In contrast, "x out of y" algorithms can be programmed to a ratio < 0.5 (e. g. programmable x out of 8 in the Biotronik Logos pacemaker). In addition, two criteria can be used, one rather stringent for small relatively small y values (e. g. 28 out of 32 = 87.5%, "strong criterion" in ELA Talent) and one less stringent for relatively large y values (e. g. 36 out of 64 = 56%, "weak criterion" in the ELA Talent pacemaker) to avoid inappropriate AMS for short periods of fast atrial rates while maintaining high sensitivity for longer periods of fast atrial rates. "X out of y" algorithms are commonly used in implantable cardioverter-defibrillators (ICD) to ensure detection of ventricular fibrillation even if fibrillation potentials are

too small to be sensed. Most designs favor a small value for "y". "X" and "y" values are usually non-programmable and come as fixed ratios such as 4/7, 5/8, 28/32, and 36/64 for SVT detection (Fig 4). Rapidity of SVT detection depends on "x" and "y" values and can be as fast as 2.3 s for a 4/7 criterion. The combination of fast reactivity with good performance even in the setting of a high degree of atrial undersensing represents a major advantage of the "x out of y" concept. Their sensitivity seems higher than that of MAR algorithms and comparable to "rate and count" algorithms (including non-consecutive short cycles). The latter need a proportion of short atrial cycles well above 50% to detect SVT, while "x out of y" algorithms often require only 1 beat above 50% (e. g. 4 out of 7, 5 out of 8) and can even be programmed to a value below 50%. For this reason, the specificity of "x out of y" algorithms appears reduced compared to MAR algorithms depending on the" x and y values."

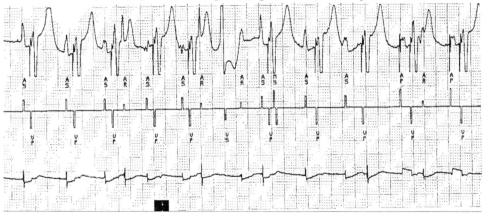

Figure 4. Automatic mode switching of Medtronic Kappa 700 triggered by multifocal atrial premature complexes. The ECG is on top, the annotated markers in the middle and the atrial electrogram at the bottom. Three premature atrial events produce 4 short intervals out of 7 thereby activating AMS (MS). AS, AR and VS abbreviations are the same as in previous figures. AP = atrial paced event, VP = ventricular paced event.

4. <u>Beat-to-beat</u>. AMS in response to one single short atrial cycle is the most sensitive and fast reacting response, but the least specific AMS concept. The first AMS algorithm (Telectronics Meta DDDR 1250) was highly unspecific in that a single sensed event within the unblanked PVARP triggered AMS.[1] The Biotronik Actros and Kairos family of DDDR pacemakers use a "retriggerable" atrial refractory period algorithm for AMS. This algorithm is simple and responds rapidly to the onset and termination of SVT.[27, 28] If the pacemaker detects a P-wave in the total

atrial refractrory period (TARP), an AV interval is not initiated and the atrial refractory period is extended by an amount equal to the TARP. If further atrial events are sensed within the new TARP (outside the atrial blanking period), the TARP is further extended, causing the pacemaker to function in the DVIR mode. This response is akin to the dual-demand function of antitachycardia pacemakers. Instantaneous resynchronization occurs when an atrial event occurs outside the TARP, or when atrial paced event is initiated at the termination of the atrial escape interval. Rapid oscillations of the paced ventricular rate may occur with intermittent atrial undersensing. Competitive (asynchronous) atrial pacing occurs during SVT. The Vitatron Diamond and Clarity DDDR pacemakers employ a physiological band to define normal versus pathological atrial rate.[29, 30] A physiological atrial rate is calculated from the running average of the actual sensed or paced atrial beats and the rate change in this moving average is limited to 2 bpm. The physiological band is defined by an upper boundary equal to the physiological rate plus 15 bpm (minimum value of 100 bpm) and the lower boundary by the physiological rate minus 15 bpm (or the sensor-indicated rate if it is higher). As the physiological rate during sensor driven pacing will be determined by the sensor, it follows that SVT detection is sensor-based when the sensor is active. If an atrial event occurs above the upper boundary of the physiological band, it is not tracked and AMS to DDIR mode will occur. The paced ventricular rate is the sensor indicated rate or lower boundary of the physiological band, whichever is higher. It seems inappropriate to activate AMS after a single atrial premature beat . For this reason, after every atrial sensed event that is not tracked secondary to AMS, the pacemaker tries to pace the atrium with an atrial " resynchronization" beat that is delivered with a safety delay after the atrial sensed beat. The mode switch feature can be programmed as either "auto" or "fixed". If the automatic mode is programmed, the SVT detection rate varies with the upper boundary of the physiological band and allows AMS to occur below the upper rate. When programmed to the fixed mode, the SVT detection rate is equal to the upper rate and AMS is allowed only when the atrial rate exceeds the upper rate.

Special considerations and future directions.

1. *Signal morphology*. Optimal discrimination between small atrial fibrillation potentials and far-field R-wave oversensing will be achieved if signal morphology criteria beyond mere amplitude are incorporated for atrial detection.

2. *Automatic adjustment of atrial sensitivity*. Intermittent atrial undersensing during atrial fibrillation is a common cause of AMS failure. While this can be partially offset by the use of a running average (MAR) algorithm, this necessarily slows the onset of AMS. A fixed atrial sensitivity setting for atrial fibrillation sensing is not optimal for AMS function because there is substantial variability of the atrial electrogram amplitude during atrial fibrillation.[31] Thus atrial sensitivity should vary throughout the atrial cycle being high at the time when an atrial signal is expected and low at the time when a ventricular far-field signal is expected.

3. *Sophisticated algorithms*. Dedicated algorithms for ventricular far-field detection (e. g. PR Logic™) may improve discrimination between far-field R-wave oversensing and SVT. The most promising algorithm for optimal SVT detection takes into account atrial rate/cycle length, AV association, AV, AA, and VA intervals, and the number of atrial events between ventricular signals. The Medtronic AT 500 pacemaker has been designed with the PR logic used in dual chamber defibrillators. The AT 500 pacemaker has a PVAB of zero after ventricular sensing and 30 ms after ventricular pacing. The atrial sensing window to activate the AMS algorithm is therefore quite large. The AMS algorithm of the AT 500 device relies on data appropriately interpreted by the PR logic of the system.

4. *Memory*. Pacemaker memory functions should provide insights into AMS performance.[32] For optimal interpretation, stored electrograms (EGMs) require the following: a). Separate channels for atrial and ventricular EGMs of sufficient resolution and duration. The summated (superimposed) atrial and ventricular EGMs in a single channel are not able to distinguish atrial premature beats or atrial flutter from far-field R-wave sensing. b). An EGM scale should be available to quantify signal amplitude c). Onset data. Stored EGMs should include a programmable number of cardiac cycles before arrhythmia onset ("pre-trigger EGM"). d. Annotations. To facilitate understanding why and how the pacemaker detected and classified an event, stored EGMs need to be annotated with

markers and intervals. An additional marker annotation (e. g. arrow, line) should indicate the exact moment when arrhythmia detection criteria were fulfilled.

5. *Manual readjustment*. This needs to be available if memory functions demonstrate that automatic parameter adjustment fails or needs to be optimized. 6. *Device intelligence and learning capability*. The pacemaker should "learn" the patient's most likely rhythms and optimize SVT detection parameters and pacing responses to individual conditions.

References

1. Mond HG, Barold SS. Dual chamber rate adaptive pacing in patients with paroxysmal supraventricular tachyarrhythmias. Protective measures for rate control. PACE 1993;16:2168-2184.
2. Barold SS. Timing cycles and operational characteristics of pacemakers. In Ellenbogen K, Kay N, Wilkoff B (Eds). Clinical Cardiac Pacing and Defibrillation. 2nd Edition, Philadelphia PA, W.B. Saunders 2000:727-825.
3. Stroobandt RX, Barold SS, Vandenbulcke FD et al. A reappraisal of pacemaker timing cycles pertaining to automatic mode switching. J Interv Card Electrophysiol 2001;5:417-429.
4. Lau CP, Leung SK, Tse HF et al. Automatic mode switching of implantable pacemakers. II. Clinical performance of current algorithms and their programming. PACE. In press.
5. Israel CW, Barold SS. Automatic mode switching. Basic concepts and overview. In Israel CW, Barold SS (Eds). Advances in the Treatment of Atrial tachycardias: Pacing, Cardioversion and Defibrillation. Armonk, NY. Futura, In press.
6. Kay GN, Bubien RS. Algorithms for management of atrial fibrillation in patients with dual chamber pacing systems. In Rosenqvist M (Ed), Cardiac Pacing. New Advances, London, England, W.B. Saunders 1997:61-82.
7. Ellenbogen KA, Wood MA, Mond HG, et al. Clinical applications of mode switching for dual-chamber pacemakers. In Singer I, Barold SS, Camm AJ (Eds); Nonpharmacological Therapy of Arrhythmias for the 21st Century. The State of the Art. Armonk NY, Futura, 1998 pp 819-844.
8. Sutton R, Stack Z, Heaven D, et al. Mode switching for atrial tachyarrhythmias. Am J Cardiol 1999; 83:202D-210D.

9. Fu EY, Ellenbogen KA. Management of atrial tachyarrhythmias in patients with implantable devices. Cardiol Clin 2000;18:37-53.

10. Johnson WB, Bailin SJ, Solinger B, et al. Frequency of inappropriate automatic pacemaker mode switching as assessed 6 to 8 weeks post implantation (Abstract). PACE 1996;19:720.

11. Fröhlig G, Kindermann M, Heisel A, et al. Mode switch without atrial tachyarrhythmias (Abstract). PACE 1996;19:592.

12. Fitts SM, Hill MR, Mehra R, et al. High rate atrial tachycardia detections in implantable pulse generators: low incidence of false-positive detections. The PA Clinical Trial Investigators. PACE 2000;23:1080-1086

13. Leung SK, Lau CP, Lam CT-F, et al. Programmed atrial sensitivity: a critical determinant in atrial fibrillation detection and optimal automatic mode switching PACE 1998;21:2214-2219.

14. Wood MA, Moskovljevic P, Stambler BS, et al. Comparison of bipolar atrial electrogram amplitude in sinus rhythm, atrial fibrillation, and atrial flutter. PACE 1996;19:150-156.

15. Brandt J, Fåhraeus T, Schüller H. Far-field QRS complex sensing via the atrial pacemaker lead. II. Prevalence, clinical significance and possibility of intraoperative prediction in DDD pacing. PACE 1988;11:1540-1544.

16. Brouwer J, Nagelkerke D, den Heijer P, et al. Analysis of atrial sensed far-field ventricular signals: A reassessment. PACE 1997;20:916-922.

17. Nowak B, Kramm B, Schwaier H, et al. Is atrial sensing of ventricular far-field signals important in single-lead VDD pacing? PACE 1998;21:2236-2239.

18. Fröhlig G, Helwani Z, Kusch O, et al. Bipolar ventricular far-field signals in the atrium. PACE 1999;22:1604-1614.

19. Brandt J, Worzewski W. Far-field QRS complex sensing: Prevalence and timing with bipolar atrial leads. PACE 2000;23:315-320.

20. Theres H, Sun W, Combs W, et al. P wave and far-field R wave detection in pacemaker patient atrial electrogram. PACE 2000;23:434-440.

21. Ellenbogen KA, Mond HG, Wood MA, et al. Failure of automatic mode switching: recognition and management. PACE 1997;20:268-275.

22. Israel CW. Automatic mode switching based on a "4 out of 7" algorithm in Medtronic Kappa 700 dual chamber pacemaker systems. Herzschr Elektrophys 1999; 10 (Suppl. 1): I/32-I/45.

23. Sutton R, Stack Z, Brüls A: Tiered management of atrial arrhythmias: The Pulsar Max™ family of pacemakers. Herzschr Elektrophys 1999; 10 (Suppl. 1): I/8-I/14.

24. Levine PA, Bornzin GA, Hauck G, et al.: Implementation of automatic mode switching in Pacesetter's Trilogy DR+ and Affinity DR pulse generators. Herzschr Elektrophys 1999; 10(suppl. 1): I/46-I/57.

25. Gencel L, Géroux L, Clementy J, et al.Ventricular protection against atrial arrhythmias in DDD pacing based on a statistical approach: Clinical results. PACE 1996; 19: 1729-1733.

26. Géroux L, Limousin M, Cazeau S: Clinical performance of a new mode switch function based on a statistical analysis of the atrial rhythm. Herzschr Elektrophys 1999; 10 (suppl. 1): I/15-I/21.

27. Barold SS, Byrd CL: Automatic mode switching variants: Dual demand pacing, retriggerable atrial refractory periods, automatic mode adaptation, and pseudomode switching. Enlightenment or obfuscation? PACE 2000; 23: 1065-1067.

28. Jayaprakash S, Sparks PB, Kalman JM, et al. Dual demand pacing using retriggerable refractory periods for ventricular rate control during paroxysmal supraventricular tachyarrhythmias in patients with dual chamber pacemakers. PACE 2000;23:1156-1163.

29. Israel CW: Automatic "beat-to-beat" mode-switch: Advantages, possible problems and recommendations to optimize programming. Herzschrittmacher 1999; 19: 88-108.

30. Boute W: Beat-to-beat mode switching for effective ventricular rate control in the presence of atrial tachyarrhythmias – how to maintain a stable ventricular rhythm. Herzschr Elektrophys 1999; 10 (suppl. 1): I/22-I/31.

31. Lam CTF, Lau CP, Leung SK et al.   Improved efficacy of mode switching during atrial fibrillation using automatic atrial sensitivity adjustment. PACE 1999;22:17-25.

32. Israel CW, Barold SS. Pacemaker systems as implantable cardiac rhythm monitors. Am J Cardiol 2001;88:442-445

16.

GUIDELINES TO THE INITIAL PROGRAMMING OF PACED (AV) AND SENSED (PV) ATRIOVENTRICULAR INTERVALS

Paul A. Levine, M.D.

St. Jude Medical CRMD, Sylmar, California USA
Loma Linda University School of Medicine, Loma Linda, California USA

In the current family pacemakers from most manufacturers, multiple programmable parameters are available for the paced and sensed atrioventricular intervals. These include independently programmable paced (AV) and sensed (PV) atrioventricular delays, Rate Responsive AV Delay and positive or negative AV/PV Hysteresis. While each pacemaker comes with nominal values for the AV and PV delays, other settings may be more effective for an individual patient. The following summarizes my approach, starting from a bedside "seat-of-the-pants" recommendation to detailed testing using either impedance cardiography (ICG) or Doppler echocardiography.

With the introduction of DDD pacing, only a single AV delay could be programmed, be it paced or sensed. The result was a significant functional difference in these two intervals which were identical in the pacemaker.[1-2] With AV sequential pacing, the AV interval starts with the atrial output pulse. The functional AV interval would be even shorter than the programmed AV delay if there was a delay between the atrial stimulus and the onset of the actual atrial depolarization (latency).[3-4] With respect to sensing, the AV delay would not begin until the intrinsic deflection of the atrial depolarization was detected by the pacemaker. As this commonly occurred some time after the onset of the atrial depolarization, the functional PV delay starting from the beginning of the P wave in the patient was significantly longer than the AV delay. An improvement introduced in the second generation of DDD pacemakers was a differential interval between the paced and sensed AV delay.[5-6] Depending on the device, this was fixed at 25 or 50 milliseconds. The next improvement was to allow the paced and sensed AV delays to be independently programmed.

At the same time, it was recognized that the PR interval was not a rigid fixed interval appropriate for all rates. The PR interval progressively shortens as the rate increased during a period of physiologic stress.[7-10] This increased velocity of conduction through the AV node is termed a positive dromotropic effect of catecholamines. Early technologic attempts

From Ovsyshcher IE. *New Developments in Cardiac Pacing and Electrophysiology.* Armonk, NY: Futura Publishing Company, Inc. ©2002.

to model the progressive PR interval shortening were relatively crude with large steps. These have been refined over the years such that the relative degree of shortening is now a programmable option.

Critical to choosing the paced and sensed AV delays is the indication for pacing. In the setting of intact AV nodal conduction with a normal ventricle and normal PR interval, it is recommended that a sufficiently long AV delay be programmed. This will enable the ventricular channel to provide back-up protection while still allowing native activation in the absence of AV block and ventricular channel inhibition. There are multiple studies [11-14] demonstrating the superiority of a normal activation sequence over a paced and hence abnormal activation sequence. In earlier generation devices, this meant programming a very long AV delay. Should first degree AV block develop, a long AV delay in the pacemaker may be counterproductive. In a study by Jutzy[15] and subsequently by a number of authors[16-19], a shorter AV delay is to be recommended if the first degree AV block is too long. The critical interval was 220 ms and a similar value was identified by Vardas[20]. Harper and colleagues[21] demonstrated that when AV nodal conduction was intact, allowing for a normal activation sequence provided the best hemodynamic results. If there was AV block, the optimal AV delay varied based on the different rates associated with an exercise test.

The value of 220 ms refers to the PR interval or the AR interval but with the R wave measured as the onset of the QRS complex and not where the R wave might be sensed by the pacemaker. There is commonly a significant difference between the PR an AR intervals as measured by the pacemaker. Examples will be shown.

In the presence of even first degree AV block, programming a very long AV delay will increase the total atrial refractory period, limit the maximum tracking and maximum sensor rate and may be hemodynamically deleterious. While the rules may be changing with the advent of biventricular pacing, (as this may normalize the ventricular activation sequence), this is not an option with the currently implanted "mono-ventricular" pacing systems nor with most of the pulse generators which are being implanted for standard indications. As a first-order approximation, I program a sufficiently long AV delay so that there is a 40 to 80 ms isoelectric interval between the end of the native or paced P wave to the ventricular stimulus.

It is necessary to be aware that the PR interval measured by the clinician from a surface ECG is NOT the same interval as measured by the pacemaker. (Figure 1)

PR Interval

Clinically, the PR interval is measured from the beginning of the P wave to the beginning of the QRS complex as assessed on the surface ECG. As a portion of the P wave or QRS may be isoelectric in a given lead, this should be measured using a multichannel ECG recording from the earliest activation of a P wave recorded in multiple simultaneous leads to the earliest activation of the QRS.

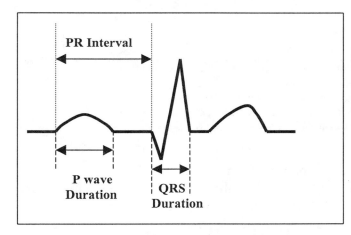

Figure 1:
Schematic diagram of the "normal" P-QRS-T complex with critical intervals identified.

The PR interval for the pacemaker starts with the intrinsic deflection of the atrial depolarization. This is the point within the P wave that the pacemaker detects the atrial depolarization. This commonly occurs between 20 to 60 ms after the onset of the P wave on the surface ECG. The pacemaker PR interval ends when the QRS complex or "R wave" is detected by the pacemaker. This may be relatively late within the QRS complex. This is illustrated on the next two panels (Figure 2a, b) recorded from a patient with intact AV nodal conduction and sinus bradycardia.

Vagal tone may affect spontaneous AV nodal conduction and the "normal PR" interval may vary from time to time. Hence, the AV delay must be programmed sufficiently long to accommodate these fluctuations if one wants to achieve functional single chamber atrial pacing with back-up ventricular protection.

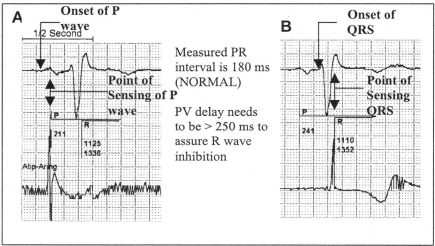

Figure 2: A is a simultaneous surface ECG and atrial electrogram combined with telemetered event markers identifying the point of sensing. B is a comparable tracing but with the bipolar ventricular electrogram. Both the markers and electrogram identify the point of sensing within each complex.

AR interval

With atrial pacing, there is commonly a small delay between the delivery of the atrial stimulus and the onset of the evoked P wave. This delay is called latency. (Figure 3) With atrial sensing, the atrial depolarization has already begun while the timing of the PV interval in the pacemaker starts from the point of atrial sensing. With atrial pacing, the AV interval starts with release of the atrial output pulse. The first level of accommodation was a fixed shortening of the PV interval compared to the AV interval to account for this difference. However, each patient may differ depending on the degree of latency, the location of the atrial lead and integrity and conduction velocity of the atrial tissue.

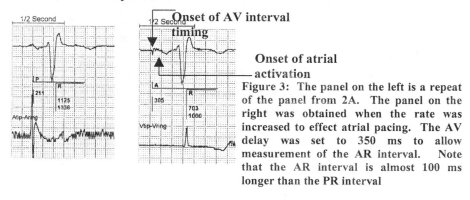

Figure 3: The panel on the left is a repeat of the panel from 2A. The panel on the right was obtained when the rate was increased to effect atrial pacing. The AV delay was set to 350 ms to allow measurement of the AR interval. Note that the AR interval is almost 100 ms longer than the PR interval

In this example from the same patient, the PR interval as measured by the physician is 180 ms while it is 211 (or as shown in Figure 2B, 240) ms as measured by the pacing system. The AR interval must take into account both the latency from the atrial stimulus to the onset of the P wave and then full ventricular activation (remember ventricular sensing starts someplace within the R wave). The result is an AR interval that is significantly longer than either the "clinical" PR interval or the pacemaker's PR interval.

If one wanted to achieve full ventricular output inhibition, it would be necessary to program the AV delay > 305 ms. Allowing for fluctuations in parasympathetic (vagal) tone, a slightly longer functional AV delay should be selected. In this case, it might be 325 or 350 ms.

Yet, based on the clinical literature, if the PR interval is > 220 ms, hemodynamics will be compromised by pacing at a longer PV or AV delay. This assumes that the resultant AR or PV interval is really greater than 220 ms. To address this issue, manufacturers have introduced a feature called AV/PV Hysteresis[22-25] and by a number of other names from different manufacturers. This feature allows for a long functional AV or PV delay when AV nodal conduction is intact facilitating native AV conduction and a shorter AV or PV delay should AV block develop. This is achieved by selecting AV and PV delays that would be optimal in the presence of AV block and then adding a preset or programmable delta. On a periodic basis during AV or PV pacing, the AV delay will be extended by the programmed delta. If a native R wave is detected during the extended AV interval, the ventricular output will be inhibited and the AV delay will remain long resulting in functional single chamber atrial pacing. Should even transient first degree AV block develop such that there is a single cycle of either AV or PV pacing at the very long AV delay, the hysteresis delta will be canceled and on the next cycle, the system will be functioning at the programmed AV or PV delay. (Figure 4) This will continue for either a programmable set number of cycles or duration of time. At the end of that time, the search mechanism will be invoked to again extend the AV/PV delay looking for the return of intrinsic AV nodal conduction. (Figure 5) This feature is particularly valuable in the patient who is only thought to need AAI pacing, where one wishes to use a dual chamber pacemaker to protect the patient should transient AV block develop. It is also indicated in the patient with known intermittent AV block as may occur with Stokes Adams Syncope but who has totally normal AV nodal conduction between spells.

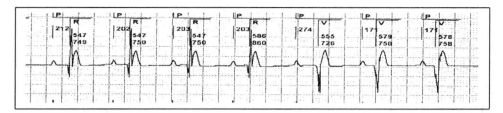

Figure 4: Development of AV block results in one cycle of pacing at a long AV delay followed by shortening to the programmed AV delay for a period of time. At the end of that time period, the AV delay will be extended by the programmed delta . If an R wave is detected within the extended AV delay, the hysteresis delta will be maintained such that the functional PR or AR interval will be the programmed PV or AV interval plus the delta. Created with a simulator interfaced with St. Jude Medical's Affinity® DR model 5330.

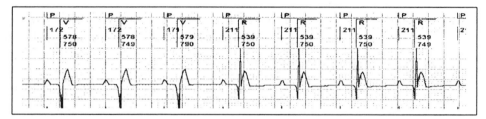

Figure 5: This shows resumption of ventricular inhibition following extension of the AV delay during the search cycle. This results in a PR interval that is longer than the programmed PV interval. Created with a simulator interfaced with St. Jude Medical's Affinity® DR model 5330.

Why not program the optimal AV delay as if AV block were present? This is fine for the patient who has persistent AV block but in the patient who has intact AV nodal conduction, this will result in forced ventricular pacing. If the resultant beat is a pseudofusion beat, the output pulse increases battery current drain and shortens device longevity without providing a direct benefit to the patient. In the presence of fusion or even full ventricular capture assuming that AV nodal conduction is otherwise intact, there is there a waste of energy, shortened device longevity and a disordered ventricular activation sequence. The abnormal activation sequence will compromise the hemodynamics by the loss of a normal ventricular activation sequence, which may compromise hemodynamics. Pavia[26] and associates made an interesting observation with respect to the recently introduced dual chamber ICDs. A 37% incidence of worsening symptoms was identified in a series of patients who had received a dual chamber ICD. This far exceeded a corresponding group of patients who had received a single chamber ICD (9%) yet the baseline ventricular function was similar, as were other demographic variables.   The difference between the two groups was the forced ventricular pacing in the DDD-ICD group as compared to the single chamber ICD group. In the single chamber ICD group, the ventricular pacing rate was programmed very low to provide back-up protection and the pacemaker portion was basically inhibited. In the dual chamber group, often implanted based on a "what if" scenario (What if AV block developed? What if sinus node slowing occurred due to concomitant pharmacologic therapy?), the AV or PV delays were left at the nominal settings forcing ventricular pacing when AV nodal conduction was intact. The authors postulated that the disordered activation sequence induced by ventricular pacing contributed to the exacerbation of congestive heart failure and symptoms. ICD patients tend to have severe ventricular dysfunction. If AV pacing is needed, an optimal AV delay is essential. If ventricular pacing is not necessary while AV nodal conduction and the QRS morphology are normal, then forcing ventricular pacing may be deleterious. In this setting, a sufficiently long AV delay to allow for full ventricular inhibition would be preferred. If AV block develops, the AV delay can be programmed to a shorter value, preferably with the assistance of Doppler echocardiography or impedance cardiography.

AV Block

In the presence of overt persistent AV block, even first degree AV block, there is nothing to be gained by programming a very long AV delay or enabling AICS. In these patients, an initial AV delay of 220 and a PV delay of 170 ms is recommended. It is essential to examine the surface ECG (not EGM) looking for a 40-80 ms isoelectric interval (flat baseline) between the end of the visible P wave and the onset of the paced ventricular complex. In some cases, there is a marked inter-atrial conduction delay such that the paced P wave is very wide. A standard PV or AV delay in these patients in the left atrial depolarization and contraction coinciding with left ventricular contraction with significant adverse hemodynamic consequences. In these patients, a very long AV delay is required. These patients commonly have a dimpled P wave (two distinct waves) and the only way that this is initially identified is to program as long an AV delay as possible and examine multiple leads of a 12 lead ECG. The AV delay needs to be programmed to a sufficient interval to allow for completion of left atrial activation before starting ventricular depolarization. (Figure 6a, b and Figure 7 a, b)

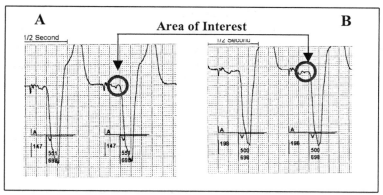

Figure 6: This concerns the paced AV delay. In A, the programmed AV delay of 150 ms is too short as the P wave virtually fuses with the QRS. In B, the AV delay was extended to 200 ms.

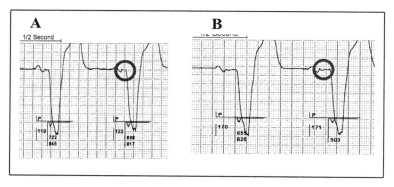

Figure 7 are examples of sensed AV delay (PV). A is too short. B is reasonable.

Figure 8: The QRS is narrow suggesting fusion beats implying atrial capture with intact conduction. The atrial depolarization was not visible within the AV interval. The AV delay was increased to 350 ms (Figure 9) in order to confirm atrial capture.

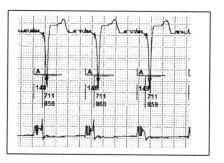

The examples with AV and PV pacing shown in Figures 6 and 7 were obtained in a patient with complete heart block. Another patient was seen recently who had a dual chamber pulse generator implanted for sinus node dysfunction. When seen, she was complaining of a sense of fullness in her throat and continued pulsations in her chest. She was more dyspneic since her pacemaker had been implanted than prior to the implant. The Event Histogram reported that she was paced in the ventricle > 99% and paced in the atrium 67% of the time. Her basic rhythm was AV paced and a clearly identified evoked atrial depolarization was not visible in the lead that was being monitored. (Figure 8)

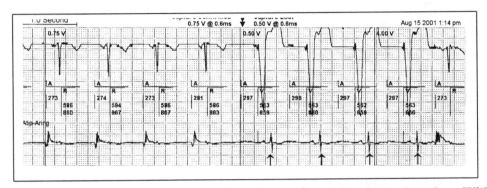

Figure 9: The atrial capture threshold is 0.75 Volts at 0.6 ms pulse duration. With the very long AV delay, there is intact AV nodal conduction. Two phenomena are readily apparent from this printout. First is a long latency (at least in this lead) between the atrial stimulus and the visible P wave. (Figure 10) The second is sensing occurs towards the end of the native QRS. With loss of atrial capture, there is also 1:1 retrograde conduction (↑) but the PVARP is sufficiently long so that a pacemaker-mediated tachycardia does not occur.

During the atrial capture threshold test, the patient remarked that the pounding sensation and fullness subsided. One of the final settings programmed at the end of this evaluation was an AV delay of 220 ms + AV hysteresis of 100 ms. The PV delay was programmed to 190 milliseconds + 100 ms PV hysteresis.

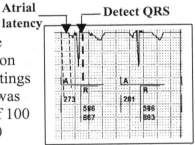

Figure 10: The latency interval and point of R wave sensing are identified. Chart speed is 25 mm/sec.

If this simple technique for selecting the AV delay does not appear to be sufficient for a given patient, a more detailed evaluation will be needed based on continued symptoms of dyspnea (shortness of breath), exercise intolerance and other signs of congestive heart failure. Doppler echocardiography or impedance cardiography[27-29] may be utilized to identify the optimal AV and PV delay for a given patient. This requires programming the pacemaker to multiple different AV delays and making repeated measurements. If Doppler echocardiography is utilized, one should look for a distinct A wave in the mitral inflow that does not fuse with the E wave and/or the largest velocity time integral (VTI) in the LV outflow tract. In using impedance cardiography, one wants the largest cardiac output. Multiple measurements at the same AV delays should be done to be reasonably certain of consistency. It is recommended that the order of AV or PV interval testing be varied and then the interval identified as being optimal be retested after all the other measurements have been made. If similar results to the first set of tests are obtained, I am comfortable as to the qualitative accuracy of the measurement. If the basic rhythm is atrial paced, the rate should then be decreased to allow identification of the optimal PV delay. If the basic rhythm is atrial sensed, the rate should be increased to allow measurement of the optimal AV delay. This may be achieved by programming the pacemaker rate 10 to 15 bpm above the intrinsic sensed rate to result in stable atrial pacing. However, if the intrinsic atrial rate is 90 bpm or higher, no attempt is made to assess the optimal paced AV delay.

There is an intrinsic limitation associated with the above measurements. Of necessity, they are all obtained with the patient at rest. If Doppler echocardiography is utilized, the patient is usually supine which may minimize some of the benefit of atrial transport. Impedance cardiography is usually performed with the patient resting comfortably on an exam table elevated to 45 to 60 degrees. As some fluid will be pooled due to the effect of gravity in this position, the importance of atrial transport may be more apparent in a semi-erect or even erect position. However, in both tests, the patient is at rest. Fluid shifts, changes in sympathetic and parasympathetic tone, heart rate and other factors may all impact cardiac function. Thus, these measurements obtained at a single physiologic state should only be considered an approximation of the optimal paced and sensed AV delay.

Intrinsic Bundle Branch Block:
Intrinsic bundle branch block is a unique condition in the setting of dual chamber pacing. When considering standard dual chamber pacing with a lead already placed in the right ventricle, the paced complex will have a left bundle branch block pattern. If the patient's native conduction is right bundle branch block, selecting the appropriate paced or sensed AV delay can force a fusion beat. Simultaneous activation of both ventricles may

result in a normalization of the QRS complex and a more synchronized ventricular contraction pattern.

A left bundle branch block pattern is more common in patients with conduction system disease who need a pacemaker. This is also the most common pattern in patients with congestive heart failure. In LBBB, the right ventricle is activated first. Placement of an epicardial lead on the LV or inserting a transvenous lead into the coronary sinus and then manipulating it into one of the cardiac veins may allow for fusion with resultant normalization of the QRS and improved hemodynamics. This was first demonstrated by de Teresa and colleagues[30] in 1983.

Rate Responsive AV Delay:
The normal response to exercise is a withdrawal of parasympathetic tone and an increase in sympathetic tone. There are increased circulating levels of catecholamines (neurotransmitters modulating sympathetic activity) that have three major effects on the heart. One is to increase the sinus rate. This is a positive chronotropic response. Another is to increase the vigor of contraction termed a positive inotropic response. The third is a positive dromotropic response. This refers to the velocity of conduction through the cardiac tissues. In a patient with normal cardiac function, the PR interval will shorten as the heart rate increases on a physiologic basis. This maintains atrial transport at progressively higher rates. If this did not occur, the P wave would begin to encroach on the T wave and ST segment of the preceding conducted QRS complex. Thus, while the intrinsic atrial activity would be driving the ventricular rate, the benefit of atrial transport to help fill the ventricle would be lost. The atrium would begin contracting against a closed mitral and tricuspid valve inducing venous regurgitation, raising pulmonary capillary wedge pressures and resulting in progressive pulmonary and systemic venous congestion. This is the major cause of symptoms in patients with persistent first degree AV block such that a dual chamber pacemaker would be indicated [16-19].

The first generation rate responsive AV delay algorithm was introduced in the mid-1980's. It utilized relative marked and abrupt changes in sensed or paced AV delay. Medtronic's Elite pacemaker had an abrupt drop in sensed AV delay from the programmed value to 65 ms when the atrial sensed rate reached 120 ppm. St. Jude Medical's Paragon (PV) and subsequently Synchrony (both PV and AV delays) family of pacemakers shortened the paced and sensed AV delays in 25 ms steps to a maximal shortening of 75 milliseconds. The degree of shortening occurred at specific rates based on the programmed maximum tracking and / or maximum sensor rates. Subsequently, the RRAVD algorithm was refined allowing for a smooth and progressive transition between the programmed AV or PV delay at base rate to the maximum tracking or sensor rates.

In patients with complete heart block who are young and healthy in whom a very high maximum tracking rate is programmed, an aggressive RRAVD algorithm (high) starting from an optimized resting paced and sensed AV delay. For most patients, the RRAVD is left at medium. If AV/PV hysteresis is enabled or a long AV delay is programmed to allow for intact AV nodal conduction, RRAVD should be disabled.

Summary:
One of the causes of continued symptoms in the presence of DDD pacing is an inappropriately programmed paced or sensed AV delay. The factors that need to be taken into account when selecting the AV delay are the patient's indication for pacing and specifically, the status of ventricular function and the integrity of the native AV conduction system. If the QRS is normal, if AV nodal conduction is normal, and ventricular function is normal, I try to maintain as long an AV delay as possible to result in functional single chamber atrial pacing. If there is any degree of AV block, the optimal paced and sensed AV delay. In view of the studies on the role of pacing in congestive heart failure, for patients with an underlying conduction abnormality, attempts should be made to place the ventricular lead in a position that will allow for fusion and normalization of the QRS pattern. In a chronic system where the leads are already in place, optimization of the AV delay using Doppler echocardiography or impedance cardiography may provide an additional incremental benefit to the patient.

As with every programmable parameter, it is appropriate to optimize the setting for the individual patient. The above guidelines might serve as a starting point but careful clinical assessment of the patient utilizing both the history and physical examination may demonstrate a need for a more detailed evaluation and modifications in the AV delay. In addition, the appropriateness of the paced and sensed AV delays that were selected initially should be periodically reviewed as the underlying disease either progresses or regresses with time.

Bibliography:

1. Ausubel K, Klementowicz P, Furman S, The AV interval in DDD cardiac pacing, Clin Prog Electrophysiol Pacing 1986; 4: 60-66.
2. Ausubel K, Klementowicz P, Furman S, Interatrial conduction during cardiac pacing, PACE 1986; 9: 1026-1031.
3. Loveland S, Maue-Dickson W, AV delay latency compensation, J Electrophysiol 1987; 1: 242-249.
4. Tyers GFO, Clark J, Mills P, Leather R, Atrial latency frequency, associations and management, PACE 1995; 18: 909 (abstract 453).
5. Janosik DL, Pearson AC, Buckingham TA, et al, The hemodynamic benefit of differential atrioventricular delay intervals for sensed and paced atrial events during physiologic pacing, J Amer Coll Cardiol 1989; 14: 498-507.
6. Alt EU, von Bibra H, Blomer H, Different beneficial AV intervals with DDD pacing after sensed or paced atrial events, J Electrophysiol 1987; 1: 250-256.
7. Frielingsdorf J, Desco T, Gerber AE, Bertel O, A comparison of quality –of-life in patients with dual chamber pacemakers and individually programmed atrioventricular delays, PACE 1996; 19: 1147-1154.
8. Sulke AN, Chambers JB, Sowton E, The effect of atrioventricular delay programming in patients with DDDR pacemakers, Eur Heart J 1992; 13: 464-472.
9. Modena MG, Rossi R, Carcagni A, et al, The importance of different atrioventricular delay for left ventricular filling in sequential pacing, clinical implications, PACE 1996; 19: 1595-1604.
10. Suntinger A, Koglek W, Wernisch M, Grimm G, Optimization of the atrioventricular interval during rest and exercise in DDDR pacing, Reblampa 1995; 8: 201-204.
11. Finney JO, Hemodynamic alterations in left ventricular function consequent to ventricular pacing, Amer J Physiol 1965; 208: 275-282.
12. Badke FR, Boinay P, Covell JW, Effects of ventricular pacing on regional left ventricular performance in the dog, Amer J Physiol 1980; 238:H858-867.
13. Rosenqvist M, Isaaz K, Botvinick EH, et al, Relative importance of activation sequence compared to atrioventricular synchrony in left ventricular function, Amer J Cardiol 1991; 67: 148-156.
14. LeClercq C, et al, Hemodynamic importance of preserving the normal sequence of ventricular activation in permanent cardiac pacing, Amer Heart J 1995; 129: 1133-1141.
15. Jutzy RV, Feenstra L, Pai R, et al, Comparison of intrinsic versus paced ventricular function, PACE 1992; 15: 1919-1922.
16. Mabo P, Cazeau S, Forrer A, et al, Permanent DDD pacing for very long PR interval alone, PACE 1992; 15: 509 (abstract).
17. Chirife R, et al, "Pacemaker syndrome" without a pacemaker, deleterious effects of first degree AV block, Revue Europeenne de Technologie Biomedicale 1990; 12: 22 (abstract).
18. Barold SS, Indications for permanent cardiac pacing in first degree AV block: Class I, II or III? (editorial), PACE 19: 747-751.

19. Bode F, Wiegand U, Katus HA, Potratz J, Inhibition of ventricular stimulation in patients with dual chamber pacemakers and prolonged AV conduction, PACE 1999; 22: 1425-1431.
20. Vardas PE, Simantrakis EN, Parthenakis FI, et al, AAIR versus DDDR pacing in patients with impaired sinus node chronotropy; An echocardiographic and cardiopulmonary study, PACE 1997; 20: 1762-1768.
21. Harper GR, Pina IL, Kutalek SP, Intrinsic conduction maximizes cardiopulmonary performance with dual chamber pacemakers, PACE 1991; 14: 1787-1791.
22. Mayumi H, Kohno H, Yasui H, et al, Use of automatic mode change between DDD and AAI to facilitate native atrioventricular conduction in patients with sick sinus syndrome or transient atrioventricular block, PACE 1996; 19: 1740-1747.
23. Stierle U, Kruger D, Vincent AM, et al, An optimized AV delay algorithm for patients with intermittent atrioventricular conduction, PACE 1998; 21: 1035-1043.
24. Bailey JR, Gayle D, Simmons TW, et al, Automated AV interval adjustment to maintain ventricular capture or prevent ventricular pseudofusion, Circ 1995; 92: I-534 (abstract).
25. Linde C. The clinical utility of positive and negative AV/PV hysteresis. In M. Santini, Ed, Progress in Clinical Pacing, Armonk, NY, Futura 1997:339-45
26. Pavia SV, Perez-Lugones A, Lam C, et al, Symptomatic deterioration postdual chamber cardioverter defibrillator implantation: A retrospective, observational study, J Amer Coll Cardiol 2001; 37: 89A (abstract).
27. Theodorakis G, Fitzpatrick A, Vardas P, Sutton R, Resting echo-Doppler estimation of cardiac output during AAI and DDD pacing, with varying AV delay at different pacing rates, Eur J Card Pacing and Electrophysiol 1992; 2: 22-25.
28. Kindermann M, Frohlig G, Doerr T, Schieffer H, Optimizing the AV delay in DDD pacemaker patients with high degree AV block: Mitral valve Doppler versus impedance cardiography, PACE 1997; 20: 2453-246.
29. Ovsyshcher IE, Toward physiologic pacing: Optimization of cardiac hemodynamics by AV delay adjustment,(editorial), PACE 1997;20: 861-865.
30. De Teresa E, Chamorro JL, Pulpon LA, et al, An even more physiological pacing: Changing the sequence of ventricular activation, in K. Steinbach, D. Glogar, A. Laszkovics (editors), Cardiac Pacing: Proceedings of the VIIth World Symposium on Cardiac Pacing, Darmstadt, Germany, Steinkopff Verlag, 1983; 395-400.

Disclosure:

The author is Vice President and Medical Director of St. Jude Medical CRMD. He continues to be clinically active at a number of hospitals in the Los Angeles area. Although all of the illustrations were obtained with either a simulator or patients implanted with SJM pacemakers, devices from other manufacturers have similar capabilities. Space did not allow for a discussion of the subtle differences between similar although not identical algorithms in different model devices.

17

WHICH ATRIAL TACHYARRHYTHMIAS CAN BE TERMINATED BY ATRIAL ANTITACHYCARDIA PACING?

Carsten W. Israel, MD, Stefan H. Hohnloser, MD, FACC FESC
Dept. of Medicine, Div. of Cardiology, J. W. Goethe University Hospital, Frankfurt, Germany

New approaches to treat atrial tachyarrhythmias (ATs) concentrate on non-pharmacological therapies such as catheter ablation, electrical cardioversion, and atrial pacing techniques. The use of an implantable device which continuously monitors the atrial rhythm and applies atrial anti-tachycardia pacing (ATP) upon AT detection, represents a promising new therapeutic avenue. Compared to electrical cardioversion, atrial ATP offers the advantage of painless termination of ATs. However, ATP will only be successful in organized ATs such as atrial flutter while disorganized ATs such as atrial fibrillation with multiple microreentrant wavelets at best seems to allow local capture and limited regional entrainment which is not sufficient to terminate the AT[1]. Therefore, several questions concerning the applicability of atrial ATP in patients with ATs arise:

1. Which degree of AT organization and which AT cycle lengths are required for successful pace-termination?,
2. How many patients with ATs reveal episodes of sufficient organization for ATP?,
3. At which time after AT onset should ATP be applied?

1. Which degree of AT organization and which AT cycle lengths are suitable for successful pace-termination?

Different criteria to classify the degree of AT organization on the basis of bipolar or multiple atrial electrograms have been proposed (Table 1). Based on electrograms derived from implanted narrow-spaced permanent pacemaker leads, we developed a classification that combines morphologic and cycle length criteria[2] (Fig. 1). Type I AT refers to a high degree of organization: The electrogram shows discrete, monomorphic potentials, intersected by a clear isoelectric baseline and an AT cycle length always above 200 ms. In contrast, type III refers to bipolar electrograms which are completely disorganized with loss of isoelectric baseline and discrete morphology; the minimal cycle length is below 200 ms. In between, type II refers to intermediately organized electrograms which do not meet criteria for type I or III. We used the terms type I-III AT and not atrial fibrillation or flutter since a single bipolar recording does not allow to reliably conclude which of these tachyarrhythmias is present, or if single or multiple reentrant circuits are present. In a prospective study, we analyzed

From Ovsyshcher IE. *New Developments in Cardiac Pacing and Electrophysiology.* Armonk, NY: Futura Publishing Company, Inc. ©2002.

	Wells	Barbaro	Konings	Israel
Type I	Discrete complexes, morphology may vary, isoelectrical baseline free of perturbations	As Wells with digital quantification of potential duration/variation and isoelectrical baseline	Single broad wavefront of activation at the right atrial free wall	Monomorphic discrete signals separated by an isoelectric line, minimal cycle length ≥200 ms
Type II	As I but with perturbations of the baseline	As Wells with digital quantification	One or two non-uniformly propagating activation wavefronts at the right atrial free wall	Meets neither type I nor type III criteria
Type III	No discrete complexes, no isoelectric intervals	As Wells with digital quantification	Multiple reentrant wavefronts simultaneously within the area of electrode array	Polymorphic or nondiscrete signals, no isoelectric baseline, minimal cycle length <200 ms
Type IV	Type III alternating with type I/II			

Tab. 1: Classification of AT organization based on atrial electrograms.

how often these types of organization occurred in 40 patients with ATs who also had a conventional indication for permanent pacing[2]. These patients were implanted with a new DDDRP pacemaker system (AT500™, Medtronic Inc, MN) which allows storage of 35 atrial electrograms with marker and cycle length annotations. During the first month, all pacing algorithms for prevention or termination of ATs were deactivated. AT episodes were stored with atrial electrograms in 21 patients during this time period. In 19 patients, correct AT onset and termination detection was confirmed upon manual analysis of stored episodes. A total of 804 atrial electrograms were available for further evaluation. Of these, 351 (43%) showed type I, 392 (47%) type II, and 81 (10%) type III degree of AT organization. Also after correcting for patients with multiple AT episodes who might have biased the analysis, an adjusted prevalence of type I of 48%, type II of 42%, and type III of 10% was found. In the second study phase, atrial ATP was activated for AT episodes lasting > 1 min. During this study phase, 361 treated AT episodes were stored by the devices and confirmed with regard to correct onset and termination detection upon manual analysis. Of 217 treated type I ATs, 135 (62%) were successfully pace-terminated. Upon the last stimulus of the ATP train, 19% terminated immediately (primary termination) and 43% terminated secondarily, i.e. ATP changed the cycle length but the AT terminated only within 30 sec after ATP (Fig. 2). Type II ATs were pace-terminated in 29 of 86 episodes (34%), all but one were secondary terminations. Type III ATs were found in 58 episodes; these could not be pace-terminated.

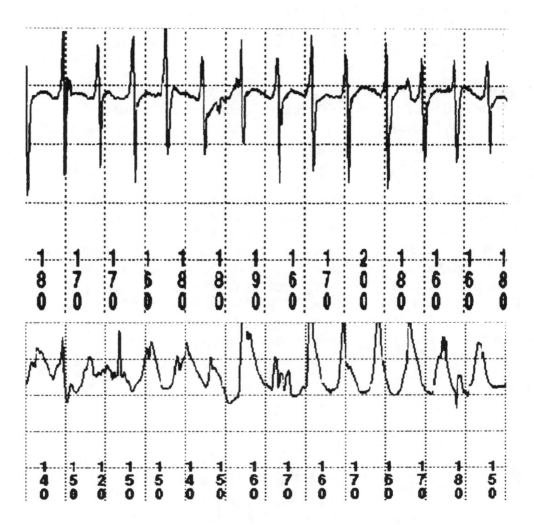

Fig. 1: Different degrees of AT organization based upon bipolar electrogram recordings. Upper panel: Type I (highly organized AT), middle panel: Type II (intermediate AT organization), lower panel: Type III (disorganized AT). Cycle length annotations in ms. See text and Tab. 1 for details.

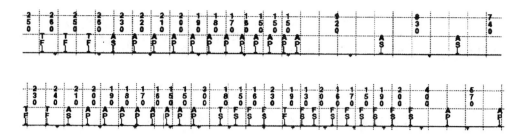

Fig. 2: Primary (upper panel) and secondary (lower panel) pace-termination of ATs by ATP (ramp). Marker annotations of device-stored treated AT episodes. AP: atrial pace, AS: atrial sense, FS: fibrillation sense, TF: tachy/fibrillation overlap zone. Cycle lengths in ms.

In another study, we analyzed if the median AT cycle length could also predict the efficacy of ATP[3]. During a follow-up of 12 months, 676 AT episodes were treated by ATP and stored with electrograms in 27 out of 62 patients (Fig. 3). Only 4 out of 58 AT episodes (7%) with a median cycle length ≤ 200 ms were terminated by ATP. In contrast, 18 out of 45 AT episodes (40%) of 210 ms, 112 of 219 AT episodes (51%) of 220-230 ms, 104 of 170 AT episodes (61%) of 240-250 ms, and 34 of 82 AT episodes (41%) of 260-270 ms median cycle length were successfully pace-terminated. In 102 AT episodes with cycle lengths of 280-360 ms, ATP success rate was much lower (28%).

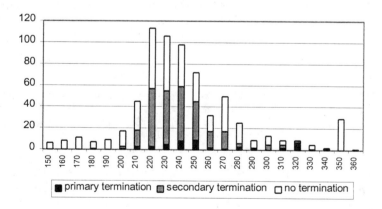

Fig. 3: ATP success rates related to AT cycle length immediately before ATP delivery. Abscissa: AT cycle length in ms, ordinate: number of AT episodes.

In conclusion, based on bipolar electrograms available from implanted pacemaker leads, AT episodes with a high degree of organization and a median cycle length of 220-270 ms show maximal ATP success rates.

2. How many patients with ATs reveal episodes of sufficient organization for ATP ?

In our study group of 40 patients[2], atrial fibrillation was the only AT documented by surface ECG before pacemaker implant in 28 patients (70%), atrial fibrillation in combination with atrial flutter was found in another 3 patients, and different types of atrial flutter in 7 patients. Two patients had ectopic atrial tachycardias. In 14 patients with atrial fibrillation as the only previously documented AT, 471 AT episodes were recorded with bipolar electrograms. These showed type I AT organization in 33%, type II in 58%, and type III in 8%. Of note, all 14 patients had type I AT episodes, either alone (4 patients) or combined with type II or III AT (10 patients). In 5 of the 12 patients with atrial flutter together with atrial fibrillation or ATs other than atrial fibrillation, 332 AT episodes were stored by the devices. In 58% of these AT episodes, type I AT was found, in 30% type II, and in 11% type III AT organization. Thus, periods of highly organized AT amenable to ATP can be found in a variety of patients with ATs, including patients with atrial fibrillation.

In a substudy of the AT500 Verification study[4], patients under treatment with amiodarone were compared to patients without class I or III antiarrhythmic drugs with regard to the number of ATP treated AT episodes and ATP success. Over a 2 months period, 20492 AT episodes occurred in patients with amiodarone (n=98) compared to 16279 AT episodes in patients without class I or III antiarrhythmic drugs (n=125). In amiodarone treated patients, significantly more of these AT episodes were treated by ATP (40%) compared to patients without class I/III antiarrhythmic drugs (35%). Since the ATP success rate was similar in both groups (49% versus 51%), the absolute number of successfully pace-terminated AT episodes and the proportion of successfully treated AT episodes to all AT episodes were higher in patients treated with amiodarone.

Thus, also in patients with atrial fibrillation, ATs show periods of high organization which may be amenable to atrial ATP. As a concept of hybrid therapy, the combination of atrial ATP with amiodarone may increase the clinical success of each of the single treatment modalities[5, 6].

3. At which time after AT onset should ATP be applied ?

If atrial ATP is applied immediately after AT detection, therapy may be unnecessary since many episodes might terminate spontaneously. In the AT500 Verification study[4], 35,785 of 52,468 AT episodes (68%) were not treated by ATP predominantly due to spontaneous AT termination within 1 minute after AT onset. On the other hand, primarily organized AT episodes may disorganize within 1 minute and then be no longer amend-able by ATP. Therefore, we looked at the type of AT organization at AT onset and 1 minute later in patients with an implanted monitoring device[2]. In 279 AT episodes, atrial electrograms were available at AT onset and 1 minute later and confirmed correct detection of AT onset and AT persistence. At AT onset, 97 episodes (35%) showed type I organization while 182 (65%) were only intermediately or not organized (types II and III). After 1 minute, the number of highly organized ATs had increased to 123, at the same time the number of type II/III ATs had decreased to 156. While 72/97 type I ATs (74%) and 131/182 type II/III ATs (72%) remained unchanged over a 1 minute period, approximately one quarter of type I ATs degenerated to a lower degree of organization, respectively organized secondarily to a higher level of organization. Therefore, a delay between AT onset detection and automatic ATP application of 1 minute does not compromise the applicability of atrial ATP due to AT degeneration during this time. Instead, it allows to withhold unnecessary therapy for AT episodes which spontaneously terminate within 1 minute.

Conclusions

Atrial ATP, automatically applied by an implanted device shortly after an organized AT has been detected, provides a new approach to treat ATs. Optimal ATP success can be achieved in AT episodes with a high degree of organization and a cycle length of 220-270 ms. Periods of a such high organization seem to be present also in most patients with atrial fibrillation and may be more frequent in patients on antiarrhythmic drug treatment. To avoid unnecessary ATP application for short lasting, spontaneously terminating AT episodes, a delay of 1 minute between AT detection and ATP application can be used without compromising ATP applicability due to degeneration of AT organization.

References

1. Kirchhof C, Chorro F, Scheffer GJ, et al.: Regional entrainment of atrial fibrillation studied by high-resolution mapping in open-chest dogs. Circulation 1993; 88:736-749.

2. Israel CW, Ehrlich JR, Grönefeld G, et al.: Prevalence, characteristics and clinical implications of regular atrial tachyarrhythmias in patients with atrial fibrillation: Insights from a study using a new implantable device. J Am Coll Cardiol 2001; 38:355-363.

3. Israel CW, Ehrlich JR, Plock KC, et al.: Degree of atrial tachyarrhythmia organization rather than cycle length predicts success of automatic atrial antitachycardia pacing. PACE 2001; 24:555.

4. Israel CW, Hügl B, Unterberg C, et al.: Pace-termination and pacing for prevention of atrial tachyarrhythmias: Results from a multicenter study with an implantable device for atrial therapy. J Cardiovasc Electrophysiol 2001; 12:1121-1128.

5. Israel CW, Ehrlich JR, Barold SS: Treatment of atrial tachyarrhythmias with pacing and antiarrhythmic drugs. In Israel CW, Barold SS (eds): Advances in the treatment of atrial tachyarrhythmias: Pacing, cardioversion and defibrillation. Armonk, NY, Futura Publishing Co, 2002, pp. 305-323.

6. Savelieva I, Camm AJ: Antitachycardia pacing for termination of atrial tachyarrhythmias. In Israel CW, Barold SS (eds): Advances in the treatment of atrial tachyarrhythmias: Pacing, cardioversion and defibrillation. Armonk, NY, Futura Publishing Co, 2002, pp. 339-368.

18.

PACING OF TRANSPLANTED HEART

Andrzej Kutarski MD, PhD

Department of Cardiology University Medical Academy, Lublin, Poland

Orthotopic heart transplantation (OHT) has already its relevant position within non-pharmacological methods for treatment of irreversible heart failure. Majority of these operations have been performed using Lower-Shumway technique (atrioatrial anastomosis). As a consequence, the patient has two connected and deformed right atria and two sinus nodes. Innervated recipient atrial remnant and dennervated donor atrium are electrically isolated from each one by surgical suture and activity both of sinus nodes reveals in ECG as two atrial rhythms[1,2].

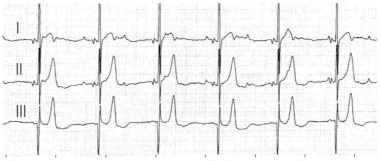

Figure 1. *Three leads of ECG of the transplanted heart patient. Visible two separate atrial rhythms.*

Bradyarrhythmias after OHT. Sinus node dysfunction (SND) (severe sinus or junctional bradycardia or episodes of sinus arrest) is the most frequent and important form of bradyarrhythmias in these patents. **Acute SND**. It is observed in most of patients within 24 hours after heart transplantation and it require support of temporary cardiac pacing or catecholamines[1,2,3]. Bradycardia during first 2-3 weeks after OHT can maintain in 14-44 % of patients[2]. **Late bradycardia.** SND is reversible in numerous patients after OHT during first year. Stafford group (556 pts) presented, that in 50% pts bradycardia disappears during 6 mth and in 75% of pts during one year after OHT[3]. In the group of McGill[4], significant SND vanished in 88% of pts. during 95 ± 75 days and in report of Houston group (245 pts.)[5] - in 56% of pts. after 3 months. **The problems related to sinus node dysfunction after OHT.** During "cyclosporine era" so dramatic manifestation of SND as cardiac arrest and sudden death is rare, but hemodynamic successions of bradycardia delays and limits early and later rehabilitation and makes that improvement is

From Ovsyshcher IE. *New Developments in Cardiac Pacing and Electrophysiology*. Armonk, NY: Futura Publishing Company, Inc. ©2002.

less than awaited[1,2]. It makes (economic aspects are important as well) that majority of patients with SND receive pacemaker before discharge from the hospital[1,2]. **How many patients after OHT needs pacemaker implantation?** In the quoted above report of Stanford group, 7,4% pts. (in 90% due to different form of sinus node disease)[3]; in McGill's one[4] - 6,4%, in Houston group[5] - 9,2%. Analysis of current literature performed by Ellenbogen[1] and Melton[2] indicates, that frequency of pacemaker implantation in patients OHT ranges between 6-23%, and most of implantations are performed usually 3 weeks after operation, in 70 - 90% due to SND. The incidence of permanent pacing due to AV block are prominently less frequent and ranged between 0-10% of pacemaker implantation[1,2,3,6]. **Selection of pacing modes in patients after OHT.** Choice of pacing system remain still controversial, in spite that the role of atrial contribution in diastolic dysfunction and the role of restoration of chronotropic competence were proved[7,8,9]. Rate responsive atrial based pacing modes are recommended[1,2,10], but a lot of patients still receive VVI or VVIR pacing system. Those authors argues, that in part of patients bradycardia may disappear during long-term observation. **Significance of atrial contribution in patients after OHT.** Midei[7] and Parry groups[8] observed decrease of cardiac output by about 11-14%, systolic, diastolic and averaged pulmonary artery pressure by about 12,9 and by 11% respectively, after change from AAI to VVI pacing mode. Roelke described increase of cardiac output from 4,9 to 6,5 l/min during inhibition of VVI pacing by NSR and explains it as result of restoration natural AV synchrony[9]. Ellenbogen[1] and Melton[2] presented complete review of papers about advantages and disadvantages of different modes of cardiac pacing in patients after OHT. In 1988 Markewitz and Osterholzer[11] described the

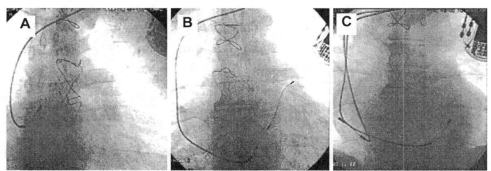

Figure 2. Atrial pacing systems implanted in patients after OHT. A: the tip of lead located in donor atrium. B: The CS designed lead (Biotrinik's) located in CS of donor heart. C: resynchronising atrial pacing system with the leads screw-in into recipient RA and donor CS ostium.

new concept of permanent pacing: recipient-donor atrial resynchronization. It allows to utilize signals of innervated sinus node of recipient atrium as natural biosensor. Additional benefits consists simultaneous contraction of recipient and donor atria. Although Parry[8] did not found significant hemodynamic effect of (donor-recipient) atrial resynchronization during rest, but Roediger showed, that such atrial resynchronization improves NYHA class, cardiac index at rest and during exercise, stroke work, pulmonary wedge pressure at exercise as well[12]. Chronic atrial fibrillation, and severe failure of sinus node of recipient atrium limited utility of this pacing mode. **Technical aspects of atrial (based) pacing in patients after OHT.** Distorted geometry and specific electrophysiological conditions of right atrium makes, that patient after OHT considered for permanent pacing consist still challenge for implanting physician.

Our experience with atrial pacing in pts after OHT

Values	Acute	Subacute	Chronic
A amplitude (mV)	**2,4** (1,4)	**2,5**(1,7)	**2,2**(1,3)
A slew rate (V/s)	0,4 (0,2)		
V amplitude (mV)	1,85 (0,9)		
A/V ratio	6,8 (10,7)		
Pacing threshold (V)	**0,87** (0,7)	**0,68** (0,4)	**1,63** (1,1)
Impedance (Ohm)	345 (52)	360,8 (58)	344,8 (57)

All reports concerning atrial based pacing in pts. after OHT (exception Woodard and Roelke's ones[10,11]) described this specific technical problems occasionally only. Roelke[9], using active fixation leads placed anteriorly in the donor right atrium, reported satisfied sensing conditions (A wave average 1,7 mV) and pacing threshold (0,5-1,8, average 0,7 V). He did not observed atrial lead dislodgement related to biopsy procedure but undersensing and pacemaker exit block he found in two out of five atrial leads[9]. Woodgard[10] as the first one, described exactly procedure of atrial lead placement in the atrium of transplanted heart. He reported experiences obtained in 11 pts. and recommended to use straight screw in lead with manually formed stylet. He pay attention that tip of lead should to be placed away from suture line to avoid oversensing of recipient atrial activity and he obtained satisfied sensing parameters (A wave aver. 3,4 mV) and pacing threshold (aver. 0,8 V) but 2 dislodged atrial leads required revision; dislodgement were independent to endomyocardial biopsy. I implanted atrial screw-in lead in 37 pts after OHT*, with SND (3 pts with coexisting additionally paroxysmal AV block received ventricular lead). Different atrial based pacing systems were implanted: AAI-R (23 pts), DDD-R (7 pts) and A_1A_2T (8 pts). In 25 pts, the lead was screwed into RA appendage or anterior wall, in 10 pts better pacing/sensing conditions were found in CS ostium region and in 2 in proximal part of CS[13]. Only in 13/37 pts native (recipient) A waves were recorded with amplitude < 0,3mV and there were no problems with recipient atrium sensing after proper programming of sensing threshold. 7 additional leads were implanted into recipient atrium for triggered pacing atrium of transplanted heart (A_1A_2T pacing). One lead dislodged required revision during postoperative period (1/44, 2%). There was not dislodgement related to endomyocardial biopsy. It seems to be interesting, that in 2 pts due to unacceptable low RA potential and/or high PTh values atrial lead was implanted to CS of allograft for sensing/pacing of its left atrium. A-wave was: 4,0 and 5,0 mV; PTh: 0,7 and 2,4 V/0,5ms respectively; recipient atrial remnant potentials were not detected. Chronic pacing/sensing conditions showed to be generally excellent and stable. One of mentioned 2 pts received AAI-R pacing system, in second one –

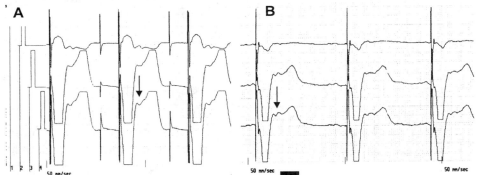

Figure 3. ECG of two transplanted patients with pacemaker's syndrome caused by erroneous location of atrial leads in recipient atrium. Retrograde conducted P waves are visible in ST-T complexes (arrows).

additional straight screw-in lead was implanted to remnant RA for A_1A_2T pacing. My experience indicates, that CS lead location in cardiac allograft for its left atrial pacing/sensing seems to be a new solution for pts after OHT with problems of RA lead placement[13].

AAI-R pacing of donor atrium. This simple pacing mode assure: natural AV synchrony, physiological ventricular activation and restores chronotropic competence[1,2,10]. Absence of ventricular lead eliminates risk of its dislodgement during RV endomyocardial biopsy[1,2]. Its disadvantages consist necessity of reoperation if AV block occurs during long term follow-up. 23 out of 37 our pts with SND received AAI-R pacing system; we found: NSR in 4 pts., sinus bradycardia in 18 pts., unstable SR with episodes of sinus arrest in 4 pts., nodal rhythm in 10 pts, retrograde atrial activation due to ventricular pacing in 1 pacemaker dependent patient.

EPS parameters		Values(SD)
Sinus rhythm (26 pts)	Frequency (bpm)	57,2 (21)
	PII wave duration (ms)	95,8 (24,5)
	P-Q interval (ms)	145,0 (21,4)
RA pacing (37 pts)	PII wave duration (ms)	101,9 (29,3)
	S-Q interval (ms)	142,9 (23,8)
	Wenckebach point (bpm)	161,7 (18,3)
RV pacing (19 pts)	Retrograde VA conduction (ms)	218,4 (67)

P wave duration in all except 2 pts. with previous long-term VVI pacing was normal. AV interval remained in normal limits in most of pts. Wenckebach point was 120/min only in 2 pts with documented AV block, 130-160/min in 15 pts and exceeded 170/min in remained 20 pts. Retrograde VA conduction was intact in 33/37 pts, but in 4 pts exceeded 260/min. During long term follow-up in no patient we observed AV conduction disturbances. In 6 pts.[14] treadmill exercise (Bruce's protocol) was repeated three times during: I) sinus (spontaneous) rhythm (average values): peak exercise 102/min, max attained workload: 6,1 MET's; II) AAI pacing 70/min, peak exercise 106/min; max attained workload: 6,2 MET's and III) AAI (DDD)-R pacing: peak exercise 138/min, max attained workload: 9,6 MET's. Duration of the exercise was significantly longer, when rate-responsive program was applied[14]. Our observation confirmed, that in pts with SND after OHT AV conduction parameters remained in normal limits; it indicates safety of rate-responsive pacing modes in this pts. Observed in some dennervated heart "supra-normal" AV conduction may to have clinical importance in case of atrial

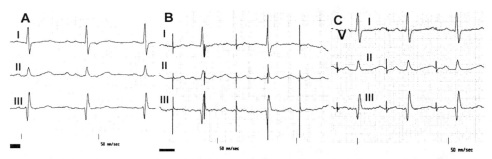

Figure 4. *ECG recorded during implantation of A₂A₂T pacing system. A: normal S.R. B: pacing of recipient atrium. C: pacing of donor atrium*

arrhythmia. **DDD-R pacing.** DDD pacing with rate modulation is the alternative pacing mode recommended for patients after OHT[1,2,5,9]. It posses all virtues AAI-R pacing. Additional ventricular lead can be useful if AV conduction disturbances occur during long term follow up. There is small (and probably overrated) risk of recently implanted lead dislodgement during endomyocardial biopsy[1,2,3]. DDD-R pacing effects of abnormal activation of the ventricles deteriorates synchrony of ventricular contraction; this fault can be eliminated by reprogramming pacemaker to AAI-R pacing mode or by programming long AV delay. The last one solution can increase possibility of endless-loop tachycardia occurrence due to usually present but frequently prolonged VA conduction in patients after OHT.

Biatrial and three-chamber pacing in heart transplant recipient. Interesting and promising alternative to AAI-R and DDD-R pacing in patients with transplanted heart consist donor and recipient biatrial pacing using triggered mode. It enables to utilise innervated recipient sinus node as sensor for triggered pacing of the atrium of transplanted heart; additional hemodynamic effect of resynchronization of atrial contraction (especially during exercise) still awaits evaluation. A_2A_2T pacing can to be obtained using single- and dual chamber pacemaker as well. Both atrial (recipient and donor) lead can be connected via Y connector to the port of SSI pacer, which is programmed to SST pacing mode. The second option consist connection of recipient atrial lead to atrial port and donor atrial

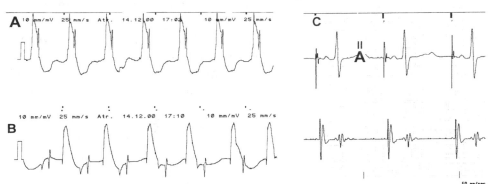

Figure 5. A: *IEGM of donor atrium recorded final lead location. B: IEGM of recipient atrium. C: Simultaneous pacing donor and recipient atria (atrial resynchronization). During operation recipient rhythm did not exceeded programmed pacemaker frequency.*

lead to ventricular port of standard DDD pacemaker; VDD or DDD program with so ultra-short AV delay permits to obtain similar effect[1,2,8,11,12,14]. In patients with co-existing AV conduction disturbances DDD pacer should be used; both atrial leads can be connected via Y connector to atrial- and ventricular lead – to ventricular port of pacemaker. Unit should have possibility of triggered pacing in atrial channel during standard DDD pacing (we used Philos DDD, Biotronik). This sophisticated pacing mode is possible only in patients with clever sinus node of recipient atrium[1,2,8,11,12,14]. In case utility of Y connector it is very important to connect cathode to donor atrium and anode to recipient atrium. This configuration enables to preserve pacing of donor atrium (using UP sensing/pacing program) if permanent AF of recipient atria occur. During implantation of pacing system in 37 pts after OHT we recognized rhythm of recipient atrium: NSR was found only in 15/37 pts. (sinus bradycardia - in 3, atrial flutter -in 3, low voltage AF - in 12 and no electrical activity - in 4 were observed in remained patients). In 3 pts. during DDD elective pacemaker replacement we found atrial lead located in recipient atrium (pts. presented symptoms of pacemaker syndrome); we implanted additional atrial lead into donor atrium and we applied A_2A_2T/D pacing system. Encouraged results and Roediger's observation[12] inspired us to wider use this pacing system, whenever it was possible. Finally we implanted eight A_2A_2T and two A_2A_2T/D-R pacing systems.

Pacing/sensing conditions in 10 pts. with atrial resynchronization		
Parameters: average (SD)	Recipient atrium	Donor atrium
Frequency of SR (bpm)	83,4 (11,3)	56,1 (19,2)
A wave amplitude (mV)	1,14 (0,8)	2,06 (0,58)
A wave slew rate (V/s)	0,2 (0,1)	0,3 (0,2)
Pacing threshold (V)	1,39 (1,07)	0,79 (0,51)
Impedance (Ohm)	354,3 (75,1)	346,1 (37,6)

Triggered pacing markedly improved mitral and tricuspid flow. Its influence on cardiac output (during rest) was less visible. All patients except one described the effect of triggered pacing as "calm" or "stillness" in the chest. 9 of them preferred AAT than AAI-R pacing program. Atrial resynchronization was possible only in about ¼ patients with SND after OHT, due to electrophysiological changes in recipient atrium; although it remain promising pacing mode for selected patients after OHT with SND.

Recapitulation. 5-15 % of patients several weeks - several months following OHT are considered for pacemaker therapy, mainly due to symptomatic SND. In spite of, that in 50% of them sinus node function may to recover during one year, early pacemaker implantation accelerates rehabilitation and improves exercise tolerance. VVI-R pacing is not recommended due to known of its unfavourable hemodynamic effects. Chronotropic incompetence and diastolic dysfunction of transplanted heart makes, that rate responsive atrial based pacing modes (AAI-R and DDD-R) are recommended, because they improves cardiac output and exercise capacity. Interesting and promising remain synchronized atrial pacing (which allows recipient-donor atrial resynchronization) but utility of this pacing mode is limited by electrophysiological condition of recipient atrium.

*) *Most of heart transplantations were performed by prof. Z. Religa and M. Zembala teams.*

References

1. Ellenboden KA: Special clinical applications and newer indications for cardiac pacing. In: Ellenboden K.A., Kay G.N., Wilkoff B.L. Clinical cardiac pacing. W.B. Saunders Company; 22: 353-366
2. Melton IC, Gilligan DM, Wood MA, Ellenbogen KA: Optimal cardiac pacing after heart transplantation. PACE 1999; 22: 1510-1527
3. DiBiase A, Tse TM, Shnittger I et al.: Frequency and mechanism of bradycardia in cardiac transplant recipient and need for pacemakers. Am J. Cardiol. 1991; 67: 1385-1389
4. Smilowitch M, Dunne C, Sirois S et al.: Sinus node dysfunction following heart transplantation: Need for permanent pacing? PACE 1991 II; 14: 264 (abstr.)
5. Maloney JD, Ragahvan R, Young J et al.: Indications for permanent pacing in post transplant patients with relative bradycardia. PACE 1995; 18 II: 96 (abstr.)
6. Miyamoto Y, Curtiss EI, Kormos RL et al.: Bradyarrhythmia after heart transplantation: incidence, time course and outcome. Circulation 1990; 82 (suppl. 4): 313-317
7. Midei MG, Baughman KL, Achuff SC et al.: Is atrial activation beneficial in heart transplant recipient? Am. J. Cardiol. 1990; 16: 1201-1204
8. Parry G, Malbut K, Dark JH et al.: Optimal pacing modes after cardiac transplantation: Is synchronisation of recipient and donor atria beneficial? Brit. Heart J. 1992; 68: 195-198
9. Roelke M, McNamara D, Osswald S: Atrial lead stability, pacemaker syndrome and ventriculo - atrial conduction in paced patients following cardiac transplantation. Eur. J.C.P.E. 1994; 2 suppl. 4: 264 (abstr.)
10. Woodard DA, Conti JB, Mills JR et al.: Permanent atrial pacing in cardiac transplant patients. PACE 1997; 20: 2398-2404
11. Markewitz A, Osterholzer G, Weinhold C et al.: Recipient P wave synchronized pacing of the donor atrium in heart transplanted patient: A case study. PACE 1988; 11: 1402-1404
12. Roediger W, Nagele H: A2A2D/T pacemaker therapy in heart transplant recipient. PACE 1997, 20, 2338 (abstr.)
13. Kutarski A, Zakliczy ski M, Oleszczak K, et al.: Coronary sinus (CS) pacing of orthotopic cardiac allograft - a new solution of donor right atrium pacing/sensing problems. 6th International Workshop on Cardiac Arrhythmias, Venice, Italy; October 5-8 1999: 25 (abstr.)
14. Kutarski A, Zakliczy ski M, Oleszczak K, et al.: Atrial based pacing modes in patients after heart transplantation (OHT) International Meeting. Atrial Fibrillation 2000, Bologna, Italy; September 16-17 1999: 159 (abstr.)

19.

PATIENT SELECTION AND LEAD POSITIONING FOR SINGLE LEAD DUAL CHAMBER PACING

I. Eli Ovsyshcher, MD, PhD, Eugene Crystal, MD*

Cardiology Department, Cardiac Research Center, Soroka University Medical Center and Faculty of Health Sciences, Ben Gurion University of the Negev, Beer-Sheva, Israel; *Department of Medicine, McMaster University, Hamilton, Ontario, Canada

Single-lead (SL) dual chamber system, with non-contact, floating in atrial (A) blood pool electrode was first tested in humans in 1973[1]. Several years later permanent SL-dual chamber systems were implanted[2,3]. Unipolar atrial sensing was sub-optimal, encouraging the development of SL systems incorporating bipolar atrial sensing[3-10]. SL systems became commercially available in Europe and USA about twelve years ago and in the last years SL has been integrated into dual chamber ICD system.[11]

Patient Selection for SL-Dual Chamber Pacing

According to the guidelines of ACC/AHA of 1998, SL-VDD pacing is indicated for patients with intact SA node function and various degrees of heart block. Such simple criteria as atrial rest rate ≥ 70, before implantation, identified patients with the low risk (0.6%-0.8%) for subsequent sinus node disease[12]. For diagnosis of SA node disease, Antonioli[9] used criteria of 60 bpm at rest and 85 bpm during exercise. On the basis of retrospective analysis of about 400 VDD implants[13], we have employed the following rule-of-thumb in evaluating patients with complete heart block (before or after temporary VVI pacemaker): the sinus rate should be ≥ 90 bpm at rest; sinus rate<90 bpm raises the suspicion of SA node dysfunction; in sinus rhythm at rest between 71-89 bpm the likelihood of chronotropic incompetence is about 10%; in sinus rhythm ≤ 70 bpm at rest probability of chronotropic incompetence is very high (about 30%). In using these criteria, nocturnal and at rest sinus bradycardia <50 bpm was observed <5% in our patients 3 years after implantation. ECG monitoring may be useful at rest and when possible during walking at maximal rate. The pre-implant right atrium (RA) volume determined by echocardiography was found an accurate predictor of atrial undersensing[14]. It may be expected that in patients with significantly dilated RA, the probability of SA node disease and atrial arrhythmias is higher than usual. To choose suitable criteria of SA node

From Ovsyshcher IE. *New Developments in Cardiac Pacing and Electrophysiology.* Armonk, NY: Futura Publishing Company, Inc. ©2002.

disease is crucial for the appropriate selection of patients for VDD pacing and should be evaluated in prospective studies. It also may be speculated that lowest incidence of chronotropic incompetence in patients selected for SL-VDD pacing may prevent appearance of AF, that may requires a change in VDD pacing to DDD or DDDR.

Paroxysmal AF is not a contra-indication for some physicians when they use VDD-system with mode switch [9,15,16]. However, it should be mentioned that patients with paroxysmal AF, prior to implantation, had significantly poorer results of VDD pacing survival for follow-up of 14±7 months[17]. We do not use any VDD systems in patients with paroxysmal AF, or any frequent premature beats, since we believe that better results may be obtained with DDD/R pacing. VDD and DDD pacing modes were recently compared in a prospective randomized study of patients with atrial tachyarrhythmia[18]. No expected benefit of DDD pacing on the recurrence of atrial arrhythmia has been demonstrated. However, in this study no antiarrhythmic therapy was a pre-requisite for inclusion, which is not the case in the majority of patients with symptomatic AF. VDD pacing should be also avoided in patients who may require administration of medication, which could lead to drug induced chronotropic incompetence.

Practical Aspects of Single Lead Positioning

SLs are available in several different lengths of atrial to ventricular apex separations: 11 cm, 13 cm, 15 cm, and 17mm with the standard separation being 13 cm for the most patients[19]. The decision to choose any AV separation may be made empirically according to the height of patients. A simple fluoroscopic technique may also be used to predict the best lead size by laying a test electrode over the chest of a supine patient and positioning it under fluoroscopy to approximate the expected intracardiac course of the lead[20].

Regarding placement of atrial electrodes there is significant controversy. The optimal position for atrial dipole should theoretically be in the SA node area. Depolarization of the atria normally begins with depolarization of the SA node area and spreads in a wave front towards the AV node. So, optimal sensing and, especially, pacing of atria (imitation of normal electrophysiology of the atria) may presumably be accomplished in the SA node area. However, non-uniformity of individual atrial anatomy due to the complex shape and boundaries of the chambers[6,9], and also due to changes related to ageing and fibrosis, could lead to complex uncoupling of transverse conduction between fibers in a muscle bundle[10]. Thus, non-uniformity of the anatomy in normal and, particularly in diseased atria, leads to multiform atrial depolarization and creates for this reason individual propagation, and so optimal place for sensing of the A-signal via the pacemaker's amplifier is absolutely random. This complexity in the anatomo-electrophysiological substrate could explain the unpredictability of the optimum location of the atrial lead and therefore recommendations of some implanters to localize atrial dipole only in some particular part of the RA (optimal from theoretical or practical points of view: compare the SA node area with RA atrial appendage or free atrial wall for placement standard atrial lead) seems unreliable from both theoretical and practical points of view.

In clinical practice there are implanters who recommend placing atrial dipole of SL in close proximity to the SA node[9,21-23], or in mid-part of RA[23]. Others, before selection of optimal place for atrial lead, strongly recommend RA mapping by atrial part of the SL[5,8,19]. In several reports (about 500 implantations of SL-devices) the optimal A-signal was most frequently found in the mid-lower and lower parts of the RA[5,7,8,11,19,24,25]. A comparative study regarding the best placement for the two types of leads (total and split rings) was conducted and no significant differences in optimal positioning or achievable atrial signal amplitude were found[26].

As expected the optimum cardiac signal is provided by contact or at least a very close position of the electrodes to the endocardium. If this is important for atrial sensing by floating electrodes, it is more important if the same leads are to provide atrial pacing.

For SL placement we use the following technique. First the lead is placed securely in the right ventricle apex in the traditional manner and adequate V-pacing and sensing performance is verified. Next, in order to obtain an optimal A-signal, it is assessed by mapping of the RA: the proximal part of the lead is either bowled to move the atrial dipole distally towards the lower part of the atrium, or straightened to relocate the dipole in a superior orientation towards the upper part of the RA. A-signal is evaluated either with a pacing system (PSA) or by one or, preferably, both of the atrial electrodes (poles) of the implanted lead to a properly grounded ECG recorder **(Figure 1B)**. One advantage of this approach is that it allows a simultaneous visual estimation of both the bipolar atrial and ventricular far-field signals as can be "seen" by the pacemaker, although in general the differential amplifiers provided in the pacemaker circuitry eliminate most of the far-field sensing signals **(Figure 1C)**.

The lead is slowly moved while assessing the A-signal amplitude after every slight change, until the location of the optimal A-signal is verified. Redundancy in the heel of the lead helps provide lead stability as well as to more closely approximate the lead electrodes to the atrial endocardial surface. At the optimal location, stability of A-signal should be assessed

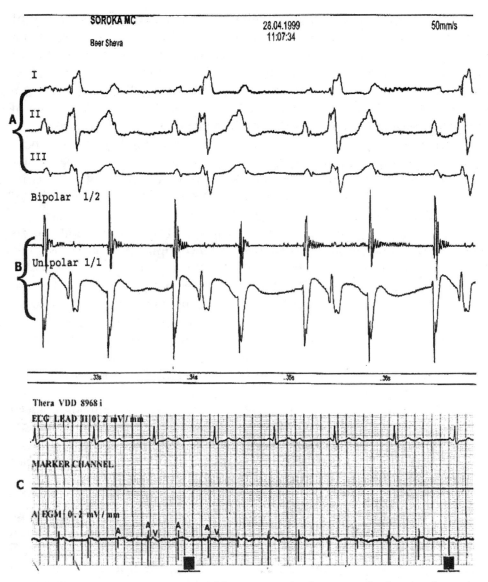

Figure 1. *Sensing of uni- and bipolar A-signals during and after implantation.*
***Panel A:** standard ECG leads.* ***Panel B:** uni- and bipolar intracardiac
electrograms (IEGM) were obtained by connecting one or both atrial electrodes
to the ECG recorder. Note: unipolar V-signal is bigger than bipolar; however
bipolar A-signal is significantly bigger than unipolar.* ***Panel C** shows the
telemetered A-signal from the VDD pacemaker. There is a high-quality A-signal
(1.4-3.4 mV) and a very low amplitude and frequency V-signal. Note the
similarity between bipolar and telemetered IEGMs: the same relationship exists
between A- and V-signals.*

using maneuvers such as deep breathing and coughing. The assessment of sensing, as well as pacing parameters should be made with the stylet withdrawn from the lead, since its presence can affect the performance of the lead quite dramatically. Caution must be exercised in order not to move the lead during fixation in the pacemaker pocket once the optimal position is found, since actions during fixation can dislocate the atrial dipole and significantly reduce A-signal.

Placing the atrial dipole near the SA node may provide an acceptable A-signal. However, the A-signal in this position is usually unstable, e.g. not optimal and its amplitude can drop drastically due to migration of the dipole to the superior vena cava during inspiration or patient movement (standing). Similarly atrial dipole placed close to the tricuspid valve will tend to be pulled distally into the ventricle by the heart's contractions, particularly if there is large redundant loop after the atrial dipole. This is particularly so in SLs, which taper to a very thin lead body distal to the atrial part.

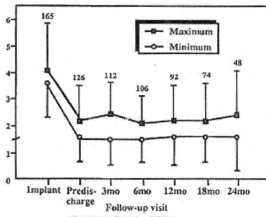

Figure 2. Mean and SD of maximum and minimum A-signal amplitude during implantation and follow-up. Note a decrease (two-fold) in A-signal in predischarge (immediately after implantation the A-signal was same as in predischarge) and the stability of A-signal over 24 months.

Another important issue during implantation of SL is the minimum acceptable amplitude of the atrial signal. As was demonstrated for the first time with Medtronic's VDD system[7] **(Figure 2)** and later with the CCS and Intermedics device[27-30], as well as in the multicenter study using the Biotronik SL-VDD system[31], there is an approximately 50% diminution in A-signal amplitude between the values obtained at implant with a PSA (measurements usually done via a ventricular channel), and the actual atrial sensing threshold detected by the pacemaker immediately after implantation. There are several reasons for diminution of atrial signal[5,7].

We do not believe that so significant a change in A-signal may be due to changes in lead positioning, because we observed a reduction in the A-signal not only in predischarge and latest follow-up measurements, but also immediately after finishing the operation. Our explanation in the drop of the A-signal is the difference in processing between the PSA measurements and telemetry signal through the pacemaker, including not only the amplifiers, but also differences in the sampling methods and blanking capabilities of the two different instruments[5,19]. Additionally, the A-signal may decrease by up to 200% during exercise or other physiological maneuvers (mean 37% ± 31%)[23,32-35]. Thus, the above-mentioned data would suggest that it is necessary to employ a large safety margin for A-signal sensing. If one assumes that pacemakers amplifiers are capable of detecting A-signals as low as 0.10-0.18 mV, the desired long-term A-signal should be minimum 0.4 mV-0.5 mV and optimum ≥ 1 mV. Therefore, during implantation of SL, for appropriate long-term survival of VDD pacing, minimally acceptable A-signal amplitude measured by the ventricular channel of the PSA should be 1-2mV, e.g. minimum 0.8 mV-1 mV and optimum ≥ 2 mV[5,7]. Thus, the desired long-term A-signal should be four to five fold than pacemaker amplifier is capable of detecting; only this safety margin still allow the prevention of significant undersensing of A-signal.

In a follow-up such diagnostic features as A-signal amplitude histograms (Saphir II, Vitatron; KAPPA 700, Medtronic) can provide further help in adequately programming atrial sensitivity.

Conclusions

1. Floating SL-VDD pacing is a reliable alternative for patients with various degrees of AV block and normal sinus node function.

2. To obtain appropriate long-term results with SL-systems, it is important to place the atrial lead at a site within the RA, where it exhibits the optimal A-signal.

3. To obtain reliable long-term results with SL-systems, it is important to use appropriate technique for placement atrial dipole. This technique is different to the placement standard contact atrial lead.

4. Difference in recognition A-signal by PSA and pacemaker amplifier and wide physiologic variation of this signal in floating atrial dipole, require high safety margin for A-signal.

References

1. Chamberlain DA, Woollons DJ, White NM, et al. Synchronous AV pacing with a single pervenous electrode. *Br Heart J* 1973; 35:559.

2. Curry PV, Raper DA. Single lead for permanent physiological cardiac pacing. *Lancet* 1978;2:757-9.

3. Antonioli G, Grassi G, Baggioni Gea. A single P-sensing ventricle stimulating lead driving a VAT generator. In: Meere C, ed. 6th World Symposium on Cardiac Pacing. Montreal, Canada, 1979:34-39.

4. Furman S, Gross J, Andrews C. Single lead VDD pacing. In: Antonioli G, Aubert A, Ector H, eds. Pacemaker leads. Amsterdam. The Netherlands.: Elsevier BV, 1991:pp. 183-197.

5. Ovsyshcher IE, Katz A, Bondy C. Clinical evaluation of a new single pass lead VDD pacing system. *PACE* 1994;17:1859-64.

6. Antonioli GE. Single lead atrial synchronous ventricular pacing: a dream come true. *PACE* 1994; 17:1531-47.

7. Ovsyshcher IE, Wagshal A. Single-lead VDD/DDD pacing. In: Vardas P, ed. Cardiac arrhythmias, Pacing & Electrophysiology. The expert view. Dordrecht-Boston-London: Kluwer Academic Publishers, 1998:389-98.

8. Tse HF, Lau CP. The current status of single lead dual chamber sensing and pacing. *J Interv Card Electrophysiol* 1998; 2:255-67.

9. Antonioli G. Single A-V lead cardiac pacing. Casalecchio (BO), Italy: Arianna Editrice, 1999.

10. Brownlee RR Toward optimizing the detection of atrial depolarization with floating bipolar electrodes. PACE 1989; 12:431-42

11. Niehaus M, Schuchert, Thamasett S, et al. multicenter experiences with single lead electrode for dual chamber ICD systems. *PACE* 2001;24:1489-1493.

12. Wiegand UK, Bode F, Schneider R, et al. Development of sinus node disease in patients with AV block: implications for single lead VDD pacing.*Heart* 1999; 81:580-5.

13. Ovsyshcher IE, Crystal E. Single-lead dual chamber pacing: how reliable and effective is it? In: Raviele A., ed., Cardiac Arrhythmias 20 0 1,Springer-Verlag, 2001, chapter 8, pp. 556-565.

14. de Cock CC, Van Campen LC, Huygens J, et al. Usefulness of echocardiography to predict inappropriate atrial sensing in single-lead VDD pacing. *PACE* 1999; 22:1344-7.

15. Nowak B, Voigtlander T, Rosocha S, et al. Paroxysmal atrial fibrillation and high degree AV block: use of single- lead VDDR pacing with mode switching. *PACE* 1998; 21:1927-33.

16. Buys EM, van Hemel NM, Jessurun ER, et al. VDDR pacing after His-bundle ablation for paroxysmal atrial fibrillation: a pilot study. *PACE* 1998;21:1869-72.

17. Ben Ameur Y, Martin E, Jarwe M, et al. VDD mode single electrode cardiac stimulation: indications, results and limitations of the method. *Ann Cardiol Angiol (Paris)* 1997; 46:585-91.

18. Gillis AM, Connolly SJ, Lacombe P, et al.. Randomized crossover comparison of DDDR versus VDD pacing after atrioventricular junction ablation for prevention of atrial fibrillation. The atrial pacing peri-ablation for paroxysmal atrial fibrillation (PA (3)) study investigators. *Circulation* 2000;102:736-41.

19. Ovsyshcher IE, Katz A, Rosenheck S, et al. Single lead VDD pacing: multicenter study. *PACE* 1996; 19:1768-71.

20. Nowak B, Voigtlander T, Liebrich A, et al. A simple method for preoperative assessment of the best fitting electrode length in single lead VDD pacing. *PACE* 1996; 19:1346-50.

21. Longo E, Catrini V. Experience and implantation techniques with a new single-pass lead VDD pacing system. *PACE* 1990; 13:927-36.

22. Ansani L, Percoco GF, Guardigli G, et al. Long-term reliability of single lead atrial synchronous pacing systems using closely spaced atrial dipoles: five-year experience. *PACE* 1994; 17:1865-9.

23. Wiegand UK, Bode F, Schneider R, et al. Atrial sensing and AV synchrony in single lead VDD pacemakers: a prospective comparison to DDD devices with bipolar atrial leads. *J Cardiovasc Electrophysiol* 1999; 10:513-20.

24. Gessman L, White M, Ghaly N, et al. U.S. experience with the AddVent VDD(R) pacing system. AddVent Phase I Investigators. *PACE* 1996; 19:1764-7.

25. Calosso E, Verzoni A, Manzo R, et al. DDD pacing by the floating electrode of a VDD single lead pacemaker. *PACE* 1997; 20:A1516.

26. Karagouz R, Guldal M, Ertas F, et al. Comparison of the optimal position of the atrial electrodes in two different single lead VDD pacing systems. *PACE* 1997; 20:A1444.

27. Wagshal AB, Ovsyshcher IE. Comparing the performance of the Unity VDD and Thera VDD pacing systems. *PACE* 1997; 20:1888-90.

28. Tse HF, Lau CP, Leung SK, et al. Single lead DDD system: a comparative evaluation of unipolar, bipolar, and overlapping biphasic stimulation and the effects of right atrial floating electrode location on atrial pacing and sensing thresholds. *PACE* 1996; 19:1758-63.

29. Palma E, Andrews C, Hanson S, et al. Atrial arrhythmia and mode survival in single pass VDD pacemakers. *PACE* 1997; 20 (II):A1538.

30. Naegeli B, Osswald S, Pfisterer M, et al. VDD(R) pacing: short- and long-term stability of atrial sensing with a single lead system. *PACE* 1996; 19:455-64.

31. Wiegand UK, Bode F, Schneider R, et al. Atrial sensing and AV synchrony in single lead VDD pacemakers: a prospective comparison to DDD devices with bipolar atrial leads. J Cardiovasc Electrophysiol 1999:10(4):513-20

32. Wiegand UK, Potratz J, Bode F, et al. Age dependency of sensing performance and AV synchrony in single lead VDD pacing. *PACE* 2000; 23:863-9.

33. Varriale P, Chryssos BE. Atrial sensing performance of the single-lead VDD pacemaker during exercise. *J Am Coll Cardiol* 1993; 22:1854-7.

34. Toivonen L, Lommi J. Dependence of atrial sensing function on posture in a single-lead atrial triggered ventricular (VDD) pacemaker. *PACE* 1996;19:309-13.

35. Langford EJ, Smith RE, McCrea WA, et al. Determining optimal atrial sensitivity settings for single lead VDD pacing: the importance of the P wave histogram. *PACE* 1997; 20:619-23.

20.

EXTRACTION OF PACING AND DEFIBRILLATOR LEAD SYSTEMS: STATE OF THE ART

Charles J. Love, MD FACC

Arrhythmia Device Services, The Ohio State University Heart Center
Columbus, OH, USA

The removal of chronic leads has evolved from the relatively primitive methods of direct traction by the operator, traction with a weight and pulley, and open heart operations. In addition, the indications for extraction of leads have developed based as the techniques have become more reliable and more safely applied to a given clinical situation. Most leads may be safely and completely extracted using transvenous extraction. The safe and effective extraction of a lead is founded on four basic concepts: 1) Preparation for complications, 2) Maintaining structural integrity of the lead during the application of traction, 3) Counter-Pressure, 4) Counter-Traction. Somewhat concerning to physicians performing lead extraction is that changes in lead and implant technologies may make lead removal more difficult. However, there are also advances that may make it fast and safe.

Indications: There is little controversy concerning extraction of the entire pacing system, including the lead(s), in the setting of pacemaker related endocarditis and/or sepsis. Failure to remove the leads in this setting will result in a failure to eradicate the infection in nearly all circumstances. Table 1 lists the indications as put forth by a panel of experts during a policy conference sanctioned by NASPE[1]. These indications now follow the well accepted "Class I-II-III" structure, and were derived from the Byrd Classification using "Mandatory-Necessary-Discretionary" guidelines[2].

Though most current indications as classified in table 1 are well accepted, removal of superfluous leads remains a most contentious issue. Many of the most experienced extraction experts prefer to remove most transvenous leads that are not necessary for the treatment of the patient. This is based on the facts that the more leads that are present and the longer these leads are in place, the more difficult and dangerous it will be to remove these leads at a later time (Fig. 1). Others feel that it acceptable to leave multiple non-functional leads in place to avoid any operative risk to the patient at the time of the proposed replacement procedure. As with all procedures, the relative risks and benefits of removing a pacing lead need to be weighed against the risks and benefits of leaving the lead in place. These will be unique to each patient and the age, medical condition, and particular

From Ovsyshcher IE. *New Developments in Cardiac Pacing and Electrophysiology.* Armonk, NY: Futura Publishing Company, Inc. ©2002.

clinical situation that is present. It will also be dependent on the competence and experience of the physician performing the extraction.

Table 1. Indications for lead extraction
Class 1(general agreement that leads should be removed)
  Sepsis and endocarditis due to infection of any part of the pacing system.
  Life-threatening arrhythmias secondary to a retained lead fragment.
  A retained lead, lead fragment, or extraction hardware posinig an immediate or imminent physical threat.
  Thromboembolic events caused by a retained lead or lead fragment.
  Obliteration or occlusion of all useable veins with the need to implant new leads.
  A lead that interferes with the operation of another pacemaker or defibrillator.
Class 2   (some divergence of opinion with respect to the benefit versus risk)
  Localized pocket infection, erosion, or chronic draining sinus that does not involve the transvenous portion of the lead system.
  An occult infection for which no other source can be found.
  Chronic pain at the pocket or lead insertion site that causes significant discomfort for the patient, and for which there is no acceptable alternative.
  A lead that, due to its design or its failure, may pose a threat to the patient.
  A lead that interferes with the treatment of a malignancy.
  Traumatic injury to the entry site of the lead interfering with reconstruction of the site.
  Leads preventing access to the venous circulation for newly required implantable devices.
  Non-functional leads in a young patient.
Class 3 (removal of leads is unnecessary)
  Any situation where the risk posed by removal of the lead is significantly higher than the benefit of removing the lead.
  A single non-functional transvenous lead in an older patient.
  Any normally functioning lead that may be reused at the time of pulse generator replacement, provided the lead has a reliable performance history.

Removal of ICD leads presents a particular challenge. This is due to the penetration of fibrous tissue into and around the shock coils. In addition, the non-isodiametric nature of these leads (the coils are wider than the lead body in most designs) forms another obstacle to lead removal. Extraction of superfluous ICD leads at an earlier time may reduce the risk to the patient at a later date. Removal also eliminates the issues of lead interaction from lead to lead contact or by shunting of current from the active lead into the inactive lead during defibrillation.

Preparation for Complications: If one performs transvenous lead extraction, complications will occur over time. The best method to prevent a patient death is to be prepared for this eventuality. Heavy fibrosis, multiple leads, very old leads, calcification around the leads as well as female gender have been associated with a higher likelihood of complications. One problem that is nearly impossible to know of in advance is a lead that does not follow the normal venous path. Leads that enter an artery, travel through a fistula, become excluded from the myocardium, perforate the heart, lie in a descending cardiac vein, or travel into the left side of the heart may result in a catastrophe upon extraction. Unfortunately, standard radiography and fluoroscopy are unlikely to identify most of these situations in advance of the operation. CT scans and echocardiography may be of some use, however most physicians do not perform these routinely prior to the operation. If the patient presents with unusual symptoms, bruit, pericardial rub, or if there is a suspicion of unusual lead location by chest radiography, further testing is warranted. Knowledge of these high risk factors prior to an attempted lead extraction should lead one to an alternate extraction approach, or a re-examination of the indication for the extraction.

In the vast majority of cases the operator cannot be certain whether or not an anatomic anomaly is present, or if a vascular tear or myocardial avulsion will occur, even for a relatively "simple" lead removal. For this reason it is imperative that certain safety precautions be present. Most importantly, this includes a competent and well-trained staff that can identify patient problems quickly and react to them instantly. Immediate access to echocardiography, pericardiocentesis, blood products and cardiovascular surgical assistance is mandatory. It is inevitable that a complication will occur, but with appropriate preparation the patient can be rescued intact. In my experience, the rapid recognition of an intra-operative problem combined with immediate steps to diagnose and resolve the problem will nearly always result in a positive outcome. A major difficulty faces the operator when the patient becomes hypotensive during or immediately following the extraction process. Most hypotension is the result of vagal reflexes combined with hypovolemia. During the traction process, the right ventricular volume may become compromised as well, due to inversion of the apex. Separating these relatively benign yet reversible issues from more serious complications can be difficult. If the patient does not respond quickly to fluid and atropine, steps must be taken to immediately diagnose and treat the problem. Extreme caution should be exercised when extracting leads from patients with high venous pressure. Any compromise of the vasculature, especially of the superior vena cava above the pericardial reflection, can result in a rapid exsanguination into the pleural cavity.

Maintaining lead integrity: During the lead extraction process, large traction forces are placed on the lead. Few leads can tolerate the amount of traction required during the extraction process without breaking or unraveling. In many cases the insulation has been broken or cut, leaving only the coil to pull on and unravel. In order to maintain structural integrity and to provide some additional stiffness that will allow the extraction sheaths to track the lead safely, stylets that lock inside the conductor coil have been developed. As can be seen in figure 2, these stylets have undergone a significant evolution over the past decade. The first iteration locking stylet (Cook Vascular, Inc.) was the precisely sized stylet requiring sizing of the inner conductor coil to .001 of an inch. A supply of variously sized locking stylets had to be maintained at a great expense. These stylets were often difficult to place into the lead, especially if any foreign material or coil irregularity was present. The second iteration (Wilkoff[TM], Cook Vascular, Inc)) utilized a thin wire inside of a hollow stylet that caused a "barb" to protrude and lock into the lead. This still required measurement of the coil diameter, but each one of these stylets spanned 3 of the original stylet sizes. The third iteration (LLD - Lead Locking Device[TM], Spectranetics Inc.) uses a stylet with a stretched wire mesh. The stylet is inserted into the lead, the mesh is released and expands to lock into the lead. Three sizes of this stylet cover all lead models. The most recent iteration is a modification of the second stylet type (Liberator[TM], Cook Vascular Inc.). A tubular stylet has a thin wire with a spring at the end. When the tubular stylet is advanced over the spring end, the spring compresses and widens locking it into the lead. With this stylet, one size fits all leads. The LLD and Liberator stylets provide a very secure lock in the lead, and allow a large amount of force to be applied to the lead without compromise of the locking mechanism or the stylet itself.

Counter-Pressure: Most lead extraction experts feel that if they can advance the extraction sheath to the tip of the lead to apply counter-traction (see below), that the lead can be safely extracted. The problem has always been getting the sheaths through the binding sites and down to the tip. The use of "counter-pressure" is the technique of advancing the sheath system along the lead body with pressure, while using counter-pressure by keeping the lead taught. With non-powered sheaths such as Teflon[TM] or polypropylene, large forces may be required to advance the sheath through or over the adherent fibrous tissues. Powered sheaths were then introduced to allow significantly less pressure to be used in order to advance through the tissues, thus less counter-pressure is required as well (figure 3). The first powered sheath was introduced by Spectranetics, Inc., and utilized excimer laser energy to photo-ablate the fibrous tissues. This type of laser has a very short depth of penetration (100 microns), such that only tissues in intimate contact with the sheath's end will be affected by the energy. This was found to be significantly more effective than non-powered sheaths (Table 2).

Table 2. Extraction results using different sheath types.[3-7]

Sheath Type	Non-Powered	Laser	EDS
Complete Removal	86-93%	94%	95.9%
Partial Removal	4-6%	2.5%	3.5%
Failure to Remove	3-6%	3.3%	0.6%
Time to Extract	22-60 min	13.9 min	8.4 min
"Power" On Time	N/A	0.83 min	2.1 min
Complication Rate	1.6-1.8%	2.6%	2.6%

More recently, Cook Vascular has introduced the Electrosurgical Dissection Sheath (EDS[TM]) that uses a standard electrosurgical cautery unit to allow localized and directional cutting of the fibrous tissue. This device has also proven to be very effective relative to non-powered sheaths (Table 2). While powered sheaths have improved the speed and success rate of the extraction process, the hope that they would enhance the safety of lead extraction has not been realized as the complication rates have remained essentially unchanged (Table 2). However, that we are now able to remove more leads without an increase in complications is important as well.

Counter-Traction: Counter-traction provides the ability to "pluck" the lead from the myocardium without causing a tear or avulsion (figure 4). This is achieved by bracing the myocardium that resides immediately around the electrode tip, and passive fixation device if applicable. The difficulty occurs when attempting to advance the sheaths to the electrode-myocardial interface during the counter-pressure phase of the procedure.

In order to advance the sheaths around the curves of the vessels and to manipulate through the adhesions, a great deal of traction force may be required on the lead. At these times the ventricle may be inverted and even pulled into the area of the tricuspid valve. The operator is usually focusing all attention to the tip of the sheath, and may not notice that the ventricle is being compromised. It is said that nearly all leads can be safely removed if one is able to get the sheath system into a position to provide counter traction. This problem applies equally (and maybe even more so) to atrial leads that are imbedded into the much thinner atrial tissue.

Conclusion: The extraction of chronic pacing and defibrillator leads has become a common procedure. It can be performed effectively, and for the most part safely, given an appropriate indication and proper patient preparation. Attention to the possibility of an anomalous course of the pacing lead should always be considered, as this represents a very high risk to the patient during extraction. The operator should be familiar with all of the tools available, including multiple types of locking stylets, non-powered sheaths and powered sheaths. The more tools that the operator has available, the more likely that a successful procedure will take place. Finally, one must always be prepared for a vascular complication, and have the trained staff and backup resources available to salvage the patient.

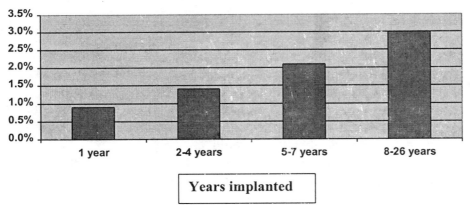

Years implanted

Figure 1a. Complication rate based on duration of implant. There is a positive correlation of higher complication rates with longer implant duration.

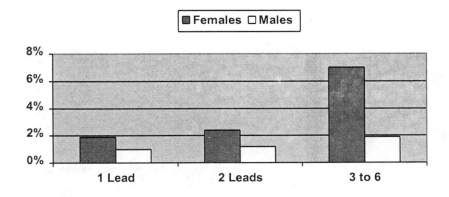

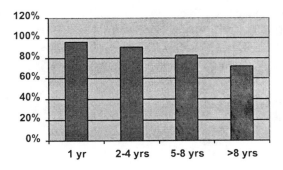

Figure 1b. Complication rate based on number of leads implanted and patient gender. More leads and female gender are correlated with higher complication rates.

Figure 1c. Success rate of total lead extraction relative to length of lead implant (pre-powered sheath era).

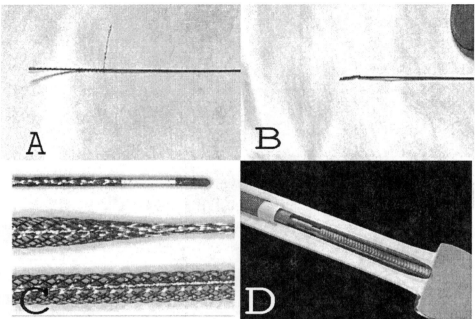

Figure 2. Different locking stylets. A) Original Cook stylet with wound wire at tip, B) "Wilkoff" stylet with barb exposed, C) Spectranetics LLD type with wire mesh, D) Cook "Liberator" with compressible spring wire at tip.

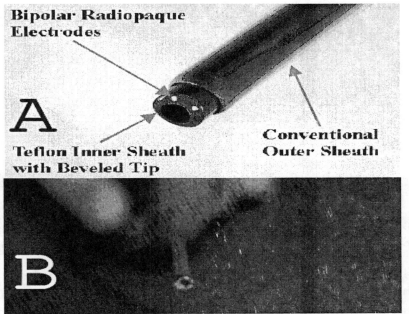

Figure 3. Powered sheaths. A) Cook Electrosurgical Dissection Sheath, B) Spectranetics Excimer Laser Sheath.

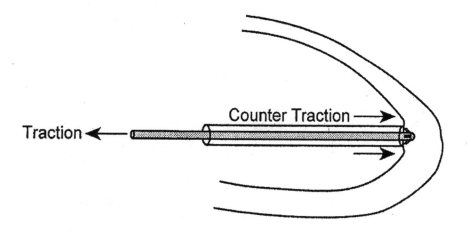

Figure 4. Traction forces on the myocardium from tension on the lead are balanced by Counter-Traction using the sheath.

References:
1. NASPE Policy conference on lead extraction.
2. Byrd CL, Schwartz SJ, Hedin N. Lead extraction: indications and techniques. Cardiol Clin 1992; 10:735-748
3. Wilkoff BL, Byrd CL, Love CJ, et al. Pacemaker Lead Extraction With the Laser Sheath: Results of the Pacing Lead Extraction With the Excimer Sheath (PLEXES) Trial. JACC 1999;33(6):1671-6
4. Love C, Byrd C, Wilkoff B, et al. Lead Extraction Using a Bipolar Electrosurgical Dissection Sheath. Europace 2001:223-228
5. Wilkoff BL, Byrd CL, Love CJ, et al. Trends in Intravascular Lead Extraction: Analysis of Data from 5339 Procedures in 10 Years PACE 1999; 22:A207
6. Byrd CL, Wilkoff BL, Love CJ, et al. Intravascular extraction of problematic or infected permanent pacemaker leads: 1994-1996. PACE 1999; 22:1346-1355.
7. Smith HJ, Fearnot NE, Byrd CL, et al. Five-years experience with intravascular lead extraction. PACE 1994; 17:2016-2020.

V. CARDIAC RESYNCHRONIZATION THERAPY
FOR PATIENTS WITH
CONGESTIVE HEART FAILURE

21

VENTRICULAR RESYNCHRONIZATION THERAPY IN HEART FAILURE: CURRENT EXPERIENCE AND FUTURE OUTCOMES

Jean-Claude Daubert, Christine Alonso, Christophe Leclercq

Department of Cardiology and Vascular Diseases, Centre Hospitalier Universitaire, Rennes, France

Whenever heart failure progresses into becoming refractory to drug treatment, clearly degrading patients' quality of life and leading to repeated hospitalisation for decompensation, pharmacological treatments are very restricted. Heart transplant remains the non-pharmacological treatment of choice. Unfortunately, it suffers from a very restricted access due to selection criteria and the increasing shortage of grafts. In 2000, only 370 transplantations where performed in France. Other non-pharmacological treatments are currently being evaluated, i.e., cellular cardiomyoplasty, (although that treatment, if validated, will only apply to ischemic heart failure with deep infarction sequelae), and left ventricular implantable assist device or artificial heart, which will always be cumbersome and costly procedures.

The need, therefore, is not questionable, for novel, simpler to implement and more economical therapeutical approaches susceptible to apply to a wider population of refractory heart failure patients, the majority of whom are elderly. Perhaps multisite pacing will meet that target, at least in certain patient categories!

I.   History of Heart Failure Electrical Treatment

Implantable pacemakers have hardly been used for more than ten years to treat heart failure. It started in 1990 when Hochleitner et al[1] reported a significant improvement of symptoms and of left ventricular systolic function indices following implantation of a standard dual chamber pacemaker (single ventricular lead sited on the apex of the right ventricle) in 17 patients with dilated cardiomyopathy and drug-refractory heart failure. None of these presented with any classic indications for cardiac pacing. Atrioventricular delay had been programmed to a short, set value of 100 ms in all cases. Despite consistency with other authors' reports[2-4], that short-term benefit was not confirmed in the mid- or long-term by either non-controlled or controlled studies[5-7]. Nishimura et al[8] in 1995 published a study with a probable explanation to that failure. These authors clearly showed that classic dual chamber pacing with individually

From Ovsyshcher IE. *New Developments in Cardiac Pacing and Electrophysiology.* Armonk, NY: Futura Publishing Company, Inc. ©2002.

optimised AV delay could improve cardiac performance only in patients with a long PR interval (> 200 ms) on surface ECG and presenting with echocardiographic signs of major mechanical AV delay in the left heart, i.e., very short ventricular filling time, A and E wave fusion on transmitral flux, evidence of the absence of atrial contribution to LV filling, diastolic mitral regurgitation... Conversely, pacing was constantly ineffective or even impaired heart performance when PR was not extended. Overall, it can be stated at this stage that classic dual chamber pacing can partially correct the deleterious consequences of major atrioventricular asynchrony secondary to prolonged PR and thus improve the clinical status of a few carefully selected patients, but can in no way be considered as a heart failure therapy per se.

A second approach was initiated in 1994 when Serge Cazeau[9] in France and Patricia Bakker[10] in the Netherlands described the first cases of DDD pacemakers implanted in patients with severe heart failure, but there again without any classic indications for permanent cardiac pacing. So the concept of *ventricular resynchronisation* by multisite biventricular pacing was born. It has since dramatically developed. This concept is mainly based upon : high prevalence of high-grade intraventricular conduction disorders in patients with chronic heart failure with, according to series, QRS duration >120 ms in 25 to 53% of cases and completel left branch block in 15 to 27% of patients[11,12] – gradual worsening of those ECG abnormalities with time and heart failure degradation[13] – their prognostic incidence: they are known to be independent predictive factors of mortality – lastly, their specific hemodynamic consequences : by desynchronising ventricular contraction et relaxation[14,15], they enhance the effects of baseline left ventricular dysfunction with additional impairment of systolic performance and ventricular filling and worsening of mitral regurgitation[14, 15].

II.   Acute Hemodynamic Studies during Temporary Pacing

The concept was validated in a large number of acute hemodynamic studies that tested the effects of atrio-biventricular pacing[16,18] and/or those of atrio left-ventricular pacing[19,21]. The results from those studies were perfectly consistent, with a significant increase in cardiac output (essentially with biventricular pacing), in systolic and differential arterial blood pressure, in left ventricular dP/dT (indirect contractility index) and a decrease in heart filling pressures (pulmonary artery and capillary pressures). Analysing pressure-volume curves showed that the improvement of left ventricular systolic performance was associated with improved ventricular filling. It is noteworthy that such an improved systolic performance was obtained without increasing O_2 myocardial consumption[22], which proves that the effects of ventricular resynchronisation are totally different from those of inotropic drugs. This acute benefit involves two complementary mechanisms:-ventricular resynchronisation, which improves coordination of the left ventricular wall contraction and relaxation - but also left atrioventricular resynchronisation, as achieved by classic dual chamber pacing in the presence of extended PR[8]. The respective contribution of each mechanism probably varies from one patient to another, but a number of experimental and clinical facts suggest that ventricular resynchronisation has the predominant role.

A bothering fact in those acute study results was the absence of a significant difference between the effects of atrio-biventricular pacing and those of left atrio-ventricular pacing, which questions the reality of the need to pace the right ventricle. Such a similarity in response was probably due to the fact that, in those patients with preserved atrioventricular conduction, atrio left-ventricular pacing induces a fusion of the intrinsic conduction which activates the RV free wall and a part of the septum within normal time and LV pre-excitation, which corrects free wall activation and contraction delay. The question remains whether such an optimised fusion can be durably sustained? The theoretical advantage of biventricular pacing is to fully capture the ventricular mass from two lead sites and to create stable activation, independent from intrinsic conduction changes (natural history and drug effects).

III.   Technical Aspects: How to Pace the Left Ventricle Safely and Efficiently ?

The main technical difficulty of that novel therapy is related to left ventricular pacing. Three different methods have been proposed to pace the left ventricle permanently. Early implantations (9, 10) used the epicardial route. But that method requires performing thoracotomy or thoracoscopy under general anesthesia, and the complicatiuon rate is still too high for progosing this approach as first intent. Some groups (22) have recently proposed to pace the left ventricle endocardially by using a screw-in lead introduced by a trans-septal approach. This technique is currently under clinical evaluation and has still to be considered as experimental.

The latter method, initially proposed by our group (23), is the most widely used. After transvenous (subclavian) insertion, a specifically-designed pacing lead is introduced into a tributary vein over the LV free wall through the coronary sinus (CS). Selective CS angiography, preferably with a ballon-tip catheter, helps to identify the target vein. There is a large consensus to-day to say that the optimal pacing site corresponds to the site of latest ventricular activation during intrinsic conduction (Figure 3). In most cases and particularly in patients with idiopathic dilated cardiomyopathy, this site is located on the lateral wall midway between the base and the apex. The target vein is indeed a lateral or postero-lateral vein. Other veins like the great cardiac vein for pacing the anterior wall or the middle cardiac vein for pacing the infero-apical region are only to be considered if there are no lateral or postero-lateral veins catheterizable.

Recent technological improvements with in particular the use of guiding sheats to facilitate CS catheterization, and new lead designs (small diameter leads, side-wire or over-the-wire technology similar to that used for coronary angioplasty) have significantly contributed to simplify the implantation procedure, increase the success rate and reduce the fluoroscopy time.

In parallel to the increasing experience of operators (with a clear learning curve), these technological advances were responsible for a dramatic decrease in the implantation - failure rate during the last few years. In our experience, the implantation success rate reached 90 % in 2000 when it was only 61 % in the very early experience before 1997 (24). The same trend was observed in the multicenter controlled studies, with an implantation success rate ranging from 87 % (Contak-CD trial) to 93 % (MUSTIC (29) and Miracle studies (30). In the two latter studies, the "target" vein i.e. a lateral or postero-lateral vein, could be reached in 75 % of cases. Furthermore the safety of the technique could be demonstrated. No peri-operative death was reported in controlled studies. In our own experience, we only observed two cases (2 %) of coronary sinus dissection or perforation, but without any significant clinical consequence.

By contrast with the left side, the optimal pacing site in the right ventricle still remains a matter of debate. In most cases the right ventricular lead is placed by facility at the apex. Further studies are needed to assess the optimal biventricular pacing configuration and to show in particular, if alternative right ventricular pacing sites like the septal wall, the anterior wall or the outflow tract are significantly better than the apex.

In patients with stable sinus rhythm, a third lead has to be implanted in the atrium, preferably at a septal site to provide more homogeneous atrial activation. The three leads are then connected to a triple-chamber pacemaker. The most recent devices have actually three independent chambers with the possibility to program pacing parameters in each chamber, but also to program a V-V delay (time interval between right and left ventricular stimulation) in order to optimize interventricular and left-intraventricular synchrony.

Finally AV synchrony in the left heart has to be optimized in each patient by using echo-Doppler techniques. Acute hemodynamic studies with temporary pacing[20,21] have clearly shown that the benefit of atrio-biventricular or atrio-LV based pacing resulted from both ventricular resynchronisation and AV resynchronisation at the left side.

IV. Clinical Experience of Permanent Biventricular Pacing

On those bases, the clinical effectiveness of *permanent biventricular pacing* was assessed in several non-controlled and controlled studies. The results from these observational studies[10,26,27] have now been published. The French pilot study[26] enrolled 53 patients between 1994 and 1996 in two centres, Rennes and Saint-Cloud ; it was the only study to report data on the long-term effects of that therapeutics[26]. The InSync study[27] enrolled 103 patients in 16 European and Canadian centres in 1997 and 1998 and confirmed the feasibility of a fully transvenous implantation technique with a 88% success rate[27]. The results from these two studies suggest that atrio-biventricular pacing significantly and durably improves symptoms (NYHA classification), exercise tolerance and the well-being (quality of life) of class III or IV patients selected because of their refractoriness to optimal medical treatment, high grade LV systolic dysfunction and spontaneous QRS duration > 150 ms on surface ECG.

Those studies also showed that the mortality rate remained high in those patients, i.e., 20% at 1 year in the InSync study, which included a majority of patients in NYHA class III and 25% (40% at 2 years) in the French pilot study which included a majority of NYHA class IV patients. Those mortality rates were close to those of control groups in major pharmacological trials performed at the same time to test the effects of beta-blockers (CIBIS II, MERIT-HF, COPERNICUS ...), spironolactone (RALES) or angiotensin receptor inhibitors (ELITE II).

Results from another four controlled studies have recently been published: PATH-CHF[28] MUSTIC[29], MIRACLE[30] and CONTAK-CD .

The data collected in the PATH-CHF[28] study are difficult to interpret because of methodological problems: too few patients recruited over a long period of almost four years; fitting of a very complex pacing system; effectiveness assessment of a so-called "optimal pacing configuration" varying between patients according to the results of an acute hemodynamic perioperative study at the origin of additional heterogeneity in the study population.

The MUSTIC[29] study used a much simpler experimental design aimed at testing the clinical effectiveness of atrio-biventricular pacing by comparison with no pacing at all during two 3-month cross-over periods. The European multicenter study enrolled 131 patients in one year to reveal that atrial biventricular pacing increased exercise tolerance (walking test) by 23% on average ($p < 0.0001$), improved quality of life by 32 % on average ($p < 0.0001$) and reduced the number of hospitalisations for decompensated heart failure to one third ($p < 0.03$). The range of effects noted (exercise tolerance and quality of life) appeared to exceed all that had previously been reported with the various drug classes, converting enzyme inhibitors in particular. MUSTIC also for the first time provided objective proof of the therapeutic interest of atrio-biventricular pacing in patients with severe heart failure without any classic indication for pacemaker implantation.

The MIRACLE study[30] included 266 patients who were selected from the same criteria as MUSTIC except for QRS duration, whose threshold was 130 ms. Transvenous implantation of an atrio-biventricular pacemaker was attempted in all patients. The implantation success rate was 93%. Successful patients were randomised into two parallel groups. In one group, pacemakers were programmed as active (atrio-biventricular mode) whereas in the other group pacing was inactivated. Patients were then followed-up for six months. The primary assessment criterion was functional tolerance, as assessed according to NYHA classification, the 6-minute walking test and quality of life score. These three parameters were significantly improved in the «active» group ($p < 0.001$ for NYHA classification, < 0.003 for the distance walked and < 0.03 for quality of life score). Additional analysis of a composite assessment criterion which combined survival rate, hospitalisations for decompensated heart failure, drug treatment modifications and functional tolerance revealed that 66% of patients were improved in the active group vs only 32% in the inactive group ($p < 0.001$). The number of hospitalisation days for decompensated heart failure was 5 times lower in the active group ($p < 0.03$). Eight deaths were recorded in the active group and 10 in the inactive group during that 6-month observation period.

The CONTAK-CD study (unpublished data, presented during the European Society of Cardiology meeting in Stockholm, August 2001) differed from the MIRACLE study in that it only included patients with chronic heart failure and an "accepted" indication for an implantable automatic defibrillator. They were all implanted with an endocavitary system which combined atrio-biventricular pacing with automatic defibrillation. Another specificity of that study was that it was possible to include patients with moderate or mild heart failure (class II, NYHA). Eighty-seven per cent of the 581 patients included could be successfully implanted and randomised into two parallel groups. Biventricular pacing was active in one group and inactive in the other one. The main study criterion was a composite one associating death from all causes, hospitalisations for decompensated heart failure and appropriate therapies for VT/VF. With a mean perspective of 4.5 months, a favourable trend (21% decrease in the number of events) can be noted in favour of active pacing, although the difference was not statistically significant due to a smaller-than-expected overall number of events. With regard to functional tolerance, as assessed from the VO_2 peak during cardio-respiratory exercise test, the distance covered in 6 minutes and the quality of life score, no significant difference could be noted between the two groups when all the patients included were taken into account. In contrast, significant benefit was noted in favour of active pacing ($p < 0.001$ for VO_2 peak; $p < 0.03$ for QOL scores) when only those patients with severe heart failure (NYHA III and IV) were taken into account.

Overall, that very significant - albeit preliminary - clinical experience, owing to the large number of patients included in controlled studies, confirmed that cardiac resynchronisation very significantly improves exercise tolerance and quality of life in patients with severe heart failure (NYHA class III or IV) who also present with ECG evidence of major ventricular asynchrony. The number of hospitalisations for decompensation is significantly reduced. The effect on mortality has yet to be elucidated, but there is no indication that biventricular pacing might induce overmortality, Lastly, beneficial effects persisted beyond one year, as confirmed by the recent publication of the MUSTIC long-term follow-up[31].

Those four studies, however, are only the first step towards clinical evaluation of this new treatment. Additional studies are necessary to determine its global impact, especially its influence on overall and sudden mortality, on morbidity, the costs of management and the cost/effectiveness ratio. Such new trials will have to compare two parallel groups of patients over long periods of time, one group being administered only the optimal medical treatment and the other receiving optimal medical treatment plus implantation of multisite pacemakers or biventricular pacemakers-defibrillators. Those studies have just been initiated. They have been named CARE – HF[32] in Europe and COMPANION[33] in North America. They should include between 800 and 2400 patients, i.e., the usual size of major drug trials. It is likely that it will take three years to secure the first results.

In the meantime, other questions yet unresolved will perhaps be answered: How can patient selection be improved and how can the degree of spontaneous ventricular asynchrony be assessed? It will probably be necessary to complement or replace classic ECG criteria (QRS duration, left bundle branch block) by new mechanical criteria provided by cardiac imaging techniques – what is the best ventricular pacing configuration : biventricular or uni left-ventricular? On which site(s): a single or several LV sites? Do biventricular or left ventricular pacing have an antiarrhythmic effect or conversely a pro-arrhythmic one (risk of tachycardia or ventricular fibrillation) in heart failure patients? Answers to that question will predominantly guide the choice of implantable devices to be developed by priority : multisite pacemakers alone or multifunction devices associating multisite pacing and automatic defibrillation...?

Conclusion

Meanwhile, the number of implantations will probably keep increasing. Hopefully, they will be performed by priority within the scope of major morbidity-mortality studies or of more specific trials designed to find answers to the above questions. Otherwise, those implantations will have to remain within the strict boundaries of the sole indication validated by the MUSTIC and MIRACLE studies, i.e., patients with severe heart failure expressed by LV systolic dysfunction (EF <35% ; telediastole diameter >55 mm), with a QRS duration >130 ms on surface ECG and who are severely impaired (NYHA class III or IV) despite optimal drug treatment, possibly including converting enzyme inhibitors or their equivalent and beta-blockers at the maximum tolerable dose.

References

1. Hochleitner M, Hortnagl H, Choi-Keung Ng, Hortnagl M, Gschnitzer F, Zechmann W. Usefulness of physiologic dual-chamber pacing in drug-resistant idiopathic dilated cardiomyopathy. Am J Cardiol 1990;66:198-202.
2. Brecker SJ, Xiao HB, Sparrow J, Gibson DG. Effects of dual-chamber pacing with short atrioventricular delay in dilated cardiomyopathy. Lancet 1992 ; 340 : 1308-11
3. Auricchio A, Sommariva L, Salo RW, Scafuri A, Chiariello L. Improvement of cardiac function in patients with severe congestive heart failure and coronary disease by dual-chamber pacing with shortened AV delay. Pacing Clin Electrophysiol 1993 ; 16 : 2034-43
4. Scanu P, Lecluze E, Michel L et al. Effets de la stimulation double-chambre temporaire dans l'insuffisance cardiaque réfractaire. Arch. Mal. Cœur 1996 ; 89 : 1643-9

5. Linde C, Gadler F, Edner M ; Nordlander R, Rosenqvist M ; Ryden L. Results of atrioventricular synchronous pacing with optimized delay in patients with severe congestive heart failure. Am J Cardiol 1995;75: 919-23

6. Gold MR, Feliciano Z, Gotdieb SS, Fisher ML. Dual-chamber pacing with a short atrioventricular delay in congestive heart failure : a randomized study. J Am Coll Cardiol 1995 ; 26 : 967-73

7. Capucci A, Romaro S, Puglisi A et al. Dual-chamber pacing with optimal AV delay in congestive heart failure. Europace 1999; 1 : 174-8

8. Nishimura RA, Hayes DL, Homes DR Jr, Tajik AJ. Mechanism of hemodynamic improvement by dual-chamber pacing for severe left ventricular dysfunction : an acute Doppler and catheterization study. J Am Coll Cardiol 1995 ; 25 : 281-8

9. Cazeau S, Ritter P, Bakdach S et al. Four chamber pacing in dilated cardiomyopathy. Pacing Clin Electrophysiol 1994 ; 17 : 1974-9

10. Bakker PF, Meijburg H, De Vries JW, et al. Biventricular pacing in end-stage heart failure improves functional capacity and left ventricular function. J Intervent Card Electrophysiol 2000;4:395-404.

11. Aaronson K, Schwartz S, Chen T, Wong K, Goin J, Mancini D. Development and prospective validation of a clinical index to predict survival in ambulatory patients referred for cardiac transplant evaluation. Circulation 1997; 95 : 2660-7

12. Farwell D, Patel NR, Hall A, Ralph A, Sulke AN. How many people with heart failure are appropriate for biventricular resynchronization ? Eur. Heart J 2000 ; 21 : 1246-50

13. Wilensky RL, Yudelman P, Cohen AI, et al. Serial electrocardiographic changes in idiopathic dilated cardiomyopathy confirmed at necropsy. Am J Cardiol 1988; 62:276-83

14. Xiao HB, Brecker SJD, Gibson DG. Effect of abnormal activation on the time course of the left ventricular pressure pulse in dilated cardiomyopathy. Br Heart J 1992 ; 68 : 403-7

15. Zhou Q, Henein M, Coats A, Gibson D. Different effects of abnormal activation and myocardial disease on left ventricular ejection and filling times. Heart 2000 ; 84 : 272-6

16. Foster AH, Gold MR, McLaughlin JS. Acute hemodynamic effects of atriobiventricular pacing in humans. Ann Thorac Surg 1995;59:294-300

17. Cazeau S, Ritter P, Lazarus A, et al. Multisite pacing for end-stage heart failure : early experience. PACE 1996; 19:1748-57

18. Leclercq C, Cazeau S, Le Breton H, et al. Acute hemodynamic effects of biventricular DDD pacing in patients with end-stage heart failure. J Am Coll Cardiol 1998 ; 32 : 1825-31

19. Blanc JJ, Etienne Y, Gilard M, et al. Evaluation of different ventricular pacing sites in patients with severe heart failure. Circulation 1997; 96: 3273-77

20. Kass DA, Chen CH, Curry et al. Improved left ventricular mechanics from acute VDD pacing in patients with dilated cardiomyopathy and intraventricular conduction delay. Circulation 1999 ; 99 : 1567-73

21. Auricchio A, Stellbrink C, Block M. et al. The effect of pacing chamber and atrio-ventricular delay on acute systolic function of paced patients with congestive heart failure. Circulation 1999; 99:2993-3001

22. Nelson GS, Berger RD, Fetics BJ, et al. Left ventricular or biventricular pacing improves cardiac function at diminished energy cost in patients with dilated cardiomyopathy and left bundle-branch block. Circulation 2000 ; 102 : 3053-9.

23. Jais P, Douard H, Shah DC, et al. Endocardial biventricular pacing. Pacing Clin Electrophysiology 1998;21: 2128-31.

24. Daubert JC, Ritter P, Le Breton H, et al. Permanent left ventricular pacing with transvenous leads inserted into the coronary veins. Pacing Clin Electrophysiology 1998 ; 21 : 239-45.

25. Alonso C, Leclercq C, Revault d'Allonnes F, et al. Six-year experience of transvenous left ventricular lead implantation for permanent biventricular pacing in patients with advanced heart failure. Heart 2001; 86:405-10.

26. Leclercq C, Cazeau S, Ritter P, et al. A pilot experience with permanent biventricular pacing to treat advanced heart failure. Am Heart J 2000;140:862-70.

27. Gras D, Mabo P, Tang T et al. Multisite pacing as a supplemental treatment of congestive heart failure: preliminary results of the Medtronic InSync study. PACE 1998; 21:2249-55

28. Auricchio A, Stellbrink C, Sack S, et al. 2000. Chronic benefit as a result of pacing in congestive heart failure : results of the PATH-CHF trial. Circulation 102 : 3352A

29. Cazeau S, Leclercq C, Lavergne T et al. Effects of multisite biventricular pacing in patients with heart failure and intraventricular conduction delay. N Eng J Med 2001 ; 344 : 873-80.

30. Abraham WT, Fisher WG, Smith AL, et al. Multicenter InSync randomized clinical evaluation (MIRACLE) : results of a double-blind, controlled trial to assess cardiac resynchronization therapy in heart failure patients. J Am Coll Cardiol 2001 ; 38 : 604-5.

31. Linde C, Cazeau S, Kappenberger L, Sutton R, Bailleul C, Daubert JC. Long-term benefits of biventricular pacing in congestive heart failure. One-year results from patients in sinus rhythm in the MUSTIC study. Eur Heart J 2001 ; 22 : 129 (Abstr.).

32. Cleland JGF, Daubert JC, Erdmann E, et al. The CARE-HF study (CArdiac REsynchronization in Heart Failure study) : rationale, design and end-points. Eur J Heart Failure 2001 ; 3 : 481-89.

33. Bristow MR, Feldman AM and Saxon LA. Heart failure management using implantable devices for ventricular resynchronization: comparison of medical therapy, pacing and defibrillation in chronic heart failure (COMPANION) trial. COMPANION Steering Committee and COMPANION Clinical Investigators. J Card Fail 2000; 6:276-85.

22

CARDIAC RESYNCHRONIZATION THERAPY: THE AMERICAN EXPERIENCE

David L. Hayes, MD

Consultant, Division of Cardiovascular Diseases and Internal Medicine, Mayo Clinic, Professor of Medicine, Mayo Medical School; Rochester, Minnesota 55905.

The American cardiology community has seemingly embraced, with enthusiasm, cardiac resynchronization therapy (CRT) for patients with congestive heart failure. Admittedly, much of the initial investigation of cardiac resynchronization was accomplished in Europe and Canada. After these earlier investigations, both observational and controlled, a number of randomized, controlled studies were undertaken in the United States.

A discussion of the "American experience" with cardiac resynchronization cannot be undertaken without some understanding of the previous and current investigations and clinical experience in Europe and Canada. This information is detailed in another chapter in this text and will not be repeated here. However, the reader is encouraged to become familiar with the data in that chapter as well.

In addition, given the rapidly evolving and changing landscape of CRT, any discussion of this topic suffers from the lag in publication and any new information that has surfaced in the interim.

American Experience to Date

The American experience with cardiac resynchronization therapy can be divided into FDA-sanctioned trials, "off-label" application of biventricular pacing, and "open-label" experience since the approval of the first cardiac resynchronization device.

In the long term, it is not known whether the device of choice for heart failure patients will be a "stand-alone" cardiac resynchronization device or one that also incorporates an implantable cardioverter defibrillator (ICD). Undoubtedly the results of ongoing trials of ICD therapy for primary prevention of sudden cardiac death in patients with heart failure or significant left ventricular dysfunction will be a deciding factor in which type of device will become most commonly used. For this reason, this manuscript will also include a brief discussion of the existing and ongoing American trials of ICD use for primary prevention of sudden cardiac death in patients with heart failure.

It should also be mentioned at the outset that the American experience has included important contributions to the understanding of

From Ovsyshcher IE. *New Developments in Cardiac Pacing and Electrophysiology.* Armonk, NY: Futura Publishing Company, Inc. ©2002.

the mechanisms of pacing in congestive heart failure. Some of this experience was with standard dual-chamber pacing[1,2] and some with CRT. In an acute hemodynamic assessment of various pacing configurations on left ventricular efficiency, Kass and colleagues[3] demonstrated that pacing only the left ventricle in patients with severe left ventricular dysfunction who have left bundle-branch block results, in some patients, in a hemodynamic response as good as or better than that to biventricular pacing. Minimizing intraventricular and interventricular dyssynchrony has been shown to improve global left ventricular function and to result in functional improvement. Pacing only from specific left ventricular sites may also reduce the abnormal left ventricular activation and improve contraction efficiency.[4]

Specific Applications and Studies

"Off-label" Application of Biventricular Pacing

On the subject of "off-label" application, no data are available. "Off-label" CRT is accomplished by utilizing a standard dual-chamber pacemaker or ICD, implanting standard right atrial and right ventricular pacing or defibrillation leads, and using some available pacing lead in a coronary venous position. As of this writing, 2 coronary sinus leads have been approved for use in the United States (Medtronic, Inc. models 2187 and 2188). Before Food and Drug Administration (FDA)-approved coronary sinus leads were available, some clinicians reported anecdotally that they used standard tined ventricular pacing leads and positioned them in the coronary venous tree, often after "trimming" the tines on the lead.

Information regarding "off-label" CRT is limited to unpublished discussions of such experience and limited case reports. At least 1 case report exists regarding "off-label" use for cardiac resynchronization and defibrillation which described abnormalities in the determination and sensing of ventricular arrhythmias occurring as a result of the "second" lead.[5]

Only 1 manufacturer makes the "Y" connector and the rumored increase in sales of this adaptor is coincident with the period of time before approval of the first cardiac resynchronization device. Nonetheless, no absolute numbers are available regarding "off-label" cardiac resynchronization in the United States.

Controlled Trials of Biventricular Pacing in the United States

A number of trials merit discussion. The trials that are included in this manuscript are those that are primarily "American."

VIGOR-CHF

This Guidant Corporation-sponsored trial was among the first resynchronization studies undertaken in the United States.[6] The VIGOR-CHF trial design is shown in Figure 1. Endpoints were improvement in functional capacity measured by peak VO_2 and 6-minute hall walk, improvement in quality of life measured by the Minnesota Living with Heart Failure score and the New York Heart Association (NYHA) class, improvement in functional status measured by left ventricular ejection fraction, Doppler-derived cardiac output, right ventricular systolic pressure, and left ventricular filling pattern. Safety was determined by the incidence of adverse events. The trial, started in 1996, antedated left ventricular pacing via the coronary veins. The study was closed after 73 patients were enrolled. Although some published data exist regarding VIGOR-CHF patients, results of the complete trial have not been published.

VENTAK-CHF/CONTAK-CD

This trial, initiated by the Guidant Corporation in 1998 as VENTAK-CHF, is the first study to evaluate the impact of CRT on the progression of heart failure, mortality, hospitalization, and ventricular tachycardia.[7] The device provided biventricular pacing and internal cardioversion/defibrillation. The trial design is shown in Figure 2. With the evolution of hardware and technique which occurred during the course of VENTAK-CHF, the transvenous CONTAK-CD device became available investigationally, and the same trial design was continued as CONTAK-CD.

The endpoints included progression of heart failure, peak VO_2, Minnesota Living with Heart Failure score, efficacy of antitachycardia pacing conversion, device safety and performance, and safety of the EASYTRAK over-the-wire coronary venous lead. Major exclusion criteria included indications for a pacemaker, presence of chronic atrial tachyarrhythmias, need for concomitant cardiac surgery, life expectancy of less than 6 months, requirement for in-hospital intravenous inotropes, and pregnancy.

As of this writing, the CONTAK-CD device had not gained FDA approval and no formal manuscript had been published. The data included here are available from the FDA website.[8]

A total of 581 patients were enrolled, of whom 248 were from an original crossover design (Phase I) and 333 patients were from the subsequent parallel design (Phase II). (The change in trial design was required by the FDA.) Of the 581 patients, 501 had the CONTAK-CD device implanted. In addition, 66 patients underwent an implant procedure but did not receive the CONTAK-CD device and 14 patients were withdrawn before having the implantation. A total of 490 patients were randomized. The demographics of the study patients were as follows:

Sex	Male 83%, female 17%
Age	66 ± 11 years
NYHA class	II 33%, III 58%, IV 9%
Ejection fraction	21 ± 7%
Conduction defect	LBBB 57%, RBBB 13%, nonspecific intraventricular conduction delay 30%
Etiology	Ischemic 69%, nonischemic 31%
QRS duration	158 ± 27 ms

The change in NYHA classification is shown in Figure 3.

When the 3 primary endpoints were assessed—death from any cause, heart failure-related hospitalization, and ventricular tachycardia/ventricular fibrillation events—they failed to achieve statistical significance either as a composite or individually, as shown in Table 1.

Table 1.—Assessment of Endpoints in VENTAK-CHF Trial

Composite endpoint event	CRT (n = 245)		NCRT (n = 245)		Overall reduction in original composite endpoint	Overall reduction in modified composite endpoint
	No.	%	No.	%		
Death from any cause	11	4.5	16	6.5	19% $P = 0.21$	23% $P = 0.11$
Hospitalizations	31	12	37	15.1		
AE for HF	15	6.1	28	11.4		
Recurrent VT/VF	33	13.5	37	15.1		

AE, adverse event; CRT, cardiac resynchronization therapy; HF, heart failure; NCRT, no cardiac resynchronization therapy; VT/VF, ventricular tachycardia/ventricular fibrillation.

When a subgroup analysis of advanced heart failure patients was performed, the "event rates" were much closer to what had been expected but still did not reach statistical significance, as shown in Table 2. However, despite the lack of statistical significance, there was a reduction in events for each of the endpoints, along with a reduction in the composite endpoint, signifying overall clinical improvement in terms of progression of heart failure.

Table 2.—Subgroup Analysis of Endpoints in VENTAK-CHF Trial

Composite endpoint event	CRT (n = 117)		NCRT (n = 109)		Overall reduction in original composite endpoint	Overall reduction in modified composite endpoint
	No.	%	No.	%		
Death from any cause	11	9.4	10	9.2	25% $P = 0.19$	29% $P = 0.11$
Hospitalizations	22	18.8	26	23.9		
AE for HF	11	9.4	17	15.6		
Recurrent VT/VF	20	17.1	19	17.4		

AE, adverse event; CRT, cardiac resynchronization therapy; HF, heart failure; NCRT, no cardiac resynchronization therapy; VT/VF, ventricular tachycardia/ventricular fibrillation.

In addition, echocardiographic data were consistent with left ventricular "reverse-remodeling," with a reduction in left ventricular internal systolic and diastolic dimension. Also noted was a significant improvement in VO_2 after CRT. The EASYTRAK coronary venous lead was shown to be safe and reliable, with a 91% first implant success rate.

Several specific manuscripts related to these initial Guidant protocols warrant discussion. An interesting substudy analysis of patients from the original VENTAK-ICD was performed by Higgins et al.[9] to determine whether the application of biventricular pacing affected the incidence of ventricular tachycardia/ventricular fibrillation. Although cardiac resynchronization may not obviate ICD therapy, it appears to significantly diminish the number of appropriate ICD therapy episodes (antitachycardia pacing + shocks).

Another widely quoted analysis combining patients from VIGOR-CHF and VENTAK-CHF assessed norepinephrine levels after biventricular pacing.[10] In this study, patients who had the greatest increase in norepinephrine levels before cardiac resynchronization demonstrated a statistically significant decrease in norepinephrine levels after 12 weeks of active therapy (Fig. 4).

Although the CONTAK-CD pulse generator had not been approved by the FDA at the time of this writing, it is expected to be approved no later than the first quarter of 2002.

COMPANION

The COMPANION (Comparison of Medical Therapy, Pacing and Defibrillation in Chronic Heart Failure) trial involves 80 centers in the United States and up to 2,200 patients.[11] It is the first controlled study to evaluate the effects of CRT on mortality and hospitalization. Inclusion criteria and trial design are shown in Figure 5. Primary endpoints are a reduction in all-cause mortality and all-cause hospitalization. Secondary endpoints are reduction in cardiac morbidity, peak VO_2 and EASYTRAK lead performance.

InSync (MIRACLE)

InSync and MIRACLE are synonymous. InSync was preceded by InSync-OUS (out of United States), a noncontrolled, open-label observational trial performed in Europe and Canada.[12] Medtronic, Inc., the sponsor of InSync-OUS, continued with a randomized, controlled, double-blind study known initially and throughout the study as MIRACLE, for Multicenter InSync Randomized Clinical Evaluation.[13] After completion of the study, it has been referred to as InSync, the name of the cardiac resynchronization pulse generator that gained approval on the basis of this investigation.

The design of the study is shown in Figure 6. Patients were initially randomized to biventricular pacing or "no" pacing for 6 months. At 6 months, patients in the control group were allowed to cross over to active therapy, and crossover was essentially 100%. Inclusion criteria included patients with NYHA functional class III or IV heart failure, left ventricular ejection fraction $\leq$ 35%, left ventricular end-diastolic dimension $\geq$ 55 mm, QRS duration > 130 ms, and a stable heart failure medical regimen for $\geq$ 1 month. Primary endpoints were 6-minute hall walk, quality of life, and NYHA class. A total of 532 patients were randomized.

The overall results of the trial have not yet been published, and data presented here were taken from the FDA website.[14] Improvement was shown in all 3 primary endpoints: quality of life (QOL) as determined by the Minnesota Living with Heart Failure questionnaire with a 9-unit improvement, $P = 0.003$; NYHA class with 1 class improvement, $P < 0.001$; and 6-minute hall walk with 30-meter improvement, $P = 0.003$ (Fig. 7). A summary of single endpoints and a combination of various endpoints in the InSync study is as follows:

	Control (%)	Treatment (%)	P value
Primary endpoints met			
NYHA functional class	37.9	67.6	< 0.001
QOL score	44.0	57.6	0.017
6-Minute hall walk	27.1	45.4	< 0.001
More than one endpoint met			
Hall walk and QOL score	18.1	32.6	0.003
Hall walk and NYHA class	14.8	37.6	< 0.001
QOL score and NYHA class	25.9	47.1	< 0.001
All 3 endpoints	12.0	29.7	< 0.001

A number of secondary endpoints were also evaluated. The study demonstrated an improvement in VO_2 max and median values of 14.2 mL/kg per minute at baseline to a 6-month median value of 13.9 mL/kg per minute in the control group versus 14.1 mL/kg per minute at baseline to a 6-month value of 16.0 mL/kg per minute in the CRT group. QRS duration improved by a median paired difference of 20 ms. Multiple echocardiographic parameters demonstrated improvement consistent with left ventricular remodeling with CRT. These included improvements in left ventricular ejection fraction (%), $P < 0.001$; left ventricular systolic volume (cm^3), $P < 0.001$; left ventricular diastolic volume (cm^3), $P < 0.001$; left ventricular mass (g), $P = 0.006$; and interventricular mechanical delay (ms) $P < 0.001$; and reduction in mitral regurgitation (cm^2, jet area), $P < 0.001$.

InSync ™ III Study

This study involves patients with NYHA class III and IV heart failure and ventricular dyssynchrony. Eligible patients may not have a standard indication for either a pacemaker or a defibrillator. The InSync™ III study evaluates safety and efficacy of cardiac resynchronization therapy but specifically assesses the potential benefit of altering V-V timing. This study is still enrolling patients, with 450 patients enrolled as of 12/2001.

InSync-ICD

This study, as the name implies, assessed the Medtronic InSync device with ICD therapy incorporated. The inclusion criteria were essentially the same as for InSync, with the addition of a disturbance in ventricular rhythm, which met accepted indications for ICD therapy. The study design was also essentially the same as that for InSync. Patients were randomized to cardiac resynchronization therapy "on" or "off," and ICD therapy was activated in all patients.

A total of 575 patients were initially enrolled in the study, and the study was then expanded for an additional 130 patients. Data have been submitted to the FDA for approval of the device, and results of the study are expected to be presented in the spring of 2002.

VecToR

The VecToR (Ventricular Resynchronization Therapy Randomized) trial is a St. Jude-sponsored study involving 40 centers worldwide and an estimated 420 patients (Fig. 8).[15] The primary objective is to evaluate the efficacy of biventricular pacing. The study will also evaluate quality of life, echocardiographic measurements, and patient mortality. Inclusion criteria include NYHA class II to IV heart failure, ejection fraction < 35%, QRS ≥ 140 ms, and left ventricular end diastolic dimension ≥ 54 mm.

PAVE

This is another St. Jude-sponsored trial, involving left ventricular post-atrioventricular nodal ablation evaluation (Fig. 9).[16] This study is not limited to the United States but involves 65 centers worldwide and an estimated 600 patients. Inclusion criteria are patients who have had atrioventricular nodal ablation, have had 3 months of stable medical therapy, are capable of a 6-minute walk, and are in NYHA class II or III. The study is powered to evaluate the effect of atrial fibrillation, patients' exercise tolerance, and quality of life with left ventricular or biventricular stimulation compared with right ventricular stimulation.

There are limited data to date regarding cardiac resynchronization in patients with chronic atrial fibrillation. If "positive," PAVE will be important in confirming the MUSTIC-AF data.[17]

Large Trials of ICD Therapy for Primary Prevention of Sudden Cardiac Death in Patients With Congestive Heart Failure

MADIT-II

The MADIT-II (Multi-center Automatic Defibrillator Implantation Trial) was a prospective, randomized, multicenter trial that enrolled more than 1,200 patients in 71 centers in the United States and 5 European centers (Fig. 10).[18] It was designed to determine whether ICDs improve survival when compared with use of drug therapy alone after myocardial infarction in patients with moderate left ventricular dysfunction. The trial was terminated early because the use of an ICD significantly reduced mortality from sudden cardiac death in this group of patients. Mortality in the group randomized to pharmacologic therapy was 19% compared with a mortality of 14% in the ICD arm, for a 30% reduction in mortality with ICD therapy.

SCD-HeFT

This study (the Sudden Cardiac Death in Heart Failure Trial) is included in this manuscript even though it, like MADIT-II, is not a study of CRT (Fig. 11).[19] It recruited patients with NYHA class II and III heart failure to evaluate whether primary prevention of ventricular tachycardia/ventricular fibrillation will reduce mortality in patients with heart failure. Like the MADIT-II trial, SCD-HEFT, if positive, would significantly alter the indications for primary prevention therapy of sudden cardiac death in the heart failure population. This would give further impetus to implantation of a device that provided both CRT and ICD therapy. SCD-HEFT enrollment is complete, and results are expected in 2003.

Conclusions

As of 2001, the American experience with cardiac resynchronization is still relatively limited. However, the paucity of the data has not prevented many American caregivers from becoming enthusiastic about the therapy. With the availability of the first FDA-approved CRT device, the number of implants in the United States is increasing and the expected approval of the first CRT/ICD devices will further increase these numbers.

On the basis of available data, the newly revised American College of Cardiology/American Heart Association/North American Society of Pacing and Electrophysiology Guidelines for Indications for Pacemakers and ICDs will update the recommendations for cardiac resynchronization devices. Although not yet endorsed by the 3 professional associations, the proposed recommendations for CRT are:

Class I – Symptomatic sinus node dysfunction, atrioventricular block, or other accepted indication for prevention of bradycardia

Class IIa – Biventricular pacing in medically refractory, symptomatic patients with cardiomyopathy (ischemic or dilated) and associated interventricular conduction delay

Given the need to learn a new technique of coronary venous permanent lead placement and the learning curve involved, training requirements for implantation of a CRT device are also being considered early in the American experience. An update of the *NASPE Training Guidelines for Cardiac Implantable Electronic Devices: Selection, Implantation, and Follow-up* is nearing completion and, once approved, will provide recommendations for training requirements in the implantation of CRT devices (Hayes DL, preliminary data, December 2001).

References

1. Nishimura RA, Hayes DL, Holmes DR Jr, et al.: Mechanism of hemodynamic improvement by dual-chamber pacing for severe left ventricular dysfunction: an acute Doppler and catheterization hemodynamic study. J. Am Coll Cardiol 1995; 25:281-288.
2. Gold MR, Feliciano Z, Gottlieb SS, et al.: Dual-chamber pacing with a short atrioventricular delay in congestive heart failure: a randomized study. J. Am Coll Cardiol 1995; 26:967-972.
3. Kass DA, Chen CH, Curry C, et al.: Improved left ventricular mechanics from acute VDD pacing in patients with delayed cardiomyopathy and ventricular conduction delay. Circulation 1999; 99:1567-1573.
4. Gerber TC, Nishimura RA, Holmes DR Jr, et al.: Left ventricular and biventricular pacing in congestive heart failure. Mayo Clin Proc 2001; 76:803-812.
5. Schreieck J, Zrenner B, Kolb C, et al.: Inappropriate shock delivery due to ventricular double detection with a biventricular pacing implantable cardioverter defibrillator. Pacing Clin Electrophysiol 2001; 24:1154-1157.
6. Saxon LA, Boehmer JP, Hummel J, et al.: Biventricular pacing in patients with congestive heart failure: two prospective randomized trials. The VIGOR CHF and VENTAK CHF Investigators. Am J Cardiol 1999; 83:120D-123D.

7. Daoud E, Hummel J, Gold M, et al.: Impact of biventricular pacing on mortality in a randomized crossover study of patients with heart failure and ventricular arrhythmias (abstract). PACE 2000; 23:569.

8. Preliminary Clinical Review of Guidant's CONTAK CD/CONTAK Renewal Heart Failure Devices and EASYTRAK Lead System PMA. Retrieved December 17, 2001, from the World Wide Web: http://www.fda.gov/cdrh/panel/briefing/071001-t1-review.pdf

9. Higgins SL, Yong P, Sheck D, et al.: Biventricular pacing diminishes the need for implantable cardioverter defibrillator therapy. VENTAK CHF Investigators. J. Am Coll Cardiol 2000; 36:824-827.

10. Saxon L, DeMarco T, Chatterjee K, et al.: Chronic biventricular pacing decreases serum norepinephrine in dilated heart failure patients with the greatest sympathetic activation at baseline (abstract). PACE 1999; 22:830.

11. Bristow MR, Feldman AM, Saxon LA: Heart failure management using implantable devices for ventricular resynchronization: Comparison of Medical Therapy, Pacing, and Defibrillation in Chronic Heart Failure (COMPANION) trial. COMPANION Steering Committee and COMPANION Clinical Investigators. J. Card Fail 2000; 6:276-285.

12. Gras D, Mabo P, Tang T, et al.: Multisite pacing as a supplemental treatment of congestive heart failure: preliminary results of the Medtronic Inc. InSync Study. Pacing Clin Electrophysiol 1998; 21:2249-2255.

13. Abraham WT: Rationale and design of a randomized clinical trial to assess the safety and efficacy of cardiac resynchronization therapy in patients with advanced heart failure: the Multicenter InSync Randomized Clinical Evaluation (MIRACLE). J. Card Fail 2000; 6:369-380.

14. Summary of Safety and Effectiveness. Retrieved December 17, 2001, from the World Wide Web: http://www.fda.gov/cdrh/pdf/p010015b.pdf

15. VecToR. Retrieved December 19, 2001, from the World Wide Web: http://www.sjm.com/5.0/5.1/ar00_6.htm

16. PAVE. Retrieved December 19, 2001, from the World Wide Web: http://www.sjm.com/5.0/5.1/ar00_6.htm

17. Witte K, Thackray S, Clark AL, et al.: Clinical trials update: IMPROVEMENT-HF, COPERNICUS, MUSTIC, ASPECT-II, APRICOT and HEART. Eur J Heart Fail 2000; 2:455-460.

18. Moss AJ, Cannom DS, Daubert JP, et al.: Multicenter automatic defibrillator implantation trial II (MADIT II): design and clinical protocol. Ann Noninvasive Electrocardiol 1999; 4(no. 1):83-91.

19. Klein H, Auricchio A, Reek S, et al.: New primary prevention trials of sudden cardiac death in patients with left ventricular dysfunction: SCD-HEFT and MADIT-II. Am J Cardiol 1999; 83:91D-97D.

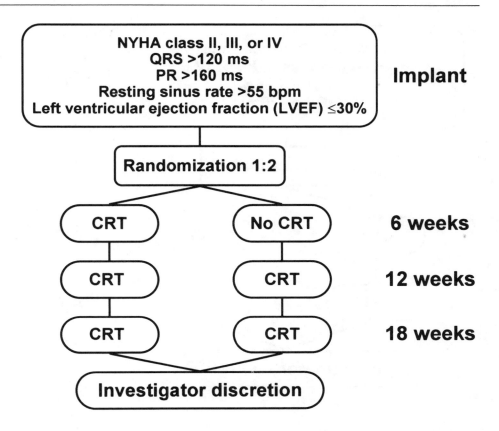

Fig. 1. Trial design for the VIGOR-CHF study. bpm = beats per minute; CRT = cardiac resynchronization therapy; NYHA = New York Heart Association.

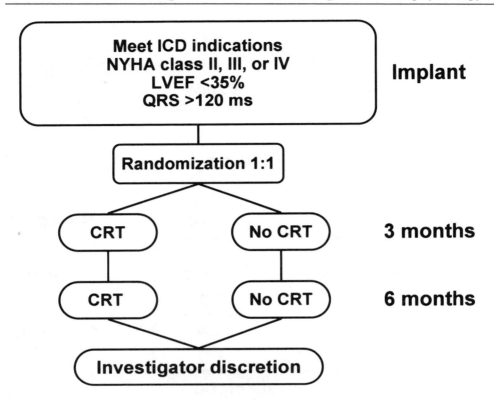

Fig. 2. Trial design for the VENTAK-CHF/CONTAK-CHF study. CRT = cardiac resynchronization therapy; ICD = implantable cardioverter defibrillator; LVEF = left ventricular ejection fraction; NYHA = New York Heart Association.

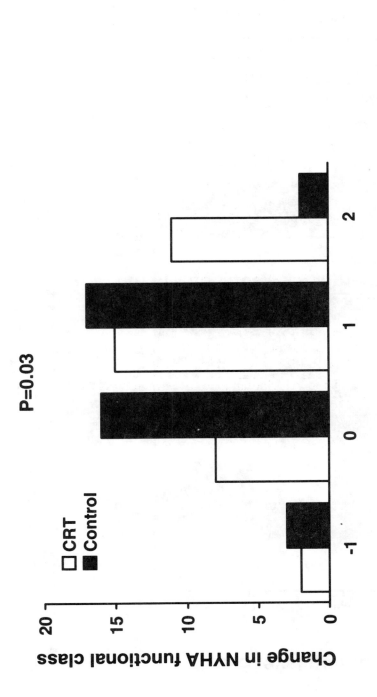

Fig. 3. Change in New York Heart Association (NYHA) functional classification in the CONTAK-CD trial. CRT = cardiac resynchronization therapy.

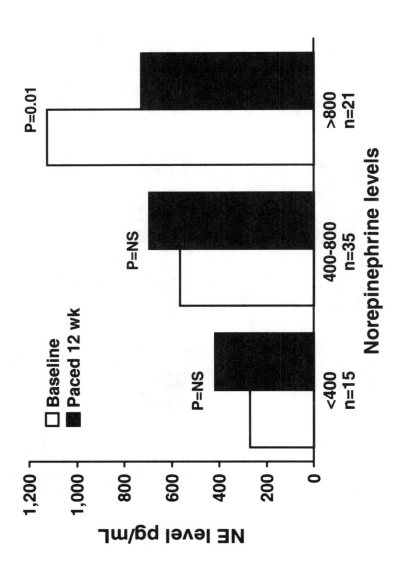

Fig. 4. Data from the VIGOR CHF, VENTAK CHF studies in which norepinephrine (NE) levels were obtained before cardiac resynchronization therapy (CRT) and after 12 weeks of CRT. Patients with the highest levels of NE before CRT had significant reduction in levels after 12 weeks of CRT. NS = not significant.

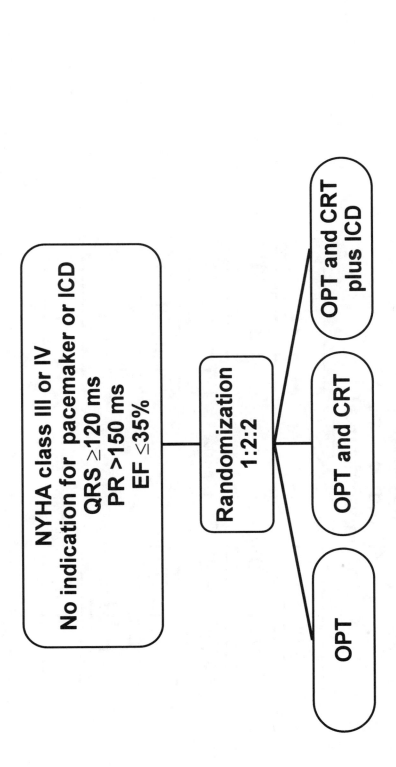

Fig. 5. Trial design for the COMPANION study. CRT = cardiac resynchronization therapy; EF = ejection fraction; ICD = implantable cardioverter defibrillator; NYHA = New York Heart Association; OPT = optimal pharmacologic therapy.

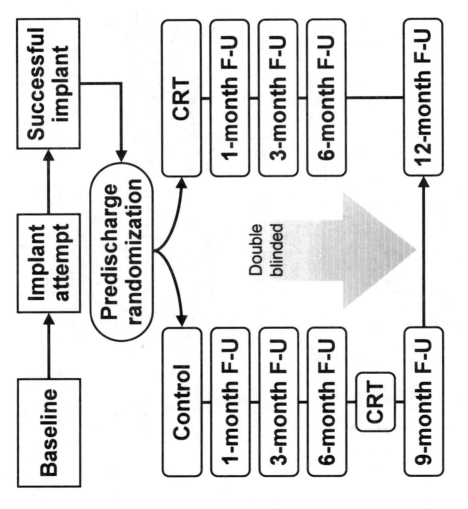

Fig. 6. Trial design for the InSync (MIRACLE) study. CRT = cardiac resynchronization therapy; F-U = follow-up.

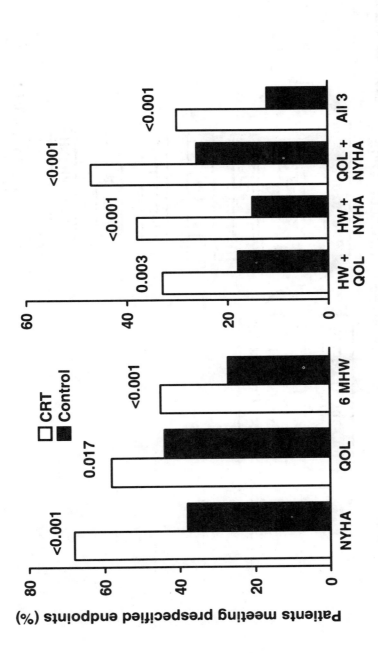

Fig. 7. Graphic representation of improvement seen in quality of life (QOL); New York Heart Association (NYHA) class, and 6-minute hall walk (MHW) in the InSync study. CRT = cardiac resynchronization therapy.

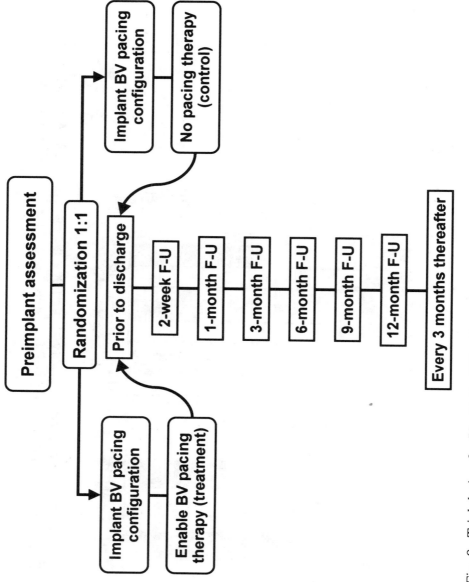

Fig. 8. Trial design for VecToR. BV = biventricular; F-U = follow-up.

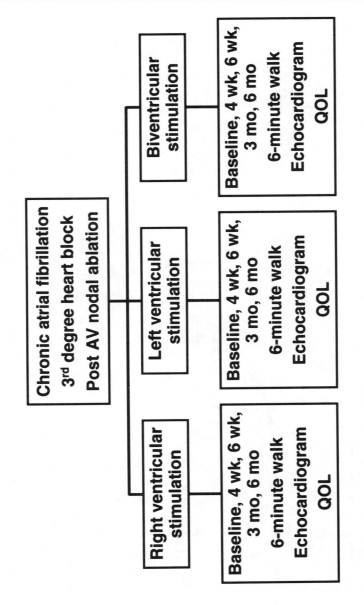

Fig. 9. Trial design for PAVE study. AV = atrioventricular; QOL = quality of life.

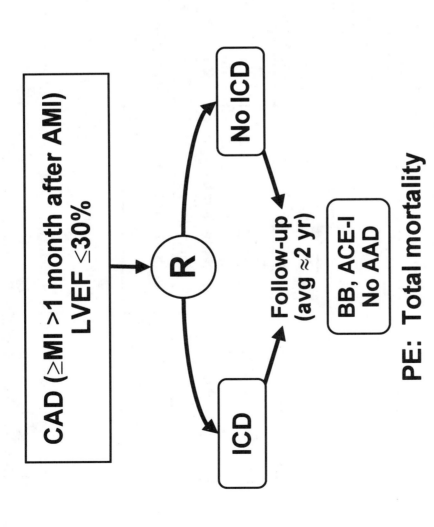

Fig. 10. Trial design for MADIT-II study. AAD = antiarrhythmic drugs; ACE-I = angiotensin-converting enzyme inhibitor; AMI = acute myocardial infarction; BB = beta blocker; CAD = coronary artery disease; ICD = implantable cardioverter defibrillator; LVEF = left ventricular ejection fraction; PE = primary endpoint; R = randomization.

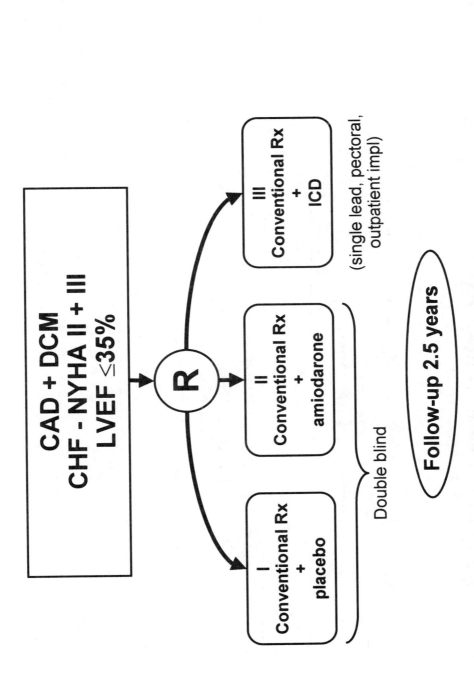

Fig. 11. Trial design for SCD-HeFT study. CAD = coronary artery disease; CHF = congestive heart failure; DCM = dilated cardiomyopathy; ICD = implantable cardioverter defibrillator; LVEF = left ventricular ejection fraction; NYHA = New York Heart Association; R = randomization.

23

LEFT VENTRICULAR REVERSE REMODELILNG AFTER BIVENTRICULAR PACING IN HEART FAILURE

Cheuk-Man Yu, MD, FRACP
Chu-Pak Lau, MD, FRCP

Division of Cardiology, Department of Medicine, Queen Mary Hospital, University of Hong Kong, Hong Kong SAR, China

Introduction

Cardiac remodeling can be defined as progressive increase in size and changes in shape resulting in deterioration of function of the heart after cardiac injury. It is secondary to genome expression, molecular, cellular and interstitial changes after the initial insult.[1] Cardiac remodeling typically occurs in the left ventricle when there are cardiac diseases causing myocardial injury, typical examples including myocardial infarction, idiopathic dilated cardiomyopathy, valvular regurgitation, and pressure overload.[2,3] Disregarding the etiology, the progression of cardiac remodeling results in decompensated cardiac enlargement and heart failure is the rule. The pathogenic mechanisms of cardiac remodeling are complex, which include the increase in hemodynamic load as a result of increase in wall tension and stress,[4] and activation of neurohormonal systems, namely the sympathetic nervous system, the renin-angiotensin-aldosterone system and possibly others yet to be identified.[5,6] Apart from the clinically-evident ventricular dilatation, histologically, the condition is characterized by progressive myocyte loss, activation of interstitial cells such as fibroblasts and deposition of collagen resulting in interstitial fibrosis.[7,8] Hypertrophy of the remaining myocytes is also evident.[9]

Prognosis Significance of Cardiac Remodeling

Progressive cardiac remodeling is an ominous sign. It has been shown that the degree of cardiac remodeling correlated with worsening of the prognosis.[10] In patients with coronary artery disease and myocardial infarction, the increase in left ventricular volume is an independent risk factor of increased mortality.[10-12] Prevention and regression of cardiac remodeling by medications against the neurohormonal activation has been shown to improve mortality, such as the use of angiotensin converting enzyme inhibitors and beta-blockers.[13-16] Interestingly, agents such as angiotensin converting enzyme inhibitors that prevent or reverse remodeling are often associated with reduction of mortality and morbidity, including hospitalization for heart failure.[15,17,18] On the other hand, agents

From Ovsyshcher IE. *New Developments in Cardiac Pacing and Electrophysiology*. Armonk, NY: Futura Publishing Company, Inc. ©2002.

such as digoxin that improve symptoms without significant change in left ventricular size or function will usually not affect the prognosis.[19] Therefore therapeutic measures targeting on reverse remodeling is a major goal of treatment nowadays.

Cardiac Remodeling in Heart Failure Patients with Widened QRS Complexes

In a subset of patients with heart failure, there is evidence of widening of QRS duration on surface electrocardiogram, either in the form of left bundle branch block or intraventricular conduction delay. It is estimated that this condition occurs in about 10-14% of patients with heart failure in the hospital setting,[20,21] and up to one-quarter in those with advanced heart failure.[22,23] Similar to cardiac remodeling, widening of QRS is a progressive condition and is also associated with significantly higher cardiovascular mortality.[22,23] Although a clear relationship between the progression of cardiac remodeling and severity of electromechanical delay has not been clearly demonstrated, it is possible that in the presence of left bundle branch block or significant intraventricular conduction delay, ventricular dilatation is exacerbated by asynchronous contraction.

Reversal of Cardiac Remodeling after Biventricular Pacing Therapy

Prevention and even reversal of cardiac remodeling in patients with heart failure was well documented by medical therapy, including angiotensin converting enzyme inhibitors, beta-blockers and recently angiotensin II receptor blockers.[13-16,24] Biventricular pacing that synchronize left ventricular contraction has been shown to improve the functional aspects of patients with advanced heart failure, although it is uncertain if it has a negative remodeling effect. This phenomenon is recently documented in two published studies.[25,26] In one study of 11 patients with wide QRS heart failure received biventricular pacing, it was reported that the left ventricular end-systolic diameter was reduced by 0.5cm, and left ventricular end-diastolic and end-systolic volumes decreased by 24% and 33%, respectively, after treatment for 3 months.[25] This was transformed into the gain in ejection fraction and cardiac output, and a reduction in the severity of mitral regurgitation.[25] Clinically, there was also significant increase in the 6-minute hall walk distance of 65 meters and improvement of the quality of life as assessed by the Minnesota Living With Heart Failure questionnaire.[25] In these subjects, the degree of remodeling is far more impressive than by medical therapy, including beta-blockers and angiotensin converting enzyme inhibitors.[15] In the Italian InSync study, 23 heart failure patients receiving biventricular pacing were followed up for a mean duration of 9 months. It was observed that there was significant reduction in the left ventricular end-diastolic and end-systolic volumes as well as gain in ejection fraction and cardiac output.[26] This was accompanied by the shortening of QRS complex duration. Therefore the reverse remodeling might be related to the minimization of electromechanical delay and hence improvement of cardiac synchronicity. Clinical and symptomatic improvement was also evident in these patients.[26] Recently, reduction of left ventricular diameter of about 0.5cm was also evident after pacing for 6 months in a large multicenter study (Abraham et al, unpublished data, MIRACLE study, 50th Annual Scientific Session of the American College of Cardiology, 2001).[27]

The question of whether pacing needs to be continued to maintain the reverse remodeling effect is addressed by our recent study.[28] In this study, 25 patients were followed up for 3 months with pacing therapy, which were followed by withdrawal of pacing for 1 month.[28] It was found that pacing is essential for the beneficial effects to be maintained (Figure 1). When pacing was withdrawn, the left ventricle enlarged progressively over the next four weeks, mitral regurgitation increased, and ejection fraction and cardiac output decreased gradually. While some benefits could lost rather immediately after withdrawal of pacing, such as the gain in diastolic filling time, the left ventricular volume remain unchanged within the first day of pacing withdrawal.[28] Therefore reverse remodeling occurs in a time and pacing dependent manner, and is critical for the maintenance of the benefits. The increase in left ventricular size to the pre-pacing level may indicate the re-occurrence of adverse hemodynamic changes in the heart when pacing was withdrawn. This could be related to the worsening of electromechanical delay resulting in ineffective systolic emptying, shortening of diastolic filling time and exacerbation of mechanical mitral regurgitation.

Predictors of Reverse Remodeling after Biventricular Pacing

Left ventricular reverse remodeling may not occur in every patient who receives biventricular pacing therapy. The proportion of patients who responds to this therapy is not clearly known. Our experience suggests that significant reverse remodeling occurs in just more than half of patients (Yu et al, unpublished data, 51st Annual Scientific Session of the American College of Cardiology, 2002). It is therefore vital to identify potential predictors of reverse remodeling. In our patients, we observed that clinical data were unable to identify responders of reverse remodeling. In the univariate model of analysis, significant predictors of reverse remodeling included prolonged pre-pacing QRS duration, large pre-pacing left ventricular end-systolic volume as well as more severe systolic asynchrony. In addition, biochemical tests may also provide adjunctive value for the prediction of remodeling. Our preliminary results showed that low neurohormonal levels were associated with more effective reduction of left ventricular volume after biventricular pacing therapy. The potential role of using these parameters, or combining multiple parameters, may prove to be a good guide for choosing appropriate therapy in these patients (Yu et al, unpublished data, 51st Annual Scientific Session of the American College of Cardiology, 2002). On the other hand, whether regression of cardiac remodeling may improve prognosis of heart failure has not been addressed. The ongoing large multicenter trials targeting on morbidity and mortality as end-points may shed some light in this regard.[29,30]

Figure 1. Progressive reduction of left ventricular end-diastolic (LVVd)

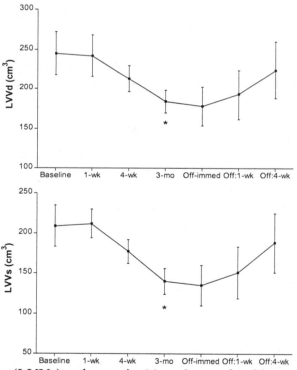

and end-systolic (LVVs) volumes in 11 patients after biventricular pacing for 3 months. When pacing was withheld, the left ventricular volumes increase over the next 4 weeks. * P < 0.05 Vs baseline.

References

1. Cohn JN, Ferrari R, Sharpe N. Cardiac remodeling--concepts and clinical implications: a consensus paper from an international forum on cardiac remodeling. Behalf of an International Forum on Cardiac Remodeling. J Am Coll Cardiol. 2000; 35:569-582
2. Sutton MG, Sharpe N. Left ventricular remodeling after myocardial infarction: pathophysiology and therapy. Circulation. 2000; 101:2981-2988
3. Gaudron P, Eilles C, Kugler I, et al. Progressive left ventricular dysfunction and remodeling after myocardial infarction. Potential mechanisms and early predictors. Circulation. 1993; 87:755-763
4. Rumberger JA. Ventricular dilatation and remodeling after myocardial infarction. Mayo Clin Proc. 1994; 69:664-674
5. Cohn JN, Levine TB, Olivari MT, et al. Plasma norepinephrine as a guide to prognosis in patients with chronic congestive heart failure. N Engl J Med. 1984; 311:819-823
6. Francis GS, Benedict C, Johnstone DE, et al. Comparison of neuroendocrine activation in patients with left ventricular dysfunction with and without congestive heart failure. A substudy of the Studies of Left Ventricular Dysfunction (SOLVD). Circulation. 1990; 82:1724-1729
7. Volders PG, Willems IE, Cleutjens JP, et al. Interstitial collagen is increased in the non-infarcted human myocardium after myocardial infarction. J Mol Cell Cardiol. 1993; 25:1317-1323
8. Yu CM, Tipoe GL, Wing-Hon LK, et al. Effects of combination of angiotensin-converting enzyme inhibitor and angiotensin receptor antagonist on inflammatory cellular infiltration and myocardial interstitial fibrosis after acute myocardial infarction. J Am Coll Cardiol. 2001; 38:1207-1215
9. Anversa P, Loud AV, Levicky V, et al. Left ventricular failure induced by myocardial infarction. I. Myocyte hypertrophy. Am J Physiol. 1985; 248:H876-H882
10. Migrino RQ, Young JB, Ellis SG, et al. End-systolic volume index at 90 to 180 minutes into reperfusion therapy for acute myocardial infarction is a strong predictor of early and late mortality. The Global Utilization of Streptokinase and t-PA for Occluded Coronary Arteries (GUSTO)-I Angiographic Investigators. Circulation. 1997; 96:116-121

11. White HD, Norris RM, Brown MA, et al. Left ventricular end-systolic volume as the major determinant of survival after recovery from myocardial infarction. Circulation. 1987; 76:44-51

12. Pfeffer MA, Braunwald E. Ventricular remodeling after myocardial infarction. Experimental observations and clinical implications. Circulation. 1990; 81:1161-1172

13. Konstam MA, Rousseau MF, Kronenberg MW, et al. Effects of the angiotensin converting enzyme inhibitor enalapril on the long-term progression of left ventricular dysfunction in patients with heart failure. SOLVD Investigators. Circulation. 1992; 86:431-438

14. Greenberg B, Quinones MA, Koilpillai C, et al. Effects of long-term enalapril therapy on cardiac structure and function in patients with left ventricular dysfunction. Results of the SOLVD echocardiography substudy. Circulation. 1995; 91:2573-2581

15. Australia/New Zealand Heart Failure Research Collaborative Group. Randomised, placebo-controlled trial of carvedilol in patients with congestive heart failure due to ischaemic heart disease. Lancet. 1997; 349:375-380

16. Metra M, Giubbini R, Nodari S, et al. Differential effects of beta-blockers in patients with heart failure: A prospective, randomized, double-blind comparison of the long-term effects of metoprolol versus carvedilol. Circulation. 2000; 102:546-551

17. The SOLVD Investigators. Effect of enalapril on survival in patients with reduced left ventricular ejection fractions and congestive heart failure. N Engl J Med. 1991; 325:293-302

18. MERIT-HF Investigators. Effect of metoprolol CR/XL in chronic heart failure: Metoprolol CR/XL Randomised Intervention Trial in Congestive Heart Failure (MERIT-HF). Lancet. 1999; 353:2001-2007

19. The Digitalis Investigation Group. The effect of digoxin on mortality and morbidity in patients with heart failure. N Engl J Med. 1997; 336:525-533

20. De Sutter J, De Bondt P, Van de Wiele C, et al. Prevalence of potential candidates for biventricular pacing among patients with known coronary artery disease: a prospective registry from a single center. Pacing Clin Electrophysiol. 2000; 23:1718-1721

21. Farwell D, Patel NR, Hall A, et al. How many people with heart failure are appropriate for biventricular resynchronization? Eur Heart J. 2000; 21:1246-1250

22. Aaronson KD, Schwartz JS, Chen TM, et al. Development and prospective validation of a clinical index to predict survival in

ambulatory patients referred for cardiac transplant evaluation. Circulation. 1997; 95:2660-2667

23. Baldasseroni S, Opasich C, Gorini M, et al. Complete left bundle-branch block (LBBB) is associated with increased 1-year mortality in patients with congestive heart failure: data from IN-CHF Registry. J Am Coll Cardiol. 2001; 37:156A

24. Konstam MA, Patten RD, Thomas I, et al. Effects of losartan and captopril on left ventricular volumes in elderly patients with heart failure: results of the ELITE ventricular function substudy. Am Heart J. 2000; 139:1081-1087

25. Lau CP, Yu CM, Chau E, et al. Reversal of left ventricular remodeling by synchronous biventricular pacing in heart failure. Pacing Clin Electrophysiol. 2000; 23:1722-1725

26. Porciani MC, Puglisi A, Colella A, et al. Echocardiographic evaluation of the effect of biventricular pacing: the InSync Italian Registry. Eur Heart J. 2000; 2 Suppl J:J23-J30

27. Abraham WT. Rationale and design of a randomized clinical trial to assess the safety and efficacy of cardiac resynchronization therapy in patients with advanced heart failure: the Multicenter InSync Randomized Clinical Evaluation (MIRACLE). J Card Fail. 2000; 6:369-380

28. Yu CM, Chau E, Sanderson JE, et al. Tissue Doppler echocardiographic evidence of reverse remodeling and improved synchronicity by simultaneously delaying regional contraction after biventricular pacing therapy in heart failure. Circulation. 2002; In press

29. Bristow MR, Feldman AM, Saxon LA. Heart failure management using implantable devices for ventricular resynchronization: Comparison of Medical Therapy, Pacing, and Defibrillation in Chronic Heart Failure (COMPANION) trial. COMPANION Steering Committee and COMPANION Clinical Investigators. J Card Fail. 2000; 6:276-285

30. Cleland JG, Daubert JC, Erdmann E, et al. The CARE-HF study (CArdiac REsynchronisation in Heart Failure study): rationale, design and end-points. Eur J Heart Fail. 2001; 3:481-489

24.

ENDOVENOUS IMPLANTATION OF THE LEFT VENTRICULAR LEAD FOR CARDIAC RESYNCHRONIZATION THERAPY IN CONGESTIVE HEART FAILURE

Philippe Ritter MD, Arnaud Lazarus MD, Gaël Jauvert MD, Christine Alonso MD, Serge Cazeau MD

InParys, Saint-Cloud - FRANCE

The endovenous approach is the reference method for the implantation of a left ventricular lead in heart failure patients. Initially performed with standard leads, the technique has improved considerably since the introduction of custom-made leads. With the leads presently available, the implantation success rate is approximately 92 %. However, this already high rate should reach 100 % with more specific materials and additional tools to be designed. The technique will only develop when the leads will allow an easy and successful implant procedure in 100 % of cases, probably at the cost of a learning curve.

The implantation procedure should be as close as possible to a conventional pacemaker implantation: the patient is awake, and is operated under local anesthesia. The concept of this technique is to reach the left lateral wall of the myocardium by catheterizing the coronary sinus and a left lateral vein.

1. Preparation of the patient.

The patient should be well prepared to this operation: he should have been informed about the different steps of the operation, and the general concept of bi-ventricular stimulation should have been explained in order to get full adhesion from the patient.

A coronary sinus angiogram should be performed prior to implant. It may help to predict catheterization difficulties (geometry of the coronary sinus, existence of valves, curves), and to select the optimal vein to be catheterized. This is a personal opinion which is not admitted by other implanters, even in our own team! Some other members of the team prefer to have the angiogram performed at the moment of the system implantation. In that case, and in my opinion, it means that a choice for a specific material has been done, which may not be correct for the individual patient.

Acute heart failure should be treated prior to the operation to get a stable condition: the implant procedure may last more than 2 or 3 hours, the patient lying on the table without being allowed to move.

From Ovsyshcher IE. *New Developments in Cardiac Pacing and Electrophysiology.* Armonk, NY: Futura Publishing Company, Inc. ©2002.

The implantation site should be perfectly free from any infectious process, skin erosion, monitoring electrode, and skin should have been prepared with application of an antiseptic solution right before entry of the patient into the operation theater.

Infection prevention should be respected in those particularly fragile patients with a limited number of persons in the room, prophylactic antibiotic; the venous line should be placed at the contralateral site.

An external defibrillator should be ready for use in the room, and an anesthesiologist should be ready to assist.

2. The Implant Procedure

The synchronizer site should be the right subclavian area. The experience showed us that the access to the coronary sinus is easier from the right subclavian vein than from the left. In addition, although longer, the length of the available leads for left ventricular pacing may be too short in tall patients with a very large left ventricle, when coming from the left subclavian site. But once again, this is a personal preference. In case of use of long sheaths (St Jude), the left side is preferable, because the sheath may have a picture at the site of venous curves, which is frequently so at the junction between the right subclavian vein and the superior cava vena.

The venous access of the left ventricular lead should be through a subclavian vein puncture, separated from the other leads: in any case a re-intervention is required, the separated access of the left ventricular lead prevents the dislocation of the others and vice versa. In case of failure of the left ventricular lead implantation, the operation may be stopped at that stage. This means that we usually start with the left ventricular lead implant before proceeding to the cephalic vein cut-down for the other leads.

2.1. The left ventricular lead

The material available. Two types of specific leads are now available. The first type is derived from the conventional leads. These are thick pre-shaped leads that may be introduced with or without a guiding catheter (first 2188, 2187 Medtronic, Situs Ela, Aescula St Jude, etc...) The lead is stabilized by its curves in relationship with the ones of the vein, or it is blocked into the vein. That means that these leads are located in the proximal part of the vein, close to the mitral annulus once in place. The second type of lead is derived from the angioplasty technology. The lead, which is very thin, is pushed along a guide wire, the whole being introduced through a guiding catheter. The guiding catheter is pushed into the coronary sinus, then the lead is introduced into the coronary sinus, and then, the guide wire goes into the targeted vein. Once the guide wire in place, the lead is slipped along the wire into the vein. The lead is stabilized when it is blocked into the vein, meaning that the lead goes deep into it, frequently close to the left lateral apex, unless the lead if blocked into a proximal branch of the targeted vein.

The entry into the coronary sinus and selection of the left vein.
Without guiding catheter. At any time, the movements given to the lead should not be abrupt. The stylet shape is essential to introduce the lead into the coronary sinus. It depends on the size of the right atrium. If the right atrium has a fairly normal size (which is a rare situation), then, a 45° angulation should be given to the stylet at approximately 5 cm from the distal tip. If the right atrium is very dilated, a large curve with an overall 90 ° angle is preferred, including the last 10 to 15 cm of the stylet. The lead with the stylet completely introduced, is oriented to the left and backwards, pushed against the isthmus. It is exceptional that the lead enters the coronary sinus immediately. The lead tip is pushed along the tricuspid annulus and the coronary ostium is most frequently found at the left border of the spinal chord in the antero-posterior view. The overall orientation of the coronary sinus is a 45 ° line between the vertical line symbolized by the spinal chord and the horizontal line symbolized by the left hemi-diaphragm. The interindividual variations are frequent and the heart geometry is frequently altered by the heart disease, and the dilatation. In addition, patients who have encountered heart surgery previously, heart geometry is frequently totally modified. The coronary sinus ostium is sometimes located much more lateral, and may have a more vertical orientation. The recording of the endocardial signals may help to better determine its location. One approaches the coronary sinus ostium when atrial and ventricular signals have similar amplitude with atrial and ventricular signals occurring at the end of the surface P and R waves respectively. The occurrence of premature ventricular beats means that the electrode tip is within the right ventricle. After several attempts, if the lead still goes towards the inferior cava vena or the right ventricle, the stylet should be withdrawn for few centimeters before starting again the same maneuvers. The left anterior oblique view can help. The orientation of the lead should be along the inferior border of the heart silhouette and backwards. The stylet exchange may help the introduction of the lead into the coronary sinus. Its shape should be adapted to the encountered difficulties. The lead is within the coronary sinus when the leftwards and upwards ascension of the lead is not accompanied with premature ventricular beats. On the endocardial recording, the atrial and ventricular

signals reveal the late depolarization of the left heart chambers compared to the corresponding surface P and R waves. Once the lead introduced, the stylet cannot be exchanged. If so, the new stylet forces the lead towards the inferior cava vena, when reintroduced into the lead, and the large buckle given to the lead in the very large atrium provokes the abrupt extraction of the lead from the coronary sinus.

Most of the time, the catheterization of the coronary sinus is easy, but can be limited by the existence of curves and valves. Rotations and push-pull maneuvers will soon force the lead to advance into the coronary sinus.

After the removal of the stylet for some millimeters or centimeters, the distal end of the lead is getting more flexible and its distal curvature is more pronounced. Depending on the lead model, it mainly depends on the relative position of the stylet tip with the lead tip. The more distal the stylet, the less pronounced the lead curvature. The long and rigid distal part of the 2188 does not help the selection of the lateral veins whose direction makes a sharp angle with the coronary sinus. In the same way, catheterization of small curved veins is not made easy. The other models which all have a more flexible distal part, give more chances to succeed in the catheterization of the small veins. The lead, still in the coronary sinus, is then oriented anteriorly is order to determine the position of the venous ostia: the lead tip frequently hits the top of the superior wall of the venous ostium. In all those maneuvers, the physician must control the lead movements in the right atrium. Every time the lead is pushed, and the lead tip is blocked somewhere, a large curve can be seen in the large right atrium and the force is loosened in a buckle. If the lead is pushed further the atrial buckle extracts the lead tip abruptly from the coronary sinus. The lead tip is frequently blocked at the selected venous ostium. The further removal of the stylet gives even more flexibility to the lead which frequently comes into the vein abruptly. In other cases, the entry into the vein is slow, needing many pushing and rotating maneuvers on the lead which progresses millimeter after millimeter. Sometimes the lead goes itself further into the vein, probably favored by the heart contractions.

If several veins can be catheterized, the left ventricular depolarization should be recorded at that stage. A correct location corresponds to a position where the left ventricular depolarization signal is the most delayed as compared with the surface QRS complex. The left atrial signal should not be visible. When the lead is in place, the tip is probably blocked into the vein.

With guiding catheter. The guiding catheter must be used very gently as its tip is very aggressive because of its stiffness. This is the reason why coronary sinus dissection had been described, that we never observed vein the pacing lead is used alone. However, the guiding catheter allows coronary sinus angiography, and is necessary when using the lead over the wire technique. It facilitates the push on the lead. However, the force applied to the lead tip may be very important.

The easiness of coronary sinus catheterization depends on the relative shapes of the guiding catheter, the right atrium and the coronary sinus ostium. Difficulties can be encountered when the right atrium is very dilated, and when the coronary sinus ostium is high in the atrium with a vertical CS initial portion. In that case, steerable EP catheters can be used to catheterize the CS, the guiding catheter being pushed over the EP catheter once into the CS. Then an angioplasty guide wire is used to select the appropriate vein, and pushed as deep as possible into the vein. Then the lead is pushed along the guide wire until it is blocked into the vein. The problem of the lead over the wire technique is that leads are very thin and very flexible, so that two major troubles may arise: to stabilize the lead, one needs to block the lead into the vein, so that the lead is frequently close to the left part of the left ventricular apex, a position which may not be as optimal as the initial portion of the vein close to the mitral annulus, a segment where the contraction is the latest (the long-term hemodynamic result may be better in this latter position); the second problem is the removal of the guiding catheter, once the lead has been fixed. This moment is critical as the guiding catheter removal may lead to the displacement of the pacing lead.

Whatever the technique and the leads used are, thresholds can then be measured. Most of the time the pacing threshold is lower than 1 Volt, but sometimes, the threshold can reach 2.5 - 3 Volts, especially in the area of a previous myocardial infarction, and at the very basal part of the ventricle, close to the mitral annulus. However these high thresholds should be accepted if the anatomical location is correct. On the contrary, the sensing has never been a problem since signal amplitudes are usually high. One another important check is to verify the absence of phrenic nerve stimulation. This adverse event is frequent and should be treated, because the patient never stands this complication for long. The unique possibility is to change the lead location, which is not always easy to perform, according to the possible previous difficulties of catheterization. Once the lead in place, it should be fix at its introduction site. The other leads can then be implanted.

2.2. The implantation of the right atrial and ventricular leads

The leads are introduced via separated accesses. Screw-in leads should be preferred because the implantation sites are frequently unconventional and the heart chambers are dilated and smoother than normal hearts. The physician should start with the right ventricular lead. An opposite position relative to the location of the left ventricular lead should be the ideal position. If the LV lead is antero-lateral, the RV lead is located at the low lateral wall. If the LV lead is at the mid-lateral wall the RV lead is implanted at the mid-lateral wall. If the LV lead is postero-lateral, the RV lead is antero-lateral. The implantation of the RV lead is frequently difficult to perform, because of frequent tricuspid valve regurgitation, and the huge dilatation of the RV. The physician must be particularly cautious in the manipulations of the lead to prevent the occurrence of life-threatening ventricular arrhythmias and the dislocation of the left ventricular lead.

In the event of a previously implanted RV lead, i.e. in a patient already implanted in the conventional VVI/DDD mode (at the conventional RV apical site), the left ventricular lead should have a high lateral site.

The main check is to control that, in spontaneous rhythm, the RV depolarization occurs at the earliest compared to the surface QRS complex, and, when pacing from the right ventricular lead, the left depolarization signal occurs at the latest in the surface QRS complex. In the bi-ventricular pacing configuration, the QRS duration should be shorter than the one obtained with all other configurations: spontaneous rhythm, RV or LV pacing. When pacing in the bi-ventricular configuration, the surface QRS should be has duration equal or shorter than the spontaneous QRS. The latter condition is obviously the best. However, in all cases, the duration of the bi-ventricular paced QRS should be much shorter than the RV paced QRS complex.

If the bi-ventricular QRS has a fairly normal axis deviation, the two ventricular are considered as being at optimal sites.

All rules above cited mean that the RV lead should be placed at different positions during the implant procedure. This is the reason why the RV lead must be a screw-in lead, at the definitive position is frequently unconventional.

The right atrial lead comes last. Once again, the implantation may be difficult due to specific characteristics: dilated right atrium, frequent high sensing/pacing thresholds, and frequent lengthening of the inter-atrial interval. In this latter situation, two options can be proposed:

the implantation of a fourth lead within the coronary sinus to resynchronize both atria. The RA lead should be located at the high RA lateral border. As far as the LA lead is considered, we never had difficulties in that situation: both coronary sinus leads stabilize each other, and we never reported any dislocation. The other possibility is to implant a screw-in lead at the coronary sinus ostium.

The other option is to implant the right atrial lead at the inter-atrial septal site. This procedure is not always feasible. Thresholds can be too high at that site. However, the implanted system is more conventional with less troubles during the follow-up.

All leads are fixed at the introduction sites and connected to the device. The pocket is then created for the device. If the device can provide bipolar stimulation, we frequently implant the device in a submuscular pocket to prevent skin erosion in those emaciated patients. When Y adapters are used, and if bipolar pacing is available, we also prefer to implant the whole material below the pectoral muscle. In case unipolar pacing is the only option, the Y adapter is placed below the muscle and the device is located in a subcutaneous pocket.

In the InSync® study, the success rate of the implantation of synchronizers is 70 % for beginners without surgical assistance. When assistance is provided, the success rate goes up to 92 %. This fact proves that a learning curve is required as for any new technique. The further improvements of the implantable material may allow a better rate in the near future. New leads and assisting tools will be furnished to facilitate the implantation and shorten it. The Bordeaux team is exploring a new approach in case the conventional endovenous approach fails: implantation of a conventional screw-in lead via a trans-septal atrial procedure. This procedure is long, but the left ventricular lead has always been implanted in their experience. The patient requires long-term anticoagulation.

3. Conclusion

The endovenous approach can be performing without major complications at the moment of the implant procedure. It requires a learning curve. The unique difficulty is the relative position of the implanted leads. The only guide is the electrophysiologic analysis of the ventricular potentials. This technique should include a simultaneous evaluation of bi-ventricular pacing during the operation. In our early experience we attempted to have echo measurements. We encountered may difficulties: the respect of asepsis was difficult, the procedure was largely prolonged, the artifacts were frequent. We should imagine to use other hemodynamic assessment means such as transthoracic bioimpedance or pressure measurements for example to guide the implanting physician. However, whatever the technique used, it should not extend the duration of the implant procedure.

VI. NEW THERAPEUTIC APPROACHES
TO PATIENTS
WITH CARDIAC ARRHYTHMIA

25.

THE APPROACH TO THE PATIENT WITH SYNCOPE WHILE DRIVING

Mark L. Blitzer, MD, Mark H. Schoenfeld, MD

Cardiac Electrophysiology and Pacer Laboratory, Hospital of Saint Raphael and Yale University School of Medicine

Background

This chapter will address two issues: first, the evaluation of a patient with syncope while driving and second, the development of a driving prescription for those who experience a syncopal event.

The occurrence of syncope (an episode of sudden and transient loss of consciousness) or near-syncope (an episode of sudden and transient altered consciousness) while driving is an important, and almost certainly, under-reported phenomenon. The evaluation of such a patient is similar to that of a patient with syncope under non-driving conditions. The etiologic diagnosis is, however, pursued with greater vigor given the life-threatening potential consequences to the affected driver, unsuspecting motorists and pedestrians if the event were to recur while driving.

Work-up: History, Physical Exam and Diagnostic Testing

The initial evaluation focuses on the history. Despite advances in technology, there are no better diagnostic tools than a well-taken history supplememted by reports from passengers, nearby motorists and the initial findings of para-medical personnel.[1] Careful probing for symptoms occurring just prior to the syncopal event or immediately after recovering from such an event can be particularly helpful. Prodromal symptoms of diaphoresis and nausea are consistent with a vaso-vagal spell. A passenger in the car may report that the patient became pale or diaphoretic just prior to the episode. This also raises the suspicion for a vaso-vagal etiology. A prior history of syncope stretching back to childhood particularly if the syncopal or near-syncopal events had previously occurred in church or in a medical setting further support a diagnosis of neuro-cardiogenic origin. It is much easier to presume the recent syncopal event reflects more of the same rather than invoke a second diagnosis. Vaso-vagal spells often repeat themselves shortly after the initial event such as when the patient first tries to stand up or in the ambulance ride to the Emergency Room.

Questions elucidating the presence of underlying structural heart disease are particularly important given the poorer prognosis in those with cardiac

From Ovsyshcher IE. *New Developments in Cardiac Pacing and Electrophysiology.* Armonk, NY: Futura Publishing Company, Inc. ©2002.

disease compared to a group without demonstrable heart abnormalities. The first group commonly suffers from malignant ventricular dysrhythmias which are often recurrent and at times, fatal. The one year mortality in patients diagnosed with "cardiac" syncope can exceed 30%.[2] This group is also more likely to manifest paroxysmal infra-hisian conduction block (Stokes-Adams attacks) or sinus node dysfunction, often in a tachy/brady type pattern. In contrast, those without structural heart disease are much more likely to have neuro-cardiogenic syndromes or supra-ventricular tachycardias (SVT) which typically have a benign prognosis.

Syncope without warning is classically thought to occur with paroxysmal atrio-ventricular block or with sustained ventricular tachycardia although numerous exceptions occur. Brief clonic jerks or loss of bladder continence may occur secondary to profound periods of hypotension due to any etiology and are not diagnostic of a preceding seizure particularly in the absence of a post-ictal state.

We and others have reported the limited yield and associated high costs of neurologic evaluation including EEG, head CT, carotid ultrasonography and MRI when a history compatible with cardiac syncope is obtainable. We have more often seen patients previously diagnosed with refractory seizures turn out to have true syncope than we have seen syncope patients found to have a neurologic cause to their events. In cases where the diagnosis remains unclear despite a comprehensive evaluation, we have noted occasional benefits to 24-hour EEG monitoring. There are reports of vertebral-basilar (V-B) insufficiency and akinetic seizures resulting in "drop attacks" but in our experience, both are extraordinarily rare. Furthermore, patients with V-B insufficiency almost always demonstrate transient focal neurologic deficits prior to the episode.

The patient's state of mind and the physical conditions inside the automobile at the moment of the event may help direct the evaluation as well. A patient who has had an episode during a long car ride home late at night after a full day at work must be questioned carefully about the possibility that he or she may have briefly fallen asleep. This is more often the case in patients with a history of "nodding off" while driving, those who have narcolepsy, those who are sleep-deprived and those who are driving in an over-heated car. The possibility of recent significant alcohol intake must always be explored.

Great diligence must be taken in the evaluation of an elderly patient who may have multiple factors contributing to his or her episode of loss of consciousness including use of vasodilating, negatively chronotropic and dehydrating drugs as well as impaired autonomic reflexes. Aggravating circumstances as benign as a recent large meal (post prandial hypotension) or failing to take off one's winter coat before getting into an over-heated car may produce sufficient hypotension to produce altered consciousness.

A directed physical exam looking for several specific physical findings can be helpful in elucidating the etiology to a spell. A displaced, dyskinetic PMI or an S_3 gallop suggest the presence of LV dysfunction and a greater likelihood of ventricular tachycardia. The presence of a bruit (carotid, femoral or abdominal) suggests systemic atherosclerosis and raises the likelihood of concomitant CAD. Carotid sinus massage should be performed, particularly in high risk subsets for carotid sinus hypersensitivity syndrome such as elderly hypertensive men or in patients who have a suggestive history of neck pressure triggering the event (i.e. syncope occurring after twisting one's neck to look at traffic behind one's car).

The EKG often provides clues to guide further investigation. Findings that connote structural heart disease such as Q waves, severe left ventricular hypertrophy or chamber enlargement raise the probability of ventricular tachycardia and mandate the need for a more invasive evaluation with an electrophysiology study. Evidence for sinus node dysfunction (sinus bradycardia, sinus exit block or sinus pauses) or AV conduction disease (incomplete or complete heart block, or bundle branch block patterns) raise the suspicion for bradyarrhythmic syncope. Nonetheless, it should be remembered that in those with bifascicular block patterns (right bundle branch block with left anterior hemi-block) and syncope, the etiology to the event is as likely to be related to ventricular tachycardia as it is to bradycardia. The EKG should also be assessed for rare but potentially life threatening conditions such as ventricular pre-excitation, long QT syndrome, right ventricular dysplasia, hypertrophic cardiomyopathy and Brugada syndrome.

Echocardiography has emerged as a critical tool to look for evidence of structural heart disease. The results of the echo have important prognostic implications and will usually suggest whether the next diagnostic test should be a tilt table test or an electrophysiology study.

Our Experience
We have looked comprehensively at our 14 year experience of treating patients with episodes of impaired consciousness (syncope or near-syncope) while driving.[3] We identified 84 consecutive patients referred to us for the evaluation of impaired consciousness while driving. In 54 patients, there was no immediately obvious etiology to the event; these formed our study cohort. All patients in the cohort received an extensive

evaluation including tilt table testing, electrophysiology studies and interrogation of pre-existing pacemakers or ICDs (where relevant) as well as EKG monitoring, echocardiography and brain imaging where appropriate. This comprehensive evaluation resulted in a diagnosis supported by both history and directed testing in 42 patients (78%). The majority of diagnoses were due to either vasovagal syncope or supraventricular tachycardia (SVT). Vasovagal syncope was diagnosed in 14 patients (26%) and SVT in an additional 14 (26%). 3 patients were diagnosed with both. Ventricular tachycardia was diagnosed in 8 (15%), advanced AV block was diagnosed in 7 (13%), vestibular syncope in 1 and seizures in 1. Of the 12 (22%) patients without a diagnosis after clinical testing, vasovagal syncope was strongly suspected in 5 (9%), sick sinus syndrome in 1, SVT in 1 and iscemia induced VT in 1. With appropriate pharmacologic, ablative or device-based therapy, there were no recurrent driving-related episodes of impaired consciousness during follow-up.

This study was interesting for several reasons. First, it demonstrated that a logical and thorough evaluation can determine the etiology of an episode of impaired consciousness in nearly four out of five cases. This is much higher than many published reports where diagnoses were only made definitively in about 50% of cases. Second, it dispelled several myths. First, vasovagal spells can definitely occur while driving. Some authors have argued that vasovagal syncope is extraordinarily uncommon while driving.   They cite the non-standing posture, the well-controlled temperatures within the car and the sense of "comfort" one normally feels in one's own car as evidence for the absence of triggers to vasovagal syncope. Our study clearly contradicts this reasoning. Although the majority of vasovagal events do occur in the presence of classic triggers such as hot, claustrophobic environments, the standing position or the presence of prior pain or anxiety, we have been impressed with the frequency of "atypical" scenarios which nonetheless, result in true vasovagal syncope. Given the high percentage of episodes of impaired consciousness (IC) while driving due to vasovagal syncope, appropriate treatment can clearly decrease the number of injuries and fatalities caused by these motorists.

We also noted a surprisingly high percentage of patients with SVT as the cause of their IC. This high incidence clearly demonstrates that SVT can have potentially serious consequences in motorists.   There are several possible mechanisms for IC during SVT including excessively rapid heart rates, underlying diastolic dysfunction leading to poor ventricular filling and subsequent poor cardiac output or, a vasodepressor reaction in response to the rapid heart rate. Like others,[4] we did not find that the episodes of IC during driving were related to tachycardia rates faster than the norm for the whole SVT cohort. Interestingly, we did note a subset of elderly patients with underlying hypertensive heart disease who had recurrent syncope without palpitations documented during episodes of induced SVT at EPS. While SVT was not initially thought to be likely in any of these instances, intensive investigation uncovered AV nodal reentrant tachycardia as the etiology. This clearly demonstrates the importance of keeping SVT in the differential diagnosis for all patients experiencing MVA when there is obvious IC preceding the event.

Driving Recommendations for Patients with Syncope
The evaluation of syncope while driving is an interesting topic; however, a related issue (i.e. the recommendations for driving in those patients with syncope occurring in other circumstances) is a much more common and difficult issue. With an explosion in the numbers of ICDs being implanted over the last decade (>100,000/yr in the US), the issue of driving restrictions in those with ICDs has sparked multiple papers and societal reviews.[5,6] Implicit in the literature is that society accepts certain risks in driving as evidenced by our allowing the elderly to continue to drive without recertification. One tries to quantify a level of risk above which society finds unacceptable. Then, one can estimate the level of risk in allowing each syncopal population to drive and can restrict driving based on whether they exceed the risk thresholds.

It must be remembered that rates of injury due to syncopal MVA remain extraordinarily low. This has been confirmed both in retrospective reviews of large cohorts of motor vehicle incidents[7] as well as with more theoretic equation-based analysis computing likely risks.[8] The latter analysis often yields annual estimates of approximately 1 in 45,000 that a recurrent arrhythmia will result in a motor vehicle related death.

Interestingly, individual states within the United States vary widely in regard to laws governing driving restrictions after a syncopal event. While 42 states have laws governing driving by patients with seizure disorders, only 26 states have laws concerning non-seizure related loss of consciousness and only 8 states have laws specifically relating to those with cardiac arrhythmias.[9] The driving restriction in those states with laws limiting people who have non-seizure syncope range from 3 – 12 months (average 4.3 months). Two realities hinder the application of these laws. The first is that physicians may be unaware of their local state's regulations.[10] Secondly, it has been repeatedly demonstrated that patients are often non-compliant with driving restrictions,[11] most commonly citing their dependence on driving for daily necessary life activities and the lack of a friend or family member who can consistently substitute.

Excellent data has recently been published by the AVID investigators which randomized a high risk group of patients with symptomatic VT or VF to cardiac defibrillator or drug treatment, most often with amiodarone.[12] Anonymous questionaires were sent out concerning driving habits, recurrent symptoms and motor vehicle accidents in this group. 88% of patients had resumed driving by the end of the first year. While driving, 2% had a syncopal spell and 11% had dizziness or palpitations necessitating stopping the vehicle. The rate of MVA in this group was 3.4% per patient year. Only 11% of these accidents were preceded by symptoms suggestive of arrhythmia. None resulted in any fatalities. Interestingly, this rate of MVA is less than half the annual accident rate of 7.1% in the general driving population of the United States.

European and American cardiology societies have published recommendations concerning driving after syncope.[5,6] Both clearly note that solid data upon which to base these recommendations are quite scant. Both emphasize that the overall rate of subsequent syncopal events leading to MVAs is quite low.

In assessing the risk of recurrent syncope in a patient after an episode of sustained ventricular tachycardia or cardiac arrest, no distinction is made between those treated with an ICD and those treated only pharmacologically. The greatest risk of recurrent events occurs in the months immediately after defibrillator implant;[13] thus, both societies have recommended a driving-free period of 6 months to assess rhythm stability and the severity of symptoms that are associated with any recurrence. An ICD shock during that monitoring period would reset the "clock" and begin a new 6 month period of abstinence. Empiric anti-arrhythmic drug therapy such as sotalol has been demonstrated to lessen the rate of subsequent events by decreasing the occurrence both of appropriate shock secondary to VT/VF as well as of inappropriate shocks from rapidly conducted SVT.[14] Further risk stratification might be possible based on the presence of monomorphic VT as opposed to VF, the degree of LV dysfunction,[15] the success of anti-tachycardia pacing algorithms and/or whether or not there is concomitant bi-ventricular pacing. Most agree that commercial drivers have greater restrictions. Their increased risk is based on a higher number of total hours behind the wheel as well as the likelihood of driving larger vehicles including trucks, usually on highways thereby incurring a much higher risk of causing substantial harm if involved in a MVA. Commercial driving with an ICD is permanently prohibited.

Patients who have ICD implants for primary prevention, (i.e. MADIT-type patients: low ejection fractions, non-sustained ventricular tachycardia and "+" EPS) clearly have lower rates of subsequent sustained dysrhythmias compared with patients who have ICDs implanted for secondary prevention purposes. Neither American nor European cardiology societies propose any restrictions on the ability of these patients to drive. This is also the case in other non-MADIT primary prevention populations such as those with hypertrophic cardiomyopathy or congenital LQTS who have ICD implants secondary to a family history of sudden cardiac death.

Recommendations for those with bradyarrhythmic syncope are much simpler than those for ventricular arrhythmias. Patients with events not clearly related to a reversible cause are prohibited from driving. Once a permanent pacemaker is placed, those who are pacer dependent should refrain from driving for 1 week to ensure good lead stability. Those who are not pacer dependent may resume driving without restriction.

Neurocardiogenic syncope remains, by far, the most common cause of syncope, particularly in a young and healthy population. Patients with mild vasovagal spells have no restrictions. Those with more severe spells particularly when multiply recurrent and occurring with minimal prodrome should refrain from driving until treatment has been instituted for 3 months and no severe episodes have recurred. There is no clear consensus on whether re-tilting patients once treatment has begun is helpful for assessing efficacy or limiting the driving-free period.

Supraventricular tachycardia may present with a broad range of symptom complexes. Studies evaluating patients who have SVT and are referred for EPS suggest approximately 25% of these patients will have experienced syncope. Radio-frequency ablation is an extremely effective treatment option for these arrhythmias. If ablation is sucessful, as it is in 95% of patients, then, driving may resume immediately. Those patients treated pharmacologically should adhere to a 1 month driving-free period to allow time to assess the drug's effect on decreasing the frequency and severity of events. Obviously, these recommendations are only broad guidelines and do not apply to every individual. Clinical judgement remains important.

Conclusions
Syncope while driving remains an important topic. An aggressive evaluation is almost always warranted given the life-threatening implications for both affected patients as well as passengers and bystanders if the event recurs. Knowledge of the most common etiologies and of their relative likelihoods is useful in the evaluation of these

patients. With a comprehensive evaluation, a specific treatable etiology can be determined in about 80%.

Driving prescriptions in those who have experienced syncope under any circumstance should be a routine part of the management of the syncopal patient. State and country laws, cardiac society recommendations and the specifics of the individual case must all be considered in arriving at a rational decision. In the vast majority of cases, personal driving can be resumed without extreme delay providing little hardship to the patient while assuaging greater societal concerns.

References

1. Linzer M, Yang EH, Estes NA, et al. Diagnosing Syncope. Part 1: Value of history, physical examination and electrocardiography. Ann Intern Med 1997; 126:989-996
2. Kapoor, WN, Karpf M, Wieand S, et al. A prospective evaluation and follow-up of patients with syncope. N Engl J Med 1983; 309:197-204
3. Ghantous AE, Saliba BC, Blitzer ML, et al. Impaired Consciousness while driving: The role of electrophysiologic evaluation [abstract]. PACE 2000; 23:666
4. Dhala A, Bremner S, Blanck, Z, et al. Impairment of driving abilities   in patients with supraventricular tachycardias. Am J Cardiol 1995; 75:516-518
5. Epstein AE, Miles WM, Benditt DG, et al. Personal and public safety issues related to arrhythmias that may affect consciousness: Implications for regulation and physician recommendations. Circulation 1996; 94:1147-1166
6. Jung W, Anderson M, Camm, AJ, et al. Recommendations for driving of patients with implantable cardioverter defibrillators. Eur Heart J 1997; 18:1210-1219
7. Christian MS. Incidence and implications of natural deaths of road users. BMJ 1988; 297:1021-1024
8. Jung W, Luderitz B. European policy on driving for patients with implantable cardioverter-defibrillators. PACE 1996; 19:981-984
9. Strickberger SA, Cantillon CO, Friedman PL. When should patients with lethal ventricular arrhythmias resume driving? An analysis of state regulations and physician practices. Ann Int Med 1991; 115:560-563
10. DiCarlo LA, Winston SA, Honoway S, et al. Driving restrictions advised by midwestern cardiologists implanting cardioverter defibrillators: Present practices, criteria utilized, and compatibility with existing state laws. PACE 1992; 15:1131-1136
11. Finch NJ, Leman RB, Kratz JM, et al. Driving safety among patients with automatic implantable cardioverter defibrillators. JAMA 1993; 270:1587-1588
12. Akiyama T, Powell JL, Mitchell LB, et al. Resumption of Driving after life-threatening ventricular tachyarrhythmia. NEJM 2001; 345:391-397
13. Larsen GC, Stupey MR, Walance CG. Recurrent cardiac events in survivors of ventricular fibrillation or tachycardia. JAMA 1994; 271:1335-1339
14. Pacifico A, Hohnloser SH, Williams JH, et al. Prevention of implantable-defibrillator shocks by treatment with sotalol. NEJM 1999; 340:1910-1912
15. Bansch D, Brunn J, Castrucci, M, et al. Syncope in patients with an implantable cardioverter-defibrillator: Incidence, prediction and implications for driving restrictions. J Am Coll Cardiol 1998; 31:608-615

26

RATE-SMOOTHING – A USEFUL TOOL FOR PREVENTION OF VENTRICULAR ARRHYTHMIAS OR A DOUBLE EDGE SWORD?

Michael Glikson, MD, Paul Friedman, MD[*], David Luria, MD, Sami Viskin, MD[**]

Heart Institute, Sheba Medical Center, Tel Hashomer, Israel, [*]Division of Cardiovascular Diseases and Internal Medicine, Mayo Clinic, Rochester, Minnesota, USA, [**]Souraski – Tel Aviv Medical Center, Israel

A rate-smoothing algorithm is used in pacemakers and implantable defibrillators (ICDs) made by Guidant Inc. to prevent sudden changes in ventricular rate.[1] When "rate-smoothing" is programmed "on," each R-R interval (whether sensed or paced) is used, as a reference value, and the next R-R interval cannot vary by more than the programmed percentage from the reference. "Rate smoothing down" and "rate smoothing up," which are programmed independently, dictate the maximal increment and maximal decrement possible in successive R-R intervals, respectively.

Although initially developed to prevent the inconvenience of sudden changes in rate in pacemaker patients, the algorithm has recently been suggested as a tool for preventing the initiation of ventricular arrhythmias, supposedly by preventing the long–short sequence that is often created by a premature ventricular contraction (PVC), which is a common trigger for ventricular tachycardia (VT). By preventing or shortening the postextrasystolic pause, rate-smoothing algorithms serve to prevent the initiation of VT. We have previously shown that this mechanism was effective in patients with long QT syndrome, in which the typical torsades de pointes is triggered by a long–short sequence.[3,4]. Preliminary results from a randomized controlled study demonstrated efficacy in decreasing the occurrence of VT in patients with ICDs implanted for other indications.[5]

Given its advantage in preventing ventricular tachyarrhythmia and in possibly controlling symptoms associated with sudden rate changes during atrial arrhythmias, the use of rate smoothing may become widespread, and many physicians tend to program it "on" routinely.

However, a recent case report[6] demonstrated a potentially dangerous absence of detection of a VT with rate smoothing "on," albeit in the setting of uncommon concomitant parameter settings. We therefore sought to determine the incidence and severity of the underdetection of

From Ovsyshcher IE. *New Developments in Cardiac Pacing and Electrophysiology.* Armonk, NY: Futura Publishing Company, Inc. ©2002.

rate-smoothing-mediated ventricular arrhythmia and to determine the critical programmable parameters that predispose to nondetection or delayed detection as a result of rate smoothing.

In this chapter we will review the literature and present our own data regarding the benefits of rate smoothing in long QT patients, as well as potential risks of routine use of this algorithm.

Benefits of Rate Smoothing in Long QT Syndrome

Cardiac pacing remains one of the most effective means for preventing torsade de pointes in patients with a long QT syndrome (LQTS).[7] This has been clearly documented for the acute treatment of arrhythmic storms related to an acquired LQTS. When antiarrhythmic drugs or bradyarrhythmias cause QT prolongation and multiple episodes of torsade de pointes,[8,9] emergency cardiac pacing through a temporary electrode can be life saving when other therapeutic measures fail.[8,9] In addition, uncontrolled studies suggest that permanent cardiac pacing reduces the frequency of symptomatic arrhythmias (during long-term follow-up) in patients with a congenital LQTS.[10-12] Nevertheless, fatal arrhythmias may occur in patients with a congenital LQTS despite combined therapy with -blockers and pacing,[13] and it is possible that failure of cardiac pacing for preventing arrhythmias in the long run is related (at least in part) to sub-optimal pacemaker programming.

Based on the mode of arrhythmia precipitation, two types of torsade de pointes are identified: "pause dependent" and "adrenergic-dependent" arrhythmias.[14,15,16]

It has been long recognized that torsade de pointes in the acquired LQTS is almost invariably "pause-dependent."[9,14,17]. However, some controversy exists regarding the importance of pauses in the genesis of arrhythmias in the congenital LQTS. Because of the long recognized association between "stress" and symptomatic arrhythmias in the congenital LQTS,[18] arrhythmias in the congenital LQTS have generally been referred to as "adrenergic-dependent."[4,19] However, we have presented data [9,14,19] suggesting that the majority of arrhythmias in the congenital LQTS -- including those related to stress -- are also pause-dependent.[15,20]. We found that age was the only independent predictor of the mode of onset of torsade de pointes in congenital LQTS. Arrhythmias in infants (3 years old) were almost *never* pause-dependent, whereas arrhythmias in adults, especially female, were generally pause-dependent.[2]

In three out of four episodes of pause-dependent torsade de pointes, the pause triggering the arrhythmia is a post-extrasystolic pause.[3,21] Typically, an extrasystole (a short cycle) generates a compensatory pause (a long cycle), which in turn is followed by a post-extrasystolic complex with bizarre QT changes from which more arrhythmias originate (the "short-long" proarrhythmic sequence). A critical role of pacing may be to prevent (or at least shorten) the post-extrasystolic pauses that facilitate the onset of torsade de pointes. Unfortunately, a normally functioning pacemaker cannot be expected to prevent the post-extrasystolic pauses that follow spontaneous extrasystoles . Therefore, unique device programming is required to effectively prevent the proarrhythmic pauses. One way of achieving this goal is to increase the lower rate limit. Pacing faster will shorten post-extrasystolic pauses, potentially reducing the risk of pause-induced torsade. However, pacing fast for long will eventually be detrimental to the left ventricle.[22] Unfortunately, the maximal pacing rate that can be used safely in the long run (without risking a iatrogenic tachycardia-induced cardiomyopathy) is not known.

An alternative method for preventing torsade de pointes is the use of pause-prevention algorithms. *Rate smoothing* is a pacing algorithm available in the *Vigor* and other Guidant-Cardiac Pacing Inc. pacemakers and defibrillators. It was originally recommended for preventing palpitations in patients in need for pacing, but we use this algorithm for preventing pause-dependent arrhythmias.

When "*rate-smoothing*" is programmed "on", each R-R interval (whether sensed or paced) is used, as reference value, and the next R-R interval cannot vary by more than the programmed percentage from the reference. "Rate smoothing down" and "rate smoothing up", which are programmed independently, dictate the maximal increment, and the maximal decrement possible in successive R-R intervals, respectively. For patients with LQTS, we program rate smoothing up "off" and rate smoothing down "on." The value most commonly used for rate smoothing down is 15%. This dictates that successive R-R intervals cannot increase by more than 15%. Thus, whenever an extrasystole creates a short cycle, pacing at a relatively fast rate for a few beats follows, with the pacing rate gradually decreasing (by 15%) until the LRL is reached or a spontaneous rhythm ensues.

So far, we have treated 12 patients with LQTS (aged 38 ± 22 years) with a pacemaker (Guidant, *Vigor*, 6 patients) or implantable cardioverter defibrillator (ICD) (Guidant, dual-chamber *Ventak AV* series, 6 patients) with rate-smoothing capabilities. Implantation followed cardiac arrest (in 7 patients) or syncope with documented torsade de pointes (in 5 patients). Implantation followed failure of -blocker therapy in all patients and failure of -blockers and ventricular pacing in one patient. The last patient experienced 8 appropriate ICD shocks (for documented pause-dependent torsade de pointes that deteriorated to ventricular fibrillation) before the use of rate smoothing.

Rate smoothing down values of 9% -20% were used and -blocker therapy was continued in all patients. After 21 ± 11 months of follow-up, all patients (except 1, who died of cancer) are alive. Two patients had recurrent arrhythmias: 1 patient with an implanted pacemaker had one episode of syncope (without documented arrhythmias) when she stopped taking her -blockers against medical advice. Another patient (with ICD) had pause-dependent torsade de pointes when rate smoothing was temporarily turned off. The patient who had previously experienced multiple appropriate ICD shocks despite ventricular pacing, remained free of arrhythmias after she underwent implantation of a dual chamber pacing with rate-smoothing. In all, 3 patients complained of palpitations. The latter were ascribed to the relatively fast pacing triggered by extrasystoles or to non-reentry persistent ventriculo-atrial synchrony. However, repeated Holter recordings did not reveal serious proarrhythmic events.

Our limited experience precludes defining the optimal rate-smoothing parameters. Documentation of repeated events of torsade helps to select the appropriate settings: The shorter the pauses that trigger torsade, the more aggressive rate smoothing should be. On the other hand, the aggressiveness of pacing should be limited to avoid pacing within the QT interval of the extrasystoles (which, on occasions, can be considerably long). This is done by programming a relatively long *upper* rate interval (like 500 msec). Accordingly, pacing will never occur before 500 msec from the last ventricular event. Long upper rate intervals like 500 msec (which is the equivalent of an upper rate limit of 120 beats/min) are well tolerated because the overwhelming majority of patients with LQTS have intact atrio-ventricular conduction.

It cannot be overemphasized that cardiac pacing should always be used in combination with beta-blocker therapy, as even rapid pacing does not mitigate the proarrhythmic effects of sympathetic stimulation. The role of cardiac pacing, when used in combination with "genotype-specific"[5] antiarrhythmic drugs remain to be defined.

Potential for Impaired Detection of Ventricular Tachyarrhythmias by a Rate-Smoothing Algorithm

In a recent report Shivkumar et al.[6] described nondetection of ventricular tachycardia due to rate smoothing algorithm. This phenomenon was observed with somewhat unusual settings of the device consisting of atrioventricular (AV) conduction interval of 300 msec, DDI mode. VT was undetected because the rate-smoothing algorithm resulted in the generation of pacing impulses during tachycardia, with subsequent tachycardia complexes falling in pace-blanking intervals [6].

We therefore sought to determine the incidence and clinical relevance of this phenomenon.

Clinical testing was performed in 16 consecutive patients undergoing PRIZM DR or PRIZM 2 DR (Guidant, Inc.) ICD implantation or device check. We programmed rate smoothing down "on" in all patients included in the study during the induction of ventricular fibrillation (VF) and VT. Other relevant parameters affecting detection in the presence of rate smoothing, such as pacing mode (DDD vs. DDI), lower and upper rates, AV conduction delay, and rate smoothing up and down percent are listed below.

Induction of both VF and VT was attempted by using "shock on T" method, manual burst, and programmed ventricular stimulation. Continuous recording of the surface electrocardiogram, endocardial electrogram, and event markers was performed during a total of 65 induced episodes of arrhythmia, looking for nondetection or delayed detection of the arrhythmia by the device. Nondetection was defined as a delay that lasted at least 20 seconds from the beginning of the episode and necessitated external shock for termination.

Sixty-five episodes of arrhythmia were induced during clinical testing. Of these, 11 were sustained monomorphic VTs (SMVTs), one was a polymorphic VT (PMVT), and 53 were episodes of VF. Most patients were tested in DDD mode with long AV delay, 3 were tested in DDD mode with normal AV delay, and 3 were tested in DDI mode with long AV delay.

Of 54 VF/PMVT episodes (ventricular rate > 240 bpm, irregular rate, and QRS morphology), there were no cases of absent detection. Detection was delayed by 1 to 2 seconds in 3 episodes (5%). These delays had no clinical significance. Figure 1 demonstrates delay of VF detection.

One induced SMVT was below the programmed VT detection cutoff. Of the 10 remaining SMVTs induced in 4 patients (VT cycle length range 270-430 msec), 6 (60%) had either delayed detection (2 patients, 1-3 seconds) or absent detection that necessitated termination by external shocks (4 episodes). All episodes with delayed or absent detection had cycle lengths between 300 and 350 msec and were induced while the ICD was programmed DDI 50 or DDD 50/60-120/145 (ranges of lower and maximal rates), AV delays between 250 and 300 msec, and rate smoothing down of 9%-12%. Slower VTs (cycle length > 350 msec) never demonstrated detection problems. Notably, there were no adverse events or consequences related to delayed or absent detection. We therefore found that rate-smoothing-induced nondetection is easily reproduced and that it occurs commonly with the use of moderate-to-long fixed AV intervals or high-pacing upper rate limits. Importantly, absent or significantly delayed detection occurred only in association with parameter interaction warnings on the programmer.

The observation of underdetection due to rate smoothing is in fact an example of the general phenomenon of underdetection when pacing at rapid rates, as has previously been described [23]. Any mechanism that will result in rapid dual chamber pacing during VT, including rate adaptive pacing, may seriously affect detection. Although we have not looked at these other mechanisms, it is conceivable that the phenomenon of undersensing is not unique to rate smoothing.

The interrelationships between various parameters and VT detection are complex and difficult to predict. Clearly, rate smoothing may seriously affect VT detection under conditions that are difficult to predict. These include, but are not limited to, VT less than 220 bpm with long AV delays and high upper rates. In order to avoid delayed detection or nondetection, we recommend using dynamic AV delay with aggressive interval shortening whenever rate smoothing is to be used, adjusting parameters to avoid programming warning messages when rate smoothing is used, and when parameters leading to interaction warnings are clinically required, performing arrhythmia induction to verify proper detection. We are currently exploring the use of simulators to reproduce clinical situations that are difficult to reproduce in the clinical setting.

Summary

Rate smoothing is an important algorithm that may prevent ventricular arrhythmia, especially those associated with long-short initiation sequence. Its value in long QT patients has been demonstrated, and there are indications from the PREVENT study that it may decrease the incidence of ventricular tachyarrhythmias in many other patients with ICDs. Nevertheless, it should be used with caution, as it may affect VT detection under specific programming settings. We recommend that warnings displayed by the programmer while programming rate smoothing be carefully considered. If the warning is intentionally ignored, extensive testing should be performed with repeated VT inductions.

References

1. Hayes DL: Pacemaker   timing   cycles   and   pacemaker electrocardiography. In: Hayes DL, Lloyd MA, Friedman PA, eds:

Cardiac Pacing and Defibrillation: A Clinical Approach. Futura Publishing Co., Armonk, 2000, pp. 201-246.

2. Marchlinski FE, Schwartzman D, Gottlieb CD, González-Zuelgaray J, Callans DJ: Electrical events associated with arrhythmia initiation and stimulation techniques for arrhythmia prevention In Zipes DP, Jalife J, eds: Cardiac Electrophysiology: From Cell to Bedside. 2nd ed. WB Saunders Co., Philadelphia, 1995, pp. 863-877.

3. Viskin S, Fish R, Roth A, Copperman Y: Prevention of torasade de pointes in the congenital long QT syndrome: use of a pause prevention pacing algorithm. Heart 1998;79:417-419.

4. Viskin S, Glikson M, Fish R, Glick A, Copperman Y, Saxon LA: Rate smoothing with cardiac pacing for preventing torsade de pointes. Am J Cardiol 2000;86 Suppl 1:K111-K115.

5. Fromer M, Wietholt D: Algorithm for the prevention of ventricular tachycardia onset: the Prevent Study. Am J Cardiol 1999;83:45D-7.

6. Shivkumar K, Feliciano Z, Boyle NG, Wiener I: Intradevice interaction in a dual chamber implantable cardioverter defibrillator preventing ventricular tachyarrhythmia detection. J Cardiovasc Electrophysiol 2000;11:1285-1288.

7. Viskin S. Cardiac pacing in the long QT syndrome. Review of available literature and practical recommendations. *J Cardiovasc Electrophysiol (in press)*.

8. DiSegni E, Klein HO, David D, Libhaber C, Kaplinsky E. Overdrive pacing in quinidine syncope and other long QT-interval syndromes. *Arch Intern Med* 1980;140:1036-40.

9. Sclarovsky S, Strasberg B, Lewin R, Agmon J. Polymorphous ventricular tachycardia: clinical features and treatment. *Am J Cardiol* 1979;44:339-345.

10. Eldar M, Griffin JC, Abbott JA, Benditt D, Bhandari A, Herre JM, Benson DW, Scheinman MM. Permanent cardiac pacing in patients with the long QT syndrome. *J Am Coll Cardiol* 1987;10:600-607

11. Eldar M, Griffin JC, Van Hare GF, Witherell C, Bhandari A, Benditt D, Scheinman MM. Combined use of beta-adrenergic blocking agents and long-term cardiac pacing for patients with the long QT syndrome. *J Am Coll Cardiol* 1992;20:830-837.

12. Moss AJ, Liu JE, Gottlieb S, Locati EH, Schwartz PJ, Robinson JL. Efficacy of permanent pacing in the management of high-risk patients with long QT syndrome. *Circulation* 1991;84:1524-1529

13. Dorostkar PC, Eldar M, Belhassen B, Scheinman MM. Long-term follow-up of patients with the idiopathic long QT syndrome treated

with combined beta-blockers and continuous pacing. *Circulation* 1999;100:2431-2436

14. Locati EH, Maison-Blanche P, Dejode P, Cauchemez B, Coumel P. Spontaneous sequences of onset of torsade de pointes in patients with acquired prolonged repolarization: quantitative analysis of Holter recordings. *J Am Coll Cardiol* 1995;25:1564-1575.

15. Viskin S, Alla SR, Barron HV, Heller K, Saxon L, Kitzis I, Van Hare GF, Wong MJ, Lesh MD, Scheinman MM. Mode of onset of torsade de pointes in congenital long QT syndrome. *J Am Coll Cardiol* 1996;28:1262-1268

16. Chinushi M, Restivo M, Caref EB, El-Sherif N. Electrophysiological basis of arrhythmogenicity of QT/T alternans in the long QT syndrome: tridimentional analysis of the kinetics of cardiac repolarization. *Circ Res* 1998; 83:614-628.

17. Kay GN, Plumb VJ, Arciniegas JG, Henthorn RW, Waldo AL. Torsade de pointes: the long-short initiating sequence and other clinical features: observations in 32 patients. *J Am Coll Cardiol* 1983;2:806-817

18. Schwartz PJ, Periti M, Malliani A. The long Q-T syndrome. *Am Heart J* 1975; 89:378-90.

19. Josephson ME. Recurrent ventricular tachycardia. In: Clinical cardiac electrophysiology. Techniques and interpretations. Pennsylvania: Lea & Febiger, 1993:417-615

20. Viskin S, Fish R, Zeltser D, Heller K, Brosh D, Laniado S, Barron HV. Arrhythmias in the congenital long QT syndrome: How often is torsade de pointes pause-dependent? *Heart* (in press).

21. Viskin S, Fish R, Zeltser D, Lesh M, Belhassen B, Dorostkar PC, Laniado S, Scheinman MM. Pause-dependent vs. non pause-dependent initiation of torsade de pointes in the congenital long QT syndrome. *PACE* 1998;21 (Part II):II-851[Abstract].

22. Shinbane J, Wood M, Jensen N, Ellenbogen K, Fitzpatrick A, Scheinman M. Tachycardia-induced cardiomyopathy: A review of animal models and clinical studies. *J Am Coll Cardiol* 1997;29:709-715.

23. Ellenbogen KA, Edel T, Moore S, et al. A prospective randomized controlled trial of ventricular fibrillation detection time in a DDDR ventricular defibrillator. PACE 2000; 23:1268-72.

27.

PACING AND PREVENTION OF ATRIAL FIBRILLATION

Luigi Padeletti, Maria Cristina Porciani, Nicola Musilli, Andrea Colella, Antonio Michelucci, Paolo Pieragnoli, Giuseppe Ricciardi, Cristina Ciapetti

Insitute of Internal Medicine and Cardiology,
University of Florence, Italy

Atrial fibrillation (AF) is the most common sustained arrhythmia and is associated with significant morbidity and mortality. As a consequence the management of patients with AF imposes significant cost to the health care system.

Long-term antiarrhythmic drug therapy is often useful in the restoration and maintenance of sinus rhythm but, however is neither uniformly effective nor uniformly safe and tolerated. A variety of non-pharmacological strategies have been investigated in the management of AF, including pacemakers, implantable atrial defibrillators, catheter ablation of the atrioventricular junction, linear atrial ablation or surgery. Newer concepts to prevent AF using atrial pacing, include algorithms which change the escape interval and stimulation rate after atrial sensed premature beats, and new different techniques of atrial pacing.

This article will focus on the following questions: Does physiologic pacing prevent the onset of AF? Are the new atrial pacing techniques more effective than right atrial appendage pacing (RAAP) in preventing AF?

Data furnished by a series of retrospective studies[1-5] and by two randomised prospective studies[6,7] indicate that the mode of pacing exerts a significant effect on the risk of developing AF and recommend atria-based pacemakers in all patients requiring pacing, especially those with sick sinus syndrome (SSS).

The combined results of observational studies comparing clinical outcome between the physiologic and single-chamber ventricular pacing modes indicate that nonphysiologic VVI pacing is consistently associated with more AF.

The Danish study[6] was the first prospective, randomised trial on the effect of the pacing mode on clinical outcomes and survival. 225 consecutive patients (83 men, 142 women) with SSS were randomised to receive either atrial 8n=110) or ventricular (n=115) pacing. At long-term follow-up[8], the cumulative incidences of AF and chronic AF (CAF) were significantly lower in the atrial group than in the ventricular group.

From Ovsyshcher IE. *New Developments in Cardiac Pacing and Electrophysiology*. Armonk, NY: Futura Publishing Company, Inc. ©2002.

In the prospective study reported by Mattioli et al.[9], 210 patients with no prior history of AF or cerebral ischemia were enrolled and randomised to receive physiologic or single–chamber ventricular pacemakers for high-degree AV block (n=100) or SSS (n=110). AF was found to develop more often in patients paced with VVI mode rather than in those with a physiologic mode.

The Canadian Trial of Physiologic Pacing (CTOPP)[10] randomised 2568 patients undergoing first pacemaker implant to ventricular-based or physiologic pacing (AAI or DDD). Patients who were prospectively found to have persistent AF lasting greater than or equal to one week were defined as having CAF. In this study physiologic pacing reduced the development of CAF by 27.1% from 3.84% per year to 2.8% per year (p=0.016).

However in these studies none or a minority of the enrolled patients had a bradycardia-tachycardia syndrome or a prior history of atrial fibrillation.

Single-chamber ventricular pacing may promote the development of AF through several probable mechanisms: 1) atrial stretch because of atrial contraction against a closed AV valve or increased valvular regurgitation; 2) asynchronous atrial activation from retrograde conduction with ventricular pacing, when introduced at a time of relative refractoriness; 3) the increased dispersion in atrial refractoriness promoted by the persistent sinus bradycardia with VVI pacing without retrograde conduction.

Atrial pacing may prevent the onset of AF because of: a) prevention of the relative bradycardia that triggers paroxysmal AF; b) prevention of the bradycardia-induced dispersion of refractoriness; c) suppression or reduction of premature atrial contractions that initiate reentry and predispose to AF; d) preservation of AV synchrony, which might prevent switch-induced changes in atrial repolarization predisposing to AF[11,12]. It was reported early this century that the area around the orifice of the coronary sinus in the rabbit possesses a high degree of rhythmicity[13]. In 1912 Zahn[14] induced tachycardia by warming the coronary sinus of the canine heart. Many later studies on animals and humans have suggested that impulses arising in the region of the coronary sinus may cause atrial extrasystoles, ectopic rhythms and tachycardias. Wit and Crenefield in 1977[15] found that there are triggerable fibers in the wall of the sinus and an automatic focus just outside its orifice.

Recent electrophysiologic studies in patients with inducible AF suggested that the posterior triangle of Koch may be a region of anisotropic conduction responsible for AF initiation. Papageorgiu et al (16) observed that inducibility of tachyarrhythmia was strongly associated with site-specific conduction delays to and within this region. Distal coronary sinus

(DCS) pacing suppresses the propensity of atrial premature depolarizations (APD) delivered at the high right atrium (HRA) to induce AF[17]. This was achieved by a decrease in APD prematurity at the posterior triangle of Koch, further supporting the concept that this region is critical in AF initiation. Yu et al.[18] investigated the effects of simultaneous HRA and DCS pacing. The successful prevention of AF by biatrial pacing was associated with less atrial conduction delay and less increase of electrogram width of the right posterior septum (RPS) caused of the early premature HRA extrastimulation. The increased atrial refractoriness reported by Sopher et al.[19], was not confirmed by the authors. However the coupling interval from the RPS atrial electrogram of the last drive train beat to the HRA extrastimulus during biatrial pacing was significantly longer than that during HRA pacing alone.

In electrophysiology laboratory dual-site right atrial pacing from the HRA and coronary sinus ostium was demonstrated to activate both atria and to suppress inducible AF or atrial flutter elicited after single-site HRA pacing in more than 50% of the cases[20]. Acute suppression was more likely in patients with greater dispersion of effective refractory period. The mechanisms suggested were an abbreviation of global atrial conduction, a change in atrial activation pattern and a reduction in right atrial dispersion of refractoriness. All these studies suggest that atrial conduction delay and non-uniform anisotropic conduction in the region of the posterior triangle of Koch play a crucial role in the initiation of AF.

Pacing the triangle of Koch or using dual wave fronts including it, may prevent recurrences of AF in patients who need to be permanently paced. Becker et al.[21] studied the effects of single-, dual-, triple- and quadruple site atrial pacing on atrial activation and refractoriness in normal canine hearts. Single-site septal, triple-site (two in the right atrium and one in the left atrium) and quadruple-site (two in the right atrium and two in the left atrium) pacing resulted similar, and were more efficient than biatrial and dual-site right atrial pacing in minimizing activation times and local recovery intervals. Yu et al.[22] showed that in patients with PAF single site pacing at either Bachmann's bundle, right posterior IAS near the coronary ostium and distal coronary sinus are similar and more effective than biatrial or dual site atrial pacing in preventing the induction of AF with RAA extrastimulation.

Recently new methods such as biatrial pacing[23], dual site right atrial pacing (24), single lead interatrial pacing at the Bachmann's bundle[25] or at the triangle of Koch[26] have been proposed in order to obtain incremental benefits relative to RAAP.

Mabo et al.[27] compared the efficacy of biatrial synchronous pacing and DDD pacing in prevention of atrial arrhythmias (SYNBIAPACE study) in 43 patients with interatrial conduction block but without conventional indications for permanent pacing. Despite a trend to a reduction in the incidence of atrial arrhythmias during biatrial pacing, no real benefit of this pacing mode was demonstrated in this selected population.

Recently Saksena et al.[28] reported that dual-site atrial pacing reduced the frequency of device-recorded atrial tachyarrhythmia events as compared to single-site atrial pacing and maintained patients in atrial pacing with fewer mode switches.

There is concern regarding some of the technical aspects of both biatrial and dual-site pacing: a) the necessity to use a Y-bifurcated connector for the atrial leads, with a consequent increase of size and potential weakness of the implanted system; b) the wide bipole between the two components of the dual site lead configuration which favours cross-talk and far-field phenomena; c) the larger resistance and the higher threshold of the coronary sinus stimulation site compared to the right atrial endocardium, need to be considered to ensure and adequate capture safety margin for both pacing sites[29,30].

Recent clinical data indicate that permanent single lead interatrial septum pacing (IASP) is safe and feasible and may provide significant benefit for prevention of paroxysmal AF (PAF) or CAF.

Our group enrolled 46 patients with sinus bradycardia and PAF[31]. Twenty four patients were randomised to traditional RAAP and 22 patients to IASP at the triangle of Koch. IASP at the triangle of Koch may prevent initiation or sustenance of AF by three mechanisms: 1) suppression of the premature beats and regularization of atrial rhythm; 2) prolongation of the coupling intervals of the premature beats in the abnormal substrate; 3) modification of the electrophysiologic properties of the substrate. The PAF episodes per month significantly decreased in both pacing modes but were significantly lower in the IASP group. PAF burden was significantly lower in the IASP than in the RAAP group.

Bailin et al.[32] randomized 120 patients with standard pacing indications to atrial pacing in either the right atrial appendage or the anterior superior interatrial septum in the Bachmann's bundle region. This second group if patients had a significantly higher rate of survival free from CAF compared with the first one at one year.

In summary, atrial and dual-chamber pacing is more effective than VVI pacing in preventing AF; IASP (single-site or dual-site), provides additional benefits for prevention of AF when compared with right atrial appendage pacing.

References

1. Feuer JM, Shandling AH, Messenger JC, et al. Influence of cardiac pacing mode on the long-term development of atrial fibrillation. *Am J Cardiol* 1989;64:1376-1379.
2. Grimm W, Langenfeld H, Maisch B, et al. Symptoms, cardiovascular profile and spontaneous ECG in paced patients: A five-years follow-up study. *Pacing Clin Electrophysiol* 1990;13:2086-90.
3. stangl K, Seitz K, Wirtzfeld A, et al. Differences between atrial single chamber pacing (AAI) and ventricular single chamber pacing (VVI) with respect to prognosis and antiarrhythmic effect in patients with sick sinus syndrome. *Pacing Clin Electrophysiol* 1990;13:2080-2085.
4. Zanini R, Facchinetti A, Gallo G, et al. Morbidity and mortality of patients with sinus node disease: Comparative effects of atrial and ventricular pacing. *Pacing Clin Electrophysiol* 1990;13:2076-2079.
5. Hesselson AB, Parsonnet V, Bernstein AD, et al. Deleterious effects on long-term single-chamber ventricular pacing in patients with sick sinus syndrome: The hidden benefits of dual-chamber pacing. *J Am Coll Cardiol* 1992;19:1542-9.
6. Andersen HR, Thuesen L, Bagger JP, et al. Prospective randomised trial of atrial versus ventricular pacing in the sick-sinus syndrome. *Lancet* 1994;344:1523-1528.
7. Rosenqvist M, Brandt J, Schuller HI. Long-term pacing in sinus node disease: Effects of stimulation mode on cardiovascular morbidity and mortality. Am Heart J 1988;116:16-22.
8. Andersen HR, Nielsen JC, Thomsen PE, et al. Long-term follow-up of patients from a randomised trial of atrial versus ventricular pacing for sick-sinus syndrome. *Lancet* 1997;350:1210-1216.
9. Mattioli AV, Castellani ET, Vivoli D, et al. Prevalence of atrial fibrillation and stroke in patients without prior atrial fibrillation: a prospective study. *Clin Cardiol* 1998;21:117-122.
10. Skanes AC, Krahn AD, Yee R, et al. Progression to chronic atrial fibrillation after pacing: the Canadian Trial of Physiologic Pacing. *J Am Coll Cardiol* 2001;38:167-172.
11. Sopher SM, Camm AJ. Atrial pacing to prevent atrial fibrillation? *J Intervent Card Electrophysiol* 2000;4(Suppl I):149-153.

12. Mehra R, Hill MRS. Prevention of atrial fibrillation/flutter by pacing techniques. In: Saksena S, Luderlitz B, editors. *Interventional electrophysiology: A Textbook*, 2nd ed. Armonk, NY: Futura Publishing; 1996. p.521-540.

13. Erlanger J, Blackman JR. A study of relative rhythmicity and conductivity in various regions of the auricles of the mammalian heart. A. *Heart Physiol* 1907;19:125-174.

14. Zahn A. Experimentelle untersuchugen uber reizbildung im atrioventrikulareknoten. *Pluegers Arch ges Physiol* 1913;151:247-278.

15. Wit AL, Cranefield PF. Triggered and automatic activity in the canine coronary sinus. *Circ Res* 1977;41:435-445.

16. Papageorgiu P, Monahan K, Boyle NG, et al. Site-dependent intra-atrial conduction delay: Relationship to initiation of atrial fibrillation. *Circulation* 1996;94:384-389.

17. Papageorgiu P, Anselme F, Kirchhof CJHJ, et al. Coronary sinus pacing prevents induction of atrial fibrillation. *Circulation* 1997;96:1893-1898.

18. Yu W-L, Chen S-A, Feng A-N, Chang M-S. Effects of different atrial pacing modes on atrial electrophysiology: Implicating the mechanism of biatrial pacing in prevention of atrial fibrillation. *Circulation* 1997;96:2992-2996.

19. Sopher SM, Murgatroyd FD, Slade AK, Waerd DE, Rowland E, Camm AJ. Dual site atrial pacing promotes sinus rhythm in paroxysmal atrial fibrillation (abstr). *Circulation* 1995;92(Suppl I):532.

20. Prakash A, Saksena S, Hill M, et al. Acute effects of dual-siye right atrial pacing in patients with spontaneous and inducible atrial flutter and fibrillation. *J Am Coll Cardiol* 1997;29:1007-1014.

21. Becker R, Klinkott R, Bauer A, et al. Multisite pacing for prevention of atrial tachyarrhythmias: Potential mechanisms. *J Am Coll Cardiol* 2000;35:1939-46.

22. Yu W-C, Tsai C-F, Hsieh M-H, et al. Prevention of the initiation of atrial fibrillation: Mechanism and efficacy of different atrial pacing modes. *Pacing Clin Electrophysiol* 2000;23:373-379.

23. Daubert C, Mabo P, Berder V, et al. Atrial tachyarrhythmias associated with high degree interatrial conduction block: Prevention by permanent atrial resynchronizations. *Eur J Card Pacing Electrophysiol* 1994;4:35-44.

24. Saksena S, Prakash A, Hill M, et al. Prevention of recurrent atrial fibrillation with chronic dual -site right atrial pacing. *J Am Coll Cardiol* 1996;28:687-694.

25. Bailin SJ, Adler SW, Giudici MC, et al. Prevention of chronic atrial fibrillation by pacing at Bachmann's bundle: Results of a randomized prospective multicenter study. *Circulation* 1999;100(Suppl I):68.

26. Padeletti L, Porciani C, Michelucci A, et al. Interatrial septum pacing: A new approach to prevent recurrent atrial fibrillation. *J Intervent Card Electrophysiol* 1999;3:35-43.

27. Mabo P, Paul V, Jung W, et al . Biatrial synchronous pacing for atrial arrhythmia prevention: the SYNBIAPACE study (abstr). *Eur Heart J* 1999;20:4.

28. Saksena S, Prakash A, Fittos S, et al. Dual site atrial pacing for prevention of atrial fibrillation (DAPPAF) trial : substudy on device based detection of recurrent atrial fibrillation (abstr). *Pacing Clin Electrophysiol* 2001;24(Suppl II):616.

29. Slade AKB, Camm AJ. Pacing to prevent atrial fibrillation. In: Oto AM, ed. *Practice and Progress in Cardiac Pacing and Electrophysiology*. Dordrecht, The Netherlands: Kluwer Academic Publishers, 1996;175-187.

30. Fahy GJ, Wilkoff BL. Pacing strategies to prevent atrial fibrillation. *Cardiol Clin* 1996;14:591-596.

31. Padeletti L, Pieragnoli P, Ciapetti C, et al. Randomized crossover comparison of right atrial appendage pacing versus interatrial septum pacing for prevention of paroxysmal atrial fibrillation in patients with sinus bradycardia. *Am Heart J* 2001;142:1047-1055.

32. Bailin SJ, Stuart A, Giudici M. Prevention of Chronic Atrial Fibrillation by Pacing in the Region of Bachmann's Bundle: Results of a Multicenter Randomized Trial. *J Cardiovasc Electrophysiol* 2001;12:912-917.

28.

THE POSTURAL TACHYCARDIA SYNDROME: A BRIEF REVIEW OF ETIOLOGY, DIAGNOSIS AND TREATMENT

Blair P. Grubb, M.D.

Division of Cardiology, Medical College of Ohio, Toledo, Ohio, USA

> *"All beginnings are hard..."*
> The Talmud

Transient episodes of autonomically-mediated hypotension and bradycardia have become a well recognized cause of recurrent syncope and near syncope.[1] The emergence of tilt table testing as a reliable method for provoking these periods of autonomic decompensation not only provided a useful diagnostic tool but has also allowed for a much better understanding of the pathophysiology of these disorders. In the course of these investigations, it became apparent that these episodic alterations in autonomic tone could result in varying degrees of systemic hypotension that, while not sufficiently large enough to cause complete loss of consciousness, were nevertheless great enough to cause symptoms such as near-syncope, lightheadedness, vertigo, and transient ischemic attacks. At the same time, we and other groups identified a large subgroup of patients who have a less severe form of orthostatic intolerance that is characterized by postural tachycardia, exercise intolerance, disabling fatigue, lightheadedness, dizziness, and blurred vision.[2] Detailed investigations of these patients have revealed that the histories, physical findings, and responses to postural change and head –up tilt were all essentially similar. This disorder has become generally known as the Postural Orthostatic Tachycardia Syndrome. The present paper will review the clinical characteristics of these patients, their responses during head upright tilt table testing, and the various therapies that appear to benefit these patients.

Physiologic Aspects

A full description of all the physiologic changes that occur in response to upright posture exceeds the scope of this review. However, briefly, approximately 25% of the body's blood is in the thorax while supine.[1] Almost immediately after assuming upright posture, gravity causes a downward displacement of about 500 ml of blood to the lower extremities and inferior mesenteric area. One-half of the amount is redistributed within seconds after standing and up to 25% of the total blood volume may be involved in the process. This causes a decrease in venous return to

From Ovsyshcher IE. *New Developments in Cardiac Pacing and Electrophysiology.* Armonk, NY: Futura Publishing Company, Inc. ©2002.

heart and stroke volume may fall by 40%. In the normal subject, orthostatic stabilization after standing is achieved in 1 min or less. Immediately after standing there is a slow progressive decline in arterial pressure and cardiac filling, which results in an activation of the high-pressure receptors of the aortic arch and the carotid sinus (as well as low-pressure cardiac and pulmonary receptors). The cardiac mechanoreceptors are joined by unmyelinated vagal effects from both the atria and ventricles. These cause continuous inhibitory actions on the cardiovascular areas of the brain stem (especially the nucleus tractus solitarii).[3] The reduced venous return caused by upright posture produces less stretch on these receptors, decreasing their discharge rates. This alteration in input to the medulla results in an increase in sympathetic outflow and there is an increase in systemic vasoconstriction. Simultaneously, the decline in arterial pressure while upright activates the high-pressure receptors in the carotid sinus, which then increase heart rate. Therefore, steady-state adaptation to upright posture causes a 10-15 beats/min increase in heart rate, an increase in diastolic blood pressure of approximately 10 mmHg, with little or no change in systolic blood pressure. More detailed descriptions of the process are available elsewhere.[4] The inability of this complex process to respond adequately (or in a coordinated fashion) can result in a failure to respond normally to sudden changes in posture (and to maintain adequate responses). Failure in this system may manifest itself as hypotension, which, if severe, may cause cerebral hypoperfusion, hypoxia and loss of consciousness.

Historical Aspects and Etiology

Beginning in the nineteenth century, physicians reported patients suffering from a condition characterized by fatigue and poor exercise tolerance that occurred without an obvious cause (such as prolonged bed rest). Some of the first reports were from the American Civil War by DaCosta who used the terms "irritable heart syndrome" and "soldier's heart" to describe the condition.[5] At the time of the First World War there were a number of reports of conditions that were variously labeled as "neurocirculatory asthenia" or "vasoregulatory asthenia" reflecting the idea that these conditions were due to a functional cardiac phenomenon caused by insufficient neural regulation of peripheral blood flow.[6] In 1944 MacLean et al. reported on a group of patients with orthostatic tachycardia that was associated with only a mild drop in blood pressure, who complained of palpitations, lightheadedness, weakness, and exercise intolerance.[7] They hypothesized that a potential mechanism for these problems might be a reduction in venous return to the heart from a disturbance at the capillary venous level.

In the 1960s, Frolich et al. reported two patients who developed a postural tachycardia (with an increase of more than 40 beats/minute on standing without hypotension) who experienced extreme postural anxiety, near syncope, and dizziness.[8] Each patient also had an exaggerated heart rate response to intravenous isoproterenol and both showed symptomatic improvement on beta-blockers. Much later, in 1982, Rosen and Cryer used the term Postural Tachycardia Syndrome to describe a patient who exhibited a greater than 44 beat/minute increase in heart rate upon standing (without orthostatic hypotension) associated with complaints of fatigue, exercise intolerance, and palpitations.[9] Shortly thereafter Fouad et al. described patients with orthostatic intolerance who demonstrated postural tachycardia and only a slight degree of hypotension, referring to the condition as "idiopathic hypovolemia."[10] Streeten et al then reported on a similar group of patients who demonstrated orthostatic tachycardia without hypotension.[11] By using gamma camera counting of sodium pertechnetate Tc 99 mm labeled erythrocytes over the calf areas of patients while supine and upright they showed evidence of extensive gravity dependent venous pooling in the lower extremities. Somewhat later, Streeten then published a report of four similar patients who additionally demonstrated a hypersensitivity to a noradrenalin infusion.[12]

Hoeldtke et al have described a total of 13 patients with near syncope, exercise intolerance, fatigue, and cognitive impairment who demonstrated evidence of postural tachycardia.[13,14] Low et al and Schondorf et al have made a comprehensive analysis of 16 patients who suffered from profound fatigue, an inability to exercise, near syncope, dizziness, and bowel hypomotility.[15,16] Many of these patients had been labeled as having psychologic problems such as chronic anxiety or panic attacks. During head upright tilt table testing these patients had markedly abnormal cardiovascular responses, with heart rates that would frequently climb to as high as 120 to 170 beats per minute often within the first two minutes of upright tilt. While some of these patients exhibited a mild reduction in blood pressure, most became hypertensive (with up to a 50 mm/Hg increase in diastolic blood pressure).

These investigators frequently employed the term Postural Orthostatic Tachycardia Syndrome (or POTS) to describe this condition and postulated that it represented an attenuated form of dysautonomia.

Khurana described a group of eight patients who had virtually identical symptoms and tilt responses who also had abnormal sudomotor function with reduced functional activity of the sweat glands of the lower extremities (presumably due to impaired innervation).[2]   Our group reported on 28 patients who presented with extreme fatigue, lightheadedness, orthostatic tachycardia, exercise intolerance, cognitive impairment, and near syncope.[2]   During upright tilt table testing each patient demonstrated an increase in heart rate of at least 30 beats/minute (which in each case exceeded 120 beats/minute) within the first 10 minutes of the test.   There was a mild fall in systolic blood pressure of approximately 20 mm/Hg during tilt (although no patient's pressure fell below 85-90 mm/Hg). A similar report from Karas et al. [17] demonstrated identical findings in a group of 35 adolescent patients, suggesting that there is a large age range affected by the disorder.

Investigators quickly noted that in some patients there was a marked familial predisposition to these disorders, raising suspicions that there was a possible genetic basis to them. This suspicion was recently confirmed by investigators at Vanderbilt, where the exact genetic basis for this disorder was determined in one severely affected family.[18] The defective gene causes a dysfunction in a norepinephrine transporter protein, producing excessive serum norepinephrine levels.   Many investigators have postulated that there are multiple genetic forms of the disorder and more detailed investigations are currently in progress.

At the same time, a large number of patients report that symptoms appear after a severe viral infection, suggesting that an immune-mediated mechanism may be involved. This concept was recently confirmed by investigators at the Mayo Clinic, who found that many patients had high serum levels of auto-antibodies to peripheral acetylcholine receptors.[19] The levels of these antibodies seemed to vary with the severity of the illness. They may be a considerable degree of overlap between POTS and "inappropriate" sinus tachycardia. Support for this concept has also come from the Mayo Clinic, which reported that radiofrequency ablation had little effect in these disorders, and sometimes made people worse.[20]

Definitions
Combining together the inform data from various investigators, these observations seem to present a fairly consistent picture of this disorder. While a number of different terms have been coined to describe this phenomena, we prefer Postural Orthostatic Tachycardia Syndrome (or

POTS) because it is a fairly descriptive term and easy to remember. These patients manifest an orthostatic intolerance in that they develop symptoms while standing that are relieved by recumbency.   POTS patients frequently present with complaints of fatigue, exercise intolerance, lightheadedness, nausea, loss of concentration and memory, tremulousness, and recurrent near syncope (and sometimes syncope). These patients may frequently be misdiagnosed as having panic attacks or chronic anxiety. Relatively simple activities such as modest exercise, showering (or sometimes even eating), may intensify these symptoms and profoundly limit even the most basic activities of daily life. Because severe autonomic failure is not present, the general physical exam is often unrevealing and patients are told that "nothing is wrong."

Currently we define POTS as the development of orthostatic symptoms that are associated with at least a 30 beat/minute increase in heart rate or a heart rate of   120 beats/minute that occurs within the first ten minutes of standing or upright tilt. With respect to age range of patients with POTS (10-60 years) this increase in heart rate exceeds the 99th percentile for control subjects 10-83 years.[23] We have tended to focus on heart rate mainly because it is the earliest, most consistent, and easiest to measure index of orthostatic intolerance. The disadvantage of focusing on the postural tachycardia is that it does not take into account the nonorthostatic symptoms such as the sudden episodes of autonomic decompensation manifested by marked fluctuations in blood pressure, sinus tachycardia, fatigue, and vasomotor symptoms that many patients experience.

Clinical Features
While the etiology of POTS is still unclear, it most likely represents a heterogenous group of disorders with similar clinical characteristics. [21] The largest group of patients appear to have a mild form of idiopathic peripheral autonomic neuropathy (a "partial dysautonomia"), in which an inability to increase peripheral vascular resistance during upright posture results in an excessive compensatory postural tachycardia. Venous pooling appears to be present that results in a reduction in ventricular preload which in turn leads to baroreceptor unloading while upright with a resultant increase in sympathetic outflow.[15,16] Some studies have looked at mean sympathetic nerve activity using microneurography in these patients, as well as heart rate variability indices, and found that they exhibit an overall enhancement of noradrenergic tone at rest and by a postganglionic sympathetic response to standing (with compensatory cardiac sympathetic over-activity). Interestingly, many of these patients

will be noted to develop a bluish discoloration of the lower extremities on prolonged standing.

A second group of patients may have a component of beta-receptor supersensitivity. Some investigators have used the term hyperadrenergic orthostatic intolerance to describe this subset. Many of these patients complain of extreme tremulousness and anxiety in addition to palpitations and tachycardia while standing. They also demonstrate exaggerated responses to low dose isoproterenol infusions while supine (it is not uncommon to see heart rate increases of 30 beats per minute or more in response to a 1 µg/minute isoproterenol infusion). Serum catecholamine levels are quite high (serum norepinephrine levels are often > 600 ng/ml). It is unclear whether this supersensitivity is primary in nature or due to a secondary denervation supersensitivity. Indeed, some of these patients appear to display excessive sympathetic activation in some distributions almost all the time. This excessively sympathetic activation is not appropriately attenuated by baroreflex mechanisms.[18] Indeed, recent genetic studies alluded to previously have demonstrated a mutation that results in a deficiency of the norepinephrine transporter that clears it from the synaptic cleft. Impairment of synaptic norepinephrine clearance could potentially produce a state of excessive sympathetic activation in response to physiologic stimuli.

While these patients share a number of characteristics with those who suffer from the partial dysautnomia form of POTS, they more often complain of tremor, migraine headache, and cold, sweaty extremities. Furthermore, detailed studies are presently under way to better understand the differences present in these two groups, and whether other subtypes may also exist.

The term "Secondary POTS" is applied to those patients with a known autonomic disorder with preserved cardiac innervation despite peripheral autonomic denervation. This can be due to diseases such as diabetes, amyloidosis, Sjogren's syndrome or lupus. In occasional patients it may be the presenting sign of more severe disorders such as Pure Autonomic Failure or Multiple Systems Atrophy.[22]

Diagnosis and Management
Initially the patient gives a detailed history and undergoes physical examination that includes a careful neurologic examination. Patients should also be evaluated for recognizable causes of orthostatic intolerance such as anemia, dehydration, or any chronic debilitating illness. Drugs

that the patient may be taking that could cause or aggravate the problem (such as vasodilators, tricyclic antidepressants, MAO inhibitors or alcohol) should be identified. Heart rate and blood pressure should be measured in the supine, sitting, and standing positions. If cardiac causes are suspected, these should be appropriately evaluated. Sinus tachycardia that is abrupt in onset and termination unrelated to posture suggests possible sinus node re-entry and may require electrophysiologic studies.

Tilt table testing is often useful as a standardized measure of response to postural change.[1]

The treatment of these patients can be somewhat of a challenge, as no single approach is uniformly successful. The first step in management of these patients is to rule out any correctable cause that might need special treatment. Conditions such as diabetes, significant weight loss, chronic debilitating disease, or prolonged immobilization are usually self-evident. One should also determine if any medications the patient may be taking could be contributing to the problem, (and in some individuals one must consider whether illicit drug use could potentially play a role). An extremely important part of therapy is educating the patient and his family as to the nature of the disorder and to avoid aggravating factors such as extreme heat, dehydration, and excess alcohol consumption. Next, we try to increase salt and fluid intake. Patients are encouraged to sleep with the head of their beds slightly elevated. Mild aerobic exercise is strongly encouraged, with an eventual goal of performing 20 minutes of aerobic activity at least three times a week. Resistance training to build up the lower extremities can be particularly helpful. Elastic support hose are useful in some patients. The hose should be waist high and provide 30 mm/Hg ankle counter-pressure. Pharmacologic therapy must be tailored to meet the needs of each individual patient and those needs will change over time. Fludrocortisone is useful in many patients, with the usual dose around 0.2 mg/day. Midodrine is quite useful, due to its peripheral vasoconstrictive action, and is usually given in 5-10 mg doses three times a day. Patients with the β-receptor hypersensitivity form may respond to either β-blocking agents or to clonidine. In patients refractory to other forms of therapy, erythropoietin may be useful. Some groups have reported that phenobarbital may be useful in selected patients. We have found the selective serotonin reuptake inhibitors useful in many patients, the most effective one being venlafaxine.[23] Frequently patients will require a combination of various therapies to be effective.   A comprehensive review of potential treatments is beyond the scope of this review and more in-depth discussions of therapy can be found elsewhere.[21]

Conclusions

POTS is a potentially recognizable and treatable disorder in which patients present with a marked orthostatic intolerance manifested by postural tachycardia, palpitations, weakness, fatigue, and exercise intolerance. The importance of this disorder goes beyond the number of people it affects, as it may cause substantial disability among young, otherwise healthy, individuals. During passive upright tilt these patients demonstrate a heart rate increase of > 30 beats/minute or a peak rate of > 120 beats/minute within the first ten minutes, reproducing the patients symptoms. Some patients may exhibit an exaggerated response to isoproterenol. Therapies directed at correcting autonomic balance can often relieve the severity of the symptoms. Greater efforts will be necessary to better understand this syndrome and its various subtypes and provide therapies that will help this group of highly symptomatic patients return to normal life. Continuing research will help provide greater insight into this and other autonomic disturbances associated with chronic orthostatic intolerance.

Acknowledgement: The author gratefully acknowledges the continuing encouragement and support of Barbara Straus, M.D., as well as the gracious support of The Sheller-Globe Foundation. This study has been supported in part by a grant from The Sheller-Globe Foundation.

References

1. Grubb BP: Neurocardiogenic syncope. In Grubb BP, Olshansy B. (eds.): Syncope: Mechanisms and Management. Armonk, NY, Futura Press, 1998, pp 73-106.
2. Grubb BP, Kosinski D, Boehm, et al.: The postural orthostatic tachycardia syndrome: A neurocardiogenic variant identified during tilt table testing. PACE 1997;20(I):2205-2212.
3. Benarroch E: The central autonomic network: Functional organization, dysfunction and perspective. Mayo Clinic Proc 1993;68:988-1001.

4. Wieling W, Lieshout J: Maintenance of postural normotension in humans. In: Low P (ed): Clinical Autonomic Disorders. Boston, MA, Little, Brown, 1993, pp. 69-73.

5. DaCosta JM: An irritable heart. Am J Med Sci 1871;27:145-163.

6. Holmgren A, et al: Low physical work capacity in suspected heart cases due to inadequate adjustment of peripheral blood flow (vasoregulatory asthenia). Acta Med Scand 1957;158:413-415.

7. MacLean AR, Allen EV, Magath TB: Orthostatic tachycardia and orthostatic hypotension: Defect in the return of venous blood to the heart. Am Heart *J* 1944;27:145-163.

8. Frolich ED, Dustan HP, Page IH: Hyperdynamic beta adrenergic circulatory state. Arch Intern Med 1966;117:614-619.

9. Rosen SG, Cryer PE: Postural tachycardia syndrome. Am J Med 1982;72:847-850.

10. Fouad FM, Tadena-Thome L, Braro EL et al.: Idiopathic hypovolemia. Ann Intern Med 1986;104:298-303.

11. Streeten DHP, Anderson GH Jr, Richardson R, et al: Abnormal orthostatic changes in blood pressure and heart rate in subjects with intact sympathetic nervous system function: Evidence for excessive venous pooling. J Lab Clin Med 1988;111:326-335.

12. Streeten DHP: Pathogenesis of hyperadrenergic orthostatic hypotension: Evidence of disordered venous innervation exclusively in the lower limbs. J Clin Invest 1990;86:1582-1588.

13. Hoeldtke RD, Dworkin GE, Gaspar SR et al.: Sympathotonic orthostatic hypotension: A report of four cases. Neurology 1989;39:34-40.

14. Holedtke RD, Davis KM: The orthostatic tachycardia syndrome: Evaluation of autonomic function and treatment with octreotide and ergot alkaloids. J. Clin Endocrinol Metab 1991;73:132-139.

15. Schondorf R, Low P: Idiopathic postural orthostatic tachycardia syndrome: An attenuated form of acute pandysautonomia? Neurology 1993;43:132-137.

16. Low P, Opfer-Gehrking T, Textor S, et al.: Postural tachycardia syndrome. Neurology 1995;45:519-525.

17. Karas B, Grubb B, Boehm K, et al.: The postural orthostatic tachycardia syndrome: A potentially treatable cause of chronic fatigue, exercise intolerance, and cognitive impairment in adolescents. Pacing Clin Electrophysiol 2000;23:344-351.

18. Shannon JR, Flattem NL, Jordan J, et al.: Orthostatic intolerance and tachycardia associated with norepinephrine-transporter deficiency. N Engl J Med 2000;342:541-549.

19. Vernino S, Low P, Fealey R, et al.: Auto-antibodies to ganglionic acetylcholine receptors in auto-immune autonomic neuropathies. N Engl J Med 2000;343:847-855.

20. Shen WK, Low P, Tahangir A, et al.: Is sinus node modification appropriate for inappropriate sinus tachycardia with features of postural orthostatic tachycardia syndrome? Pacing Clin Electrophysiol 2001;24:217-230.

21. Grubb BP, Kanjwal MY, Kosinski DJ: The postural orthostatic tachycardia syndrome: Current concepts in pathophysiology, diagnosis and management. J Intervent Cardiac Electrophysiol 2001;5:9-16.

22. Grubb BP: Dysautonomic syncope. In: Grubb BP, Olshansky B (eds)Syncope: Mechanisms and Management. Armonk, NY, Futura Publishing Co. 1998, pp.107-126.

23. Grubb BP, Karas BJ: The potential role of serotonin in the pathogenesis of neurocardiogenic syncope and related autonomic disturbances. J Intervent Cardiac Electrophysiol 1998;2:325-332.

29.

EARLY DEFIBRILLATION WITHOUT CPR CAN DOUBLE SURVIVAL FROM SUDDEN CARDIAC ARREST IN A COMMUNITY

Alessandro Capucci, MD, Daniela Aschieri, MD

Department of Cardiology, General Hospital, Piacenza, Italy.

Introduction

The key factor in fighting out-of-hospital sudden cardiac arrest (SCA) is early defibrillation.[1] In fact the majority of SCA is caused by ventricular fibrillation (VF) or pulseless ventricular tachycardia (85%)[2] and early defibrillation is the most important intervention affecting survival.[3] Survival rates have been shown to be high when early defibrillation is administered within the first few minutes following SCA.[4,5,6] After 10 minutes, very few resuscitation attempts are successful (0-2%).[7]

When defibrillation in the community rely predominantly upon the emergency medical system (EMS) ambulance service every effort to improve survival from existing levels over the past several decades has been useless.[8,9] The chance to be discharged alive from hospital is not affected by the paramedic's length of experience, or the number of trained paramedics neither in Scotland or England.[8,9] Actually only 2-5% of victims of SCA can be resuscitated with the commonly used EMS approach,[10] while two-tier systems of intervention with lay volunteers equipped with an automatic external defibrillators (AEDs) has considerable promise. In Rochester experience, for example, the use of police armed with AEDs resulted in an average response time of 6 minutes with a 45% survival rate for witnessed VF.[11]

It is still unclear what value conventional CPR holds for resuscitation[12]: it may only serve to buy time between call to 118 and the arrive of the defibrillator increasing the chance of survival by prolonging VF duration.

Starting from these concepts we have focused our effort on planning a two tiers s system with first responders in the community training the lay volunteers to perform only early defibrillation and no CPR.

Our project is called "*Piacenza Progetto Vita*" (PPV) and initiated June 6th 1999.

What is public access defibrillation?

Public access to defibrillation is the concept of placing AEDs in public and/or private settings where large numbers of people are found or where people generally considered at high risk for SCA live. There is

From Ovsyshcher IE. *New Developments in Cardiac Pacing and Electrophysiology.* Armonk, NY: Futura Publishing Company, Inc. ©2002.

unequivocal evidence showing the inverse relationship between time to first defibrillation and survival from VF as in the airline[5] and the casino experience.[6,13] These reports support the idea that defibrillators should be widely available and accessible.[14,15] The evidence of improved survival with early defibrillation coupled with important AED technological advances has lead to international action to increase public access to early defibrillation. This concept has obtained international recognition when the AHA has introduced among its major objectives public access defibrillation programs to reduce the time to defibrillation.[14]

Preliminary steps in the Piacenza Progetto Vita development
Piacenza is a mid-sized town (99,878 inhabitants in the city with 163,353 inhabitants in the surrounding region). It is characterized by the presence of few places with high population density (i.e. sky-scrapers, industries, factories, stores), but with a good road system. Since 1990 an Emergency Medical System (EMS), located in the city center, has been organized to coordinate the response to health emergencies. Once a "118" phone number alerting EMS to a possible SCA, an ambulance with physician assistance and a defibrillator is immediately dispatched.

However the"118" is different from the North America "911" phone number: while the latter is in fact the unique number for all types of emergencies, the Italian "118" is for health emergency only. For other kinds of emergency (i.e. for Police, Fireman calls) different phone numbers are used.

As an integral part of PPV, involved a public information campaign regarding the need to call for help quickly as well as a public campaign seeking donations for purchase of AEDs.

Thereafter 39 AEDs were purchased and placed in both mobile and fixed locations as dictated by a careful analysis of the city places with the highest population density identified. Twelve AEDs were placed at a single location at the main public squares, the University, the Stadium, Sporting Centers, the Post Office, and the Railway Station. AEDs in these locations were called "fixed AEDs". In addition, 15 AEDs were placed in the vehicles of policemen and firemen and a further 12 AEDs in the vehicles of volunteers of the "*Public Assistance*" i.e. the non-profit organization of volunteers participating in the assistance and transportation of sick persons. AEDs distributed in either of these manners were called "mobile AEDs". The population covered by PPV totaled 173,114 inhabitants (65% of the population of the Piacenza Region), 1 AED/4438 inhabitants.

Training Course for Lay Volunteers

All lay volunteers operated under the medical responsibility of the Chief of the EMS Department who authorized the training courses and the qualifying examination required by the first responders using AHA guidelines.[9,13] The lay volunteer training courses included 3-4 hours of theoretical and practical lessons. Four instructors trained 12 volunteers during each session and focused on the epidemiology of SCA, the objective of early defibrillation training, assessment of the patient, protocol for EMS and "Code Blue" activation (the activation of the lay volunteers integrated with EMS), orientation to the AED, protocol for AED use, small group practice with the AED, and skills' testing.

In particular participants were instructed to recognize the absence of consciousness, the absence of breathing, and to check for signs of circulation. If none was present, they were instructed to turn on the AED and to follow the voice instructions of the AED. No specific instruction for CPR was provided. A final examination (which included written-theoretical and practical parts) was performed following the AHA guidelines.[16] At 6 month intervals all lay volunteers after first certification, performed review tests.

Twenty-two instructors were certified according to AHA certification courses and, in turn, organized daily AED training courses for the lay volunteers. A total of 1.285 lay volunteers in the city were trained including policemen, financial guards, town guards, fireman, railway station personnel, ambulance personnel, post office personnel, pharmacy personnel, lifeguards, and other motivated volunteers. Trained volunteers staged mock SCA scenes at various locations in the Piacenza Region to determine the reliability and efficiency of the system and the length of time required to bring an AED to those locations.

Activation of the System: "the Code Blue"

All emergencies in the Region of Piacenza suspected to be a SCA initiated the PPV response and the "118" phone dispatcher activates the "Code Blue" which included: i) the departure of the medical ambulance ii) phone contact with the Central Phone Stations to identify the mobile patrol equipped with a "mobile AED", nearest to the location of the event, iii) identification and phone call to the lay volunteers of the nearest "fixed AED".

All out of hospital SCA from June 6th 1999 to April 30, 2001 are recorded on standardized forms.

During the first 22 months of the PPV experience, a total of 354 SCA occurred in the area covered by PPV. The mean age of the victims was 72 ± 12 years; 61% were male. SCA was witnessed in 73%.

Survival rate from VF was 44% vs. 21% (15/34 in PPV group vs. 7/33 in EMS group; $p < 0.005$) (*data in publication*). The analysis of times during "Code Blue" activation allowed us to compare the time of intervention of PPV volunteers vs. EMS staff. The intervention time to arrival from incoming 118 call was 4.8±1.2 min in PPV vs. 6.2 ± 2.3 min in EMS respectively ($p < 0.05$).

The PPV volunteers needed an average time of application of the AED of 40 ± 13 seconds.

At the retraining course of 1 hour duration performed with a practical exam, only 16 lay volunteers out of 1.285 trained (1%) failed the review test.

Conclusions

Although after a relative short time of experience of the PPV we have demonstrated that the integration of lay volunteers trained to only defibrillation with the EMS is better than a system with EMS alone. The rate of survival to hospital discharge is higher in the group of patients treated first by lay volunteers than in the patients treated first by EMS alone due to the reduction in time for defibrillation.

We consider early defibrillation by lay volunteers a priority goal over all other interventions when an AED was available. A simple method of instruction to early defibrillation without CPR instruction seems feasible, reliable, safe, and inexpensive and creates a group of competent AED operators In fact the lay volunteers are able to retain the skill of AED operation after 6 months from a short training course of only 3-4 hours.

Public awareness and support are crucial to the success of public access defibrillation programs. The development of community sensitivity and the need for a communal effort to support the dedicated task force created a campaign that energized ordinary citizens and political leaders alike. Likewise, the media served as an influential ally.

Thus, in a middle size European city this method can be proposed in order to increase survival from SCA.

References

1. Cobb LA, Fahrenbruch CE, Walsh LTR, et al. Influence of cardiopulmonary resuscitation prior to defibrillation in patients with out-of-hospital ventricular fibrillation. JAMA 1999; 281:1182-1188.
2. Chambless L, Keil U, Dobson A, et al. For the WHO MONICA project 1985-1990. Population versus clinical view of case fatality from acute coronary heart disease. Results from the WHO MONICA project 1985-1990. Circulation 1997;96:3849-3859.
3. Bayes de Luna A, Coumel P, Leclercq JF. Ambulatory sudden cardiac death mechanisms of production of fatal arrhythmia on the basis of data from 157 cases. Am Heart J 1989;117:151-9.
4. Eisenberg MS, Bergner L, Hallstrom A. Cardiac resuscitation in the community: importance of rapid provision and implications of program planning. JAMA 1979;241:1905-7.
5. Page RL, Joglar JA, Kowal RC et al. Use of automated external defibrillators by a US Airline. N Engl J Med 2000;26343:1210-6.
6. Valenzuela TD, Roe DJ, Nichol Clark LL, et al. Outcomes of rapid defibrillation by security officers after cardiac arrest in casinos. N Eng J Med 2000;343:1206-9.
7. Cummins RO. From concept to standard-of-care? Review of the clinical experience with automated external defibrillators. Ann Emerg Med 1989;18:1269-75.
8. Mackintosh AF, Crabb ME, Granger R, et al. The Brighton resuscitation ambulances: review of 40 consecutive survivors of out-of-hospital cardiac arrest. BMJ 1978;1:1115-8.
9. Guly UM, Mitchell RG, Cook R, et al. Paramedics and technicians are equally successful at managing cardiac arrest outside hospital. BMJ 1995;310(6987):1091-4.
10. Norris RM on behalf of the UK Heart Attack Study Collaborative Group. Fatality outside hospital from acute coronary events in three British health districts 1994-5. BMJ 1998;316:1065-70.
11. White RD, Asplin BR, Bugliosi TF, et al.. High discharge survival rate after out- of- hospital ventricular fibrillation with rapid defibrillation by police and paramedics. Ann Emerg Med 1996;28:480-485.
12. Becker LB, Berg RA, Pepe PE, et al. A reappraisal of mouth-to-mouth ventilation during bystander-initiated cardiopulmonary resuscitation. Circulation 1997 ;96(6):2102-12.
13. Karch SB, Graff J, Young S, et al. Response time and outcome for cardiac arrest in Las Vegas casinos. Am J Emerg Med 1998;16:249-53.

14. Weisfwldt ML, Kerber RE, McGoldrick RP, et al Public access defibrillation: a statement for healthcare professionals from the American Heart Association Task Force on the Automatic External Defibrillation Circulation 1995;92:2763.
15. Kloeck W, Cummins R.O, Chamberlain D et al. ILCOR Advisory Statement. Early defibrillation: An Advisory Statement From the Advanced Life Support WORKING Group of the International LIASON committee on Resuscitation. Circulation 1997;95:2183-84.
16. Cummins RO, Hazinski MF, Kerber RE, et al. Low-energy biphasic waveform defibrillation: evidence-based review applied to emergency cardiovascular care guidelines: a statement for healthcare professionals from the American Heart Association Committee on Emergency Cardiovascular Care and the Subcommittees on Basic Life Support, Advanced Cardiac Life Support, and Pediatric Resuscitation. Circulation. 1998; 97(16):1654-67.

AUTHORS INDEX